Basic Forensic Psychiatry

Second Edition

Malcolm Faulk

BSc, MB, BS, MPhil, FRCP, FRCPsych
Medical Inspector, HM Inspectorate of Prisons
Formerly Consultant Forensic Psychiatrist
and Director of Wessex Regional Secure Unit

OXFORD
BLACKWELL SCIENTIFIC PUBLICATIONS
LONDON EDINBURGH BOSTON
MELBOURNE PARIS BERLIN VIENNA

© Malcolm Faulk 1988, 1994

Blackwell Scientific Publications
Editorial Offices:
Osney Mead, Oxford OX2 0EL
25 John Street, London WC1N 2BL
23 Ainslie Place, Edinburgh EH3 6AJ
238 Main Street, Cambridge,
  Massachusetts 02142, USA
54 University Street, Carlton,
  Victoria 3053, Australia

Other Editorial Offices:
Librairie Arnette SA
1, rue de Lille
75007 Paris
France

Blackwell Wissenschafts-Verlag GmbH
Düsseldorfer Str. 38
D-10707 Berlin
Germany

Blackwell MZV
Feldgasse 13
A-1238 Wien
Austria

First edition published 1988
Reprinted 1991
Second edition published 1994

Set by DP Photosetting, Aylesbury, Bucks
Printed and bound in Great Britain by
Hartnolls Ltd, Bodmin, Cornwall

DISTRIBUTORS

Marston Book Services Ltd
PO Box 87
Oxford OX2 0DT
(*Orders:* Tel: 0865 791155
    Fax: 0865 791927
    Telex: 837515)

USA
Blackwell Scientific Publications, Inc.
238 Main Street
Cambridge, MA 02142
(*Orders:* Tel: 800 759-6102
    617 876 7000)

Canada
Times Mirror Professional Publishing, Ltd
130 Flaska Drive
Markham, Ontario L6G 1B8
(*Orders:* Tel: 800 268-4178
    416 470-6739)

Australia
Blackwell Scientific Publications Pty Ltd
54 University Street
Carlton, Victoria 3053
(*Orders:* Tel: 03 347-5552)

British Library
Cataloguing in Publication Data
A Catalogue record for this book is available
from the British Library

ISBN 0–632–03321–5

Library of Congress
Cataloging in Publication Data
Faulk, Malcolm.
    Basic forensic psychiatry/Malcolm
Faulk.—2nd ed.
    p. cm.
    Includes bibliographical references and
index.
    ISBN 0–632–03321–5
    1. Forensic psychiatry. I. Title.
    [DNLM: 1. Forensic Psychiatry.
W 740 F263b 1994]
RA1151.F36   1994
614'.1—dc20
DNLM/DLC
for Library of Congress   93-41796
                                      CIP

Contents

Preface   iv
1 The Forensic Psychiatric Services   1
2 Legal Aspects: The Courts and their Sentences   11
3 Legal Aspects: The Law and the Mentally Abnormal Offender   28
4 Legal Aspects: Appeals and Protection   54
5 Criminological Facts and Theories   67
6 Offences Against Property and Forensic Psychiatry   83
7 Offences Against the Person and Forensic Psychiatry   101
8 Mental Illness and Forensic Psychiatry: The Functional
  Psychoses and Neuroses   148
9 Mental Illness and Forensic Psychiatry: Organic Brain
  Syndromes   174
10 Psychopathic Disorder and Forensic Psychiatry   193
11 Mental Retardation and Forensic Psychiatry   213
12 Sexual Disorders and Forensic Psychiatry   227
13 Women and Juvenile Offenders   253
14 Dangerousness   271
15 Writing a Report   287
16 Ethics and Forensic Psychiatry   315
17 Management of Patients within Secure Psychiatric Institutions   332
18 The Civil Courts and Forensic Psychiatry   353
Index   372

Preface

I hope that this book will prove a useful introduction and practical guide to psychiatrists (especially those in training) and also to other health professionals, such as nurses, psychologists, social workers and occupational therapists. It contains material which will also be helpful to non-healthcare professionals whose work brings them into contact with forensic psychiatry, such as probation officers and lawyers.

This new edition incorporates the changes from the Criminal Justice Act 1991 and the Criminal Procedures (Insanity and Unfitness to Plead) Act 1991, the 1993 Code of Practice for Psychiatry, the Royal College of Psychiatrists' publication on the Ethics of Psychiatric Care in Prison, the setting up of the Special Hospital Services Authority and proposals of the Reed Committee. The text has been updated generally, and there are over 20 new sections, including a section on false confessions, multiple homicides, the sexual abuse of children, Munchausen's syndrome by proxy, the role of serotonin in violent behaviour, and the value of the reconviction prediction score. In addition, this edition has been expanded to include a chapter on the civil courts and forensic psychiatry.

I have used the tenth edition of the International Classification of Disease (ICD 10) and the revised third edition of the Diagnostic and Statistical Manual of Mental Disorders (DSM IIIR) for guidance in the definitions of mental disorders. I am grateful to the World Health Organization for permission to quote from the ICD 10 Classification of Mental and Behavioural Disorders. I am also grateful to the Controller of Her Majesty's Stationery Office for permission to reproduce the Reconviction Prediction Score Table in Chapter. 14.

I must also express my very grateful thanks to my wife, Barbara, for her continued support and supply of refreshments.

Malcolm Faulk,
Winchester, July 1993.

References

American Psychiatric Association (1987) *Diagnostic and Statistical Manual of Mental Disorders* (third edition, revised). American Psychiatric Association, Washington DC.

Ward, D. (1987) The validity of the reconviction prediction score. *Home Office Research Study No. 94.* HMSO, London.

World Health Organization (1992) *The ICD 10 Classification of Mental and Behavioural Disorders: Clinical Descriptions and Diagnostic Guidelines.* World Health Organization, Geneva.

Chapter 1

The Forensic Psychiatric Services

Introduction

This chapter gives an outline of the areas in which forensic psychiatry is practised and covers the penal system, special hospitals, regional secure units, local psychiatric hospitals and community facilities. More detailed descriptions of these institutions are given in Chapter 17.

Definition

'Forensic' means pertaining to, connected with, or used in, courts of law. A forensic psychiatrist's work may be said to start with the preparation of psychiatric reports for the court on the mental state of offenders suspected of having a mental abnormality. The psychiatrist will then be expected to provide or arrange treatment for the mentally abnormal offender where appropriate. Other psychiatrists, and other professionals seeing the sort of patient the forensic psychiatrist is looking after, will refer similar patients who may not actually have reached the court or broken the law. In practice, all psychiatrists may, at some time or another, have to prepare psychiatric reports on their own patients. Some general psychiatrists have a special interest or responsibility in forensic psychiatry. The term 'forensic psychiatrist' is used to describe those for whom this is their principal work.

Where is forensic psychiatry practised?

The penal system

The large majority of the prisons are run by the Prison Service (an agency service to the Home Office), although there is an increasing move to contract out the running of the prisons to private companies answerable directly to the Director General of the Prison Service. The penal system is divided into facilities for prisoners on remand (awaiting trial) and facilities for convicted offenders. At the present time there are some 45 000 people in prison including some 10 000 awaiting trial. The numbers have been rising steadily over the years.

There are prisons for adults over 21, convicted or remanded and Young Offender Institutions and Remand Centres for young people aged 17–21. The system is currently segregated into female prisons and male prisons. Remand facilities for adults are generally centred in old prisons in the centre of county towns. Remand centres for young people are often separate new buildings. Whilst on remand the inmate has many rights (which are lost after conviction); own clothes may be worn, and frequent visitors are permitted, etc. Once convicted, the imprisoned offender is placed with other convicted offenders, prison clothes must be worn (although this rule is being relaxed), visitors are restricted, and prison rules governing discipline and management apply. The adult convicted prisoner will subsequently be allocated to a prison with security appropriate to the case. The young adult (17–21) will be allocated to a young offender institution. All prisoners on ordinary custodial sentence serve only a proportion of their sentence in prison with a proportion in the community (the longer sentenced offenders on supervision). After a certain time, people on long sentences and life sentences have their case reviewed at set intervals by the parole board.

Advice on policy, standards and staffing relating to the health care of prisoners within the Prison Service is now the responsibility of the Health Care Service for Prisoners – a department (or directorate) of the prison service with its own director. Each prison governor is responsible for seeing that there is proper healthcare for the inmates in his establishment. Each prison has a Health Care Centre (varying from the equivalent of a general practice office in the smaller establishments, to a building and service for inpatients beds in the larger establishments) staffed by doctors and nursing staff responsible to the governor of the prison. Inmates with physical or mental illness will have to be cared for there until such time as they recover or can be transferred to the National Health Service (NHS). From a psychiatric point of view, it is important to realize that the health care centre is not recognized as a hospital within the meaning of the Mental Health Act and that the doctors are therefore unable to treat any patient against his will except in certain emergencies. This means, for example, that floridly psychotic patients may have to remain untreated until they can be transferred to the NHS unless they are willing to cooperate or their condition deteriorates so that treatment becomes imperative.

The prison medical staff is made up of some 130 doctors who have been employed directly by the Home Office to work full-time in the penal system. They are complemented by a similar number of practitioners employed to work sessions within the prisons. The present prison medical officers come from varied backgrounds, some will have higher degrees in psychiatry, others will have acquired the bulk of their experience in psychiatry whilst in post. At the present time, following various criticisms and a review of the prison medical service, there is a plan to gradually contract out the provision of medical services to doctors in the community when there are sufficient funds and staff to provide the service.

Should a convicted prisoner become mentally disturbed then this will be brought to the attention of the prison doctor, who, depending on the degree of disturbance, may arrange transfer to the prison hospital for further observation. If a serious mental disturbance is diagnosed, requiring treatment in a psychiatric hospital, then the prison doctor will recommend to the Home Office that the prisoner be transferred to an NHS hospital. The prison doctor may try to involve the patient's local psychiatric hospital directly by inviting the consultant to see the prisoner so that both the local consultant and the prison doctor can together write to the Home Office. In practice, prisons have often found considerable difficulty in obtaining a place in NHS hospitals. The psychiatric hospital's anxiety will revolve around the possible dangerousness of the inmate, the difficulties he is likely to provide in terms of management, the ability of the hospital to prevent absconding, and shortage of resources. However, this situation does seem to be easing now, although there are still some floridly psychotic patients who have to be looked after in prison for weeks or even months while a bed is found for them in the NHS.

Nevertheless many inmates with mental disorder will be treated in prison by the prison medical officer or by visiting psychiatrists employed on a sessional basis. Minor disorders can be treated in the local prison hospital but there are also specialized prisons or wings which concentrate on treating particular disorders. For example, Grendon Prison has a therapeutic community treatment programme for personality disorder; 'C' wing in Parkhurst Prison runs a programme for inmates with severe personality problems; and Feltham Youth Custody Centre specializes in the care of psychiatrically disordered young adults.

The other main psychiatric task for the prison medical officer is the provision of psychiatric reports for courts, parole boards, life sentence boards and reports to the governor on the mental state of men accused of prison disciplinary offences. When a person is remanded in custody and the court requires a psychiatric report then the prison medical officers will receive this request and will make the initial assessment of the inmate. In most cases, if treatment in a psychiatric hospital is deemed necessary, then the prison medical officer will contact the appropriate NHS colleague and invite him to make a second assessment in order that a joint opinion can be made available to the court. The prison medical officer will often take responsibility for collecting the psychiatric report from the NHS and advising the court about the appropriate details.

Special hospitals

The 'Special Hospitals' are those hospitals in England and Wales run (since 1989) by the Special Hospital Services Authority which provide treatment for psychiatric patients who need to be nursed in high security because of their potential dangerousness. The three special hospitals in England are: Broadmoor Hospital, Berkshire, Rampton Hospital, Nottinghamshire and, in Merseyside, Ashworth Hospital (formed in 1989 from unifying Moss Side Hospital and the recently built Park Lane Hospital). Carstairs Hospital in Perthshire is the equivalent hospital in Scotland, and Dundrum Hospital in Dublin is the equivalent for Southern Ireland. The first special hospitals in England were originally linked to the Home Office but all came under the Department of Health in 1948–49. Broadmoor originally took only offenders who had been sentenced by the court to have psychiatric treatment or criminals who had become psychiatrically disordered in prison. Rampton, like Moss Side, came to be covered by the Mental Deficiencies Acts, and could take non-offender subnormal patients. The Mental Health Act 1959 made it possible to transfer any detained psychiatric patient, including those detained on a civil section, from an ordinary psychiatric hospital to any special hospital on the grounds of dangerousness. This arrangement thus allowed non-offender patients to be transferred to a special hospital.

Special hospitals give a great deal of attention to the level of their physical security in order to prevent patients from absconding. This involves a perimeter fence or wall, well established routines of locking, and of checking the movements of patients. Within the restrictions imposed by these security measures the hospitals endeavour to incorporate all modern psychiatric techniques. The hospital is staffed by psychiatrists and nurses (although because of the historical link with the Home Office many of the nurses belong to the Prison Officers' Association).

Admission to a special hospital is controlled by each hospital's admission panel to which psychiatric reports about the patient must be submitted with the request. The patient must be detainable under the Mental Health Act 1983 and must be sufficiently dangerous to require conditions of special security. The patient must first have been considered for admission to a 'Regional Secure Unit' with whom the special hospitals work closely. In practice, it is often sensible to seek the opinion of a special hospital consultant about the case before making the application. This opinion, if favourable, can then be used with the application. The Special Hospital Services Authority runs a central panel to rule on difficult cases, e.g. those refused by a hospital admission panel.

Patients detained in special hospital will have reports prepared on them during their stay for a number of bodies. When the patient becomes ready to leave, the psychiatrist will also be required to write assessments, first, to convince the Home Secretary, in the case of restricted patients, that transfer or discharge is appropriate, and, second, to convince the receiving doctors in the catchment area hospital that the patient is ready to move on.

Regional secure units

The change in mental hospitals from closed secure institutions to open conditions which occurred in the 1950s onwards, made people aware that a small group of patients would not be provided for under the new arrangements. The recommendation by the Secure Hospital Working Party in 1961[1] that regional secure units be provided for these patients met with very little response. The request was repeated in 1974 by the Interim Butler Committee[2] and Glancy Committee[3] and on this occasion received considerably more support from the authorities, with the result that there has been a slow development of regional secure units[4].

These units vary in size from providing 30 beds to 100 beds. They have the function, in each Regional Health Authority, of caring for those patients who are too difficult or dangerous for the ordinary hospitals but not so disturbed as to require care in a special hospital. They are said to provide medium security, by which is meant that they have the capacity to prevent patients absconding as necessary but at the same time run a treatment programme which will include, as the patient improves, parole outside the unit. Thus, on such a unit some patients will be virtually as secure as in a special hospital whilst others will have unescorted freedom of movement into the local community. All regional secure units have an area which is physically secure and all aim to provide a good range of therapeutic facilities within their campus. They are highly staffed on the assumption that this will produce greater therapeutic efficacy and greater security.

The patients in the unit will almost all be detained under the Mental Health Act 1983 and the bulk will have been through the courts, though a sizeable number will have been referred from local psychiatric hospitals. The task of the psychiatrist attached to the unit will include preparing psychiatric reports on offenders at the request of the court, the prison medical service, solicitors, or the probation service. Other tasks include assessing patients in local psychiatric hospitals to advise on further management or placement (particularly placement in the regional secure unit), and the assessment, for transfer, of patients in special hospitals. At the regional secure unit the psychiatrist and the team will be concerned with inpatient treatment and, in a number of cases, day- and outpatient care. During the patient's stay on the unit the psychiatrist will have to prepare reports for the Mental Health Review Tribunal, the Home Office, The Mental Health Act Commission and the managers of the hospital.

When the patient is ready to leave the unit, the psychiatrist (in the case of restricted patients) will have to write reports to convince the Home Office of the safety of the patient, and to convince the psychiatrists in local hospitals that the patient can be safely managed there. The regional secure units, in terms of the total number of patients admitted to psychiatric hospitals in a region, admit a minute percentage of the total but this should be those few patients who are causing considerable anxiety or difficulty in management. The units form a centre for a forensic psychiatric service which includes the psychiatric assessments of offenders in the community (on bail, in hostels, on probation) as well as consultations and advice to other psychiatrists on difficult cases.

Originally the regional secure units were directly financed and protected by the Regional Health Authorities with money top-sliced from the regional budget. The 1990 NHS and Community Care Act will lead to the distribution of that money to the District Health Authorities who can then choose whether or not to spend it on regional secure unit care or develop or buy alternatives.

The services for the mentally disordered offender were reviewed by the Reed Committee[5]. Deficiencies were described in the number of medium-secure beds provided, and an increase from the present 600 to 1500 beds nationally was recommended. Attention was also drawn to the need for longer-term medium-secure beds in order to allow the transfer of patients from special hospital who no longer needed high security. Whether these beds will now be developed in regional secure units or in locally developed units or in the private hospitals remains to be seen.

Specialized private hospital services

There has been a development in the private sector of medium-secure services for detained patients. They are generally used for those patients for whom a bed cannot be found in the NHS hospitals or social services due either to local facilities being full or unable to provide for certain problematical cases (e.g. patients with behaviour disorder or brain damage). The fees of the hospital are met by the purchasing authority. Under the new NHS arrangements it may be that such hospitals, being cheaper than some regional secure units, will grow at the expense of these units.

Local hospital inpatient services

From time to time each psychiatrist responsible for a catchment area will find that patients in his area are in trouble with the law and a psychiatric report is required on their mental state. The psychiatrist must know how to write a report for a court, and he must be aware of the legal possibilities and their implications for his hospital, his patient and his own responsibility in the matter.

The majority of hospital orders made by the court for the seriously mentally ill result in the patient going to local hospitals – an indication, in the majority of these cases, that the offences are minor and the patient can be easily looked after. Nevertheless, hospitals vary enormously in their willingness or ability to accept such patients, few though they are. At one end of the spectrum are hospitals that provide a ward to cope with difficult patients employing a high staff ratio for greater therapeutic efficacy and a degree of physical security ('an intensive care ward'). To encourage this, consultant posts are being created for general psychiatrists with a special interest in forensic psychiatry. At the other end of the spectrum are hospitals that are unable to do this, either through lack of will or lack of facilities. There is a dearth of research in this area to show what effect these differences have on the service available to patients.

The local hospital psychiatrist is expected therefore to receive some patients with a forensic history from a variety of sources: courts, prisons, regional secure units, special hospitals, the community. The psychiatrist will be involved in the preparation of reports associated with all these situations. The work differs from a forensic psychiatrist at the regional secure unit only in its extent as the cases in the catchment area will be relatively few and less problematic and will form a small proportion of the workload of the general psychiatrist.

Diversion schemes and outpatient and community services

It has become clear in the last few years that it is possible to divert the mentally ill from the legal system more quickly using 'diversion schemes'. The aim is to provide a service to the police and the courts which rapidly identifies and transfers those offenders who require psychiatric treatment. In certain cases the Crown Prosecutor may then choose not to proceed with the prosecution (e.g. lesser offences with clear psychiatric illness and good psychiatric care). Encouraged by the Department of Health and the Home Office various schemes have been developed[6]. In all areas the police should have ready access to psychiatric advice about people they have arrested who appear mentally disturbed. The diversion schemes are in addition to this.

In large metropolitan areas a psychiatrist or community psychiatric nurse might regularly attend or make himself available to a busy court or police station for an immediate consultation on an offender suspected of being mentally disordered. Arrangements can then be made for immediate transfer to hospital if required. In some places the emphasis has been on developing a multidisciplinary committee to consider the placement and aftercare of problematic cases which might involve probation, social services, housing and a variable psychiatric input. Overall, the results seem very encouraging with a reduction in the time taken to get the mentally abnormal offender into proper care[7]. Joseph[8] points out, however, that to do the job properly for the 25% of most difficult patients there must be secure hospital facilities.

Patients who have broken the law may be remanded on bail and a report be sought from local psychiatric facilities. People on probation may require psychiatric assessment and these too will be referred to local psychiatric facilities. Arrangements for these facilities vary from region to region. In some, the forensic psychiatrists attached to the regional secure unit have outpatient clinics that cope with the majority of these cases. This arrangement is particularly suitable for densely populated metropolitan areas. In other regions, where the workload is more evenly distributed, it is shared with the local psychiatrists, although the regional secure unit psychiatrist may have an outpatient clinic to serve local courts.

Hostels and probation officers may find themselves with an offender who is beginning to show a mental abnormality. Easy access to a psychiatric service considerably facilitates the work of these services. Some local psychiatrists, particularly those with a special interest in the problems of the mentally abnormal offender, may become a consultant to a local probation hostel or voluntary hostel. Their function will be to give advice and guidance to the staff of the hostel as well as psychiatric opinions on inmates.

All local psychiatrists will find themselves as part of a chain in the management of the potentially dangerous patient. As the patient improves so transfer to lesser security is expected. This transfer, using the 'care programme' approach should be in conjunction with the local authority services as part of the community health services generally. There will need to be continued supervision on an outpatient basis (especially in the case of the restricted patient) so that treatment will be continued and re-entry to hospital will be facilitated if necessary. *It is essential that the community workers are fully briefed and aware of the clinical facts. As the community workers change (social workers leaving etc.) so a dangerous loss of awareness can occur. A formal regular link between the original team and the community workers is essential.*

Inter-connection of the services

Reed[5] enunciated 5 principles which should govern the care of the mentally abnormal offender:

(1) Care should be based on individual need,
(2) Care should, as far as possible, be in the community,
(3) Care should be near the patient's home,
(4) Care should only be at the level of security justified by the patient's dangerousness,
(5) Care should be aimed at maximizing rehabilitation and the prospect of independent living.

Psychiatric services for the mentally abnormal offender can only work if *all* the above institutions are in place and working together so there can be a continual flow of patients through the system according to their psychiatric need.

The total numbers are relatively small (e.g. some 600–700 patients per annum are sent by the courts to hospital for treatment under Section 37 and around 300 under section 37/41 of the Mental Health Act). The majority will be sent to ordinary psychiatric hospital, a minority to regional secure units and a smaller number still to special hospital. Nevertheless there have been considerable difficulties. Special hospitals and regional secure units often have problems in getting their patients accepted by catchment area hospitals. Prisons, including remand prisons, can experience similar difficulties. Coid[9,10] found that one in five mentally abnormal offenders remanded in prison were rejected by local psychiatric services. Local mental hospitals did best, while district general hospitals and academic units performed worst. In a comparison of two similar regions, he found that the one with a regional secure unit provided the better service. What evidence there is suggests that the problems reflect a shortage of resources and negative professional attitudes to difficult, sometimes dangerous, and uncooperative patients.

References

(1) Ministry of Health (1961) *Special Hospitals. Report of Working Party.* HMSO, London.
(2) Home Office and Department of Health and Social Security (1974) *Interim Report of the Committee on Mentally Abnormal Offenders* (Interim Butler Report). Cmnd. 5698. HMSO, London.
(3) Department of Health and Social Security (1974) *Revised Report of the Working Party on Security in National Health Service Hospitals* (Glancy Report). Unpublished.
(4) Bluglass, R. (1985) The development of secure units. In Gostin, L. ed. *Secure Provision.* Tavistock Publications Ltd, London.
(5) Department of Health and Home Office (1992) *Review of Health and Social Services for Mentally Disordered Offenders and Others Requiring Similar Services.* (Chairman: Dr John Reed) Final Summary Report. CM 2088. HMSO, London.
(6) Blumenthal, S., & Wessely, S. (1992) National survey of current arrangements for diversion from custody in England and Wales. *British Medical Journal* **305**, 1322–5.
(7) James, D.V., & Hamilton, L.W. (1991) The Clerkenwell scheme: assessing efficacy and cost of a psychiatric liaison service to a magistrates court. *British Medical Journal* **303**, 282–5.
(8) Joseph, P.L.A., & Potter, M. (1993) Diversion from custody. II: effect on hospital and prison resources. *British Journal of Psychiatry* **162**, 330–4.
(9) Coid, J.W. (1988) Mentally abnormal prisoners on remand 1: Rejected or accepted by the NHS? *British Medical Journal* **296**, 1779–82.

(10) Coid, J.W. (1988) Mentally abnormal prisoners on remand II: Comparison of services providing Oxford and Wessex regions. *British Medical Journal* **296**, 1783–5.

Chapter 2

Legal Aspects: The Courts and their Sentences

Introduction

The courts of law in this country are divided according to function. The forensic psychiatrist is concerned with the criminal court (adult and juvenile) primarily but, from time to time, may also be involved with the civil courts (see Chapter 18), the courts of appeal and the coroner's court. The courts, in sentencing, have to consider the safety of the public, retribution for the offence, the general deterrent effect of the sentence on the offender and on others, and, finally, the interests of the offender. This chapter introduces the types of offences and the concept of responsibility in law. The structure of the courts and an outline of the sentences available to them is described, as is the probation service and its relationship to psychiatry.

The Crown Prosecution Service

The police are responsible for investigating crime and referring the case to the Crown Prosecution Service. This service (set up by the Prosecution of Offences Act 1985) then takes over the conduct of criminal proceedings including the decision to prosecute. The Director of Public Prosecutions heads the service and deals with the most difficult cases. England and Wales are divided into areas each with a chief crown prosecutor and subdivided into branch offices each with a branch crown prosecutor in charge. The Crown Prosecution Service may contact a psychiatrist to prepare a psychiatric report on an offender either to rebut a defence report or because an offender's mental state is in doubt. In general, under the Code for Crown Prosecutors, there is a presumption against prosecuting a person who was mentally disordered at the time of the offence unless over-ridden by public interest as in serious cases. This is particularly so where the psychiatrist can offer appropriate care. Where prosecution has been started the crown prosecutor will pay serious attention to any report which says that continuing the prosecution will worsen the mental condition. This will be balanced by the knowledge that some mental conditions may have been brought on by the fact of prosecution.

It is also possible for individuals or organizations (e.g. shops) to prosecute (a private prosecution). The latter happens, for example, where local police custom is not to proceed on shoplifting offences and the shop prosecutes instead.

Offences and the court

The offences which bring an offender before the criminal court are divided into three types:

(1) Minor offences which can be dealt with in a magistrates' court ('summary offences') (e.g. minor criminal damage, common assault, minor motoring offences, begging, drunkenness.)
(2) Offences which are triable in either a magistrates' court or in a crown court, e.g. theft, burglary, indecent assault. The decision as to which court rests both with the magistrates and with the accused, although the law may be changed to limit the decision to the magistrates.
(3) More serious offences are known as indictable offences (e.g. murder, rape, robbery) because the offender has to be indicted (accused) before a jury in a crown court.

Concepts of responsibility and mental disorder

In all offences it must be proven that the accused physically did the act (known as the *actus reus*). In most offences it must also be proven that the defendant's intention or attitude of mind was as required for the crime in question (known as having the necessary *mens rea*). For a crime to have been committed, therefore, it is not only necessary for the accused to have done the act but there must also have been intent to do it or negligence about the consequences of the behaviour. A plea of not-guilty may be based on an absence of *mens rea* – e.g. the act may have been carried out in a state of distraction, at which time the person may not have formed the necessary intent. There are a few crimes which require no proof of *mens rea*, i.e. where the act itself is sufficient for an offence to have been committed. These are known as offences of strict liability and include certain statutory offences such as driving through a red traffic light.

The concept of responsibility in law concerns the degree to which the accused is held accountable for the act committed. To be found guilty means to have done the act and deserve punishment. Full responsibility goes hand in hand with full rationality and consciousness (or will). Impairment of either is taken to alter responsibility. Automatism (see Chapter 3) implies the absence of conscious control and therefore there is no guilt. Rationality may be so impaired by mental disorder that the offender is not held responsible for his acts resulting in the finding of not guilty by reason of insanity (see Chapter 3). Less severe mental disorder will often mitigate the sentence of the court, which will, generally, seek to give a more merciful sentence aimed at assisting the offender rather than providing punishment and deterrence. In infanticide (see Chapter 3) a disturbed balance of mind reduces responsibility.

The term 'diminished responsibility' is a technical term in law specifically related to a defence against the charge of murder (see Chapter 3). In such cases the defendant admits the act and the intent but claims that his mind at the time was so disturbed by an abnormality of mind that his mental responsibility for his act was substantially impaired. If the court is convinced of the defendant's claim then the defendant will be found guilty of manslaughter rather than of murder. Apart from this very specific example of deciding to what extent responsibility is diminished, with all other charges the psychiatrist is generally not asked to comment on 'responsibility' and use of the term may lead to confusion. The court is very much more pragmatic and requires simply an account of the patient's mental abnormality, its effect on the patient, its prognosis and the treatment arrangements which can be made. Without mentioning the word 'responsibility' the legal representatives of the offender will hope to use the psychiatric report as mitigation, in any particular case.

The accusatorial system

In criminal and civil courts in England the accusatorial system is adopted in which first the evidence of the prosecution is heard and then the evidence of the defence. On the strength of this evidence the decision about guilt is made. Similarly, a psychiatrist will be asked by one side to prepare a report. It may be found that the other side is represented by a psychiatrist taking a different point of view. The court has to decide which of the psychiatric views it will accept, if any, and also whether or not to take up the suggestions made by the psychiatrists. For example, the court may agree with the psychiatrist that the defendant is mentally disordered, but disagree about the disposal, believing that the protection of the public overrides the defendant's needs for treatment.

Magistrates' courts

There are two sorts of magistrates. The commonest is a lay person who has been accepted as a Justice of the Peace, to sit (generally with two others) in a magistrates' court. Their task is to hear the evidence, in the case of summary offences, decide the question of guilt and sentence the offender when guilty. The magistrates will be guided on the legal aspects of the case by the clerk of the court. The other sort of magistrate is the paid professional lawyer who may sit alone and is known as a stipendiary magistrate (he receives a salary as opposed to the non-stipendiary magistrate who works voluntarily). Stipendiary magistrates are only employed in metropolitan areas. The defendant is usually represented by a solicitor in a magistrates' court. The magistrates' courts deal annually with some 2 million offenders whilst the crown courts deal with some 100 000 offenders.

The prosecution services have discretion (granted by the Attorney General) about prosecuting where the alleged offender has a mental abnormality and thus may choose not to prosecute or to drop proceedings. However, if a person has been charged and detained in a police cell he must be produced before a magistrate within 24 hours (longer at weekends and Bank Holidays) and the charge repeated in court. If, after arrest, the man is allowed to go home he may later be summonsed to the court. At that first appearance the court may deal with the matter there and then but in more serious offences the case is set back to allow the accused to prepare a defence with his legal advisers. Similarly, time will be required by the prosecution to prepare their evidence.

The accused will then be remanded for up to three weeks when the accused, or his representatives, will have to appear again and the position reviewed. These remands continue until both parties are ready to present their evidence. The magistrates' court will then deal with those cases within its powers but in the case of indictable offences, at this point, the magistrates' court will decide whether there is a case to be answered against the accused. The magistrate can dismiss the case at that point but if there is a case to be answered then it is 'committed' to a crown court to be heard by a judge and jury. The accused will be remanded again, in custody or on bail, and there may be a wait of some months until the crown court case can be heard. The sentencing powers of a magistrates' court are severely limited. They may only give a maximum of six months' imprisonment for any one offence with a total sentence up to 1 year. There are certain offences which may require a longer or more severe sentence than this in which case the magistrates, having found the man guilty, may refer the case to crown court for sentencing.

Psychiatric reports may be requested by solicitors (defence or prosecution) or by the courts in order to check the defendant's fitness to plead or to stand trial, or to consider whether there are any psychiatric conditions which may affect sentence. The psychiatric reports are heard after the finding of guilt. A solicitor may have the report prepared before the final court appearance but if the magistrate requests the report it will always be after the finding of guilt to assist them with the sentencing, except in cases where fitness to plead and stand trial is an issue.

Crown courts

In the crown court the case for the prosecution and the defence is usually argued by barristers. The decision about guilt, if contested, is made by a jury, and the judge ensures that the rule of law is followed during the trial. The judge also has the task of summing-up the evidence for the jury and finally of sentencing the man if he is found guilty. Crown courts are ranked into three levels according to the seriousness of the offences which they try. The most serious offences, e.g. murder go to tier 1 courts. The judges are high court judges, circuit judges or recorders, depending on the seriousness of the offence. Psychiatric reports for the crown court may be requested by the prosecution, defence or court in relation to fitness to plead or stand trial, the need for treatment during the trial or the state of mind of the offender at the time of the offence.

The crown court also acts as a court of appeal on decisions made in the magistrates' court. The accused may appeal against conviction, sentence, or both. In the case of an appeal, the judge sits with magistrates but without a jury. At the end of an appeal, the judge, if the accused is still found guilty, has the power to increase or decrease the original sentence within the limits available to magistrates. Psychiatric reports may play a part in the appeal.

Court of Appeal (Criminal Division)

The Court of Appeal (Criminal Division) is held in London. Hearings on appeals against crown court decisions occur before three judges (known as Justices of Appeal) and including a senior Lord Justice of Appeal. Before an accused can have his case heard in the appeals court he must present his reasons to that court who will decide whether there are sufficient grounds to allow an appeal. Psychiatrists may be involved where the defendant claims that the crown court sentence did not give proper weight to psychiatric opinion at the time. The psychiatrist will be expected to provide a report and give evidence in the court in the hope of having the crown court sentence amended.

The House of Lords

This is the court of appeal against the decisions of the Court of Appeal. The House of Lords will only hear cases after giving consent to do so based on a study of the case put forward by the defendant. An appeal to the House of Lords will generally be on a point of law and will not affect the sentence directly.

Juveniles and responsibility

Juveniles are defined by the Criminal Justice Act 1991 as young people below the age of 18 years. They are divided into 'young persons' (14–17 years inclusive) and 'children' (under 14 years). Children are considered criminally responsible from the age of 10. From age 10 to 13 years the prosecution must prove the child knew what he did was wrong. Above that age the court will assume that the young offender has that understanding. Children and young offenders are tried in youth courts except in those rare cases where the offence is very serious when they must be tried and sentenced in a Crown Court. This occurs (1) when the charge is homicide, (2) when the offence carries a maximum sentence of 14 years in an adult, (3) when the offence was carried out with an adult and they are charged jointly and the adult has to go to crown court, and (4) possibly when the charge arises as a result of circumstances connected with an adult being charged.

Youth courts

The youth court arises from the Criminal Justice Act 1991. The courts are held by three magistrates from a special youth court panel. They deal with all 'children' (aged 10–13 years) and 'young persons' (aged 14–17 years, inclusive) who have broken the law, except in certain very serious cases. The 1991 Act extends 'young persons' to include 17-year-olds.

The Criminal Justice Act 1991 holds parents responsible for their children's behaviour. They must attend court with their child unless the court considers it unreasonable. If the offender is 16 or over, the court may require the parents to attend. If the child is in care then the local authority with parental responsibility must send a representative.

Coroners' courts

The coroner is generally a doctor or lawyer. The functions of the court include enquiring into the cause of death when someone dies in prison or dies from violent or unnatural causes or where the cause of death is unknown. A jury is empanelled to give a verdict on the facts. Psychiatrists may have to give evidence about their own patients who have died in such circumstances.

Sentences of the court

The Criminal Justice Act 1991 is the principle Act governing the court's powers for criminal cases. It is designed to reduce the number of minor offenders sent to custody and places the emphasis on non-custodial sentences for this group. Very good reasons have to be given to justify custodial sentences.

It is important to know the range of sentences that a criminal court can impose. They can be divided into:

(1) Simple non-custodial sentences, e.g. discharges, binding over, financial penalties.
(2) Community sentences and
(3) Custodial sentences.

Three age groups have to be considered, 'adult' (21 years and older), 'Young adult' (18–21 years), and offenders under 18 years. Below 10 years a child is not considered criminally responsible and cannot be prosecuted.

Mentally abnormal offenders will be considered separately.

Adults: simple non-custodial

(1) Absolute discharge: In this case the defendant has been found guilty but the court has decided not to punish him at all, either because of the triviality of the offence or the circumstances of it.
(2) Conditional discharge: The court chooses not to punish the offender provided that the offender does not re-offend within a set period (usually up to three years). If within that time there is a further offence then the old crime as well as the new one will be considered.
(3) Binding over: The court chooses not to punish but instead requires the offender to comply with certain conditions otherwise he will forfeit a stipulated sum of money and have the original offence dealt with. The offender can be brought back to court if he breaches the conditions which may include keeping the peace and being of good behaviour.
(4) Fines: The size of the fine in a magistrates' court (not a crown court) is now related not only to the offence and any mitigating factors but also to the disposable income of the offender. Repayment of fines can be deducted directly from Department of Social Services (DSS) payments.
(5) Compensation order: Compensation must be considered by the court when there has been loss, damage or personal injury. This order may be the only sentence or it may be combined with any other. A compensation order may be given preference over a fine though an offender can be required to pay both.
(6) Criminal bankruptcy order: This gives the court the power to make the offender bankrupt and turn his assets over to the court. It is a way of dealing with offenders who have made substantial financial gains from their offending.
(7) Disqualified from driving: This is used as a punishment for a number of driving offences.

(8) Exclusion order: The court may prohibit an offender, who was violent in licensed premises, from entering specific premises for 3–24 months.

Adults: community sentences

(1) Probation order: In appropriate cases – i.e. 16-year-olds and older (where supervision in the community is desirable for rehabilitation or prevention of offending or harm to others) – the court may choose to place the offender on probation from six months to three years. The offender must be willing to comply with the order before it can be made and a probation officer consulted. Failure to comply once the order is made may constitute a breach of probation which may lead to re-sentencing for the offence. However, a new offence in itself does not constitute a breach to any community sentence. The court will deal with it on its merits.

The order can be reviewed (and terminated for good behaviour) at the request of the supervising officer or the offender.

Various requirements can be attached to the order, such as:
(a) to live in a particular place, e.g. a probation hostel,
(b) to attend a probation centre where there may be groups (e.g. sex offender groups, anger management groups) or other therapies aimed at dealing with the offender's behaviour,
(c) to attend at a specified place to take part in various schemes or activities organized by the probation service,
(d) to attend for treatment for substance abuse (residential or non-residential),
(e) to refrain from doing particular things during a particular time,
(f)   to have psychiatric treatment (see below).
The order may be combined with a fine or other community sentence.
(2) Community service order: In this case the offender (aged 16 or older), convicted of an imprisonable offence, is required to complete a period (40–240 hours over 12 months) doing a job organized by the probation service for the benefit of the community. The offender has to be accepted by the probation community service organizer, who will write a report to the court on the suitability of the offender for such an order (the offender must consent). If the offender fails to complete his community service then he can be taken back to court and re-sentenced.

The order may be combined with a fine for the same offence.
(3) Combination order: This new penalty combines a probation order with a community order for offenders aged 16 years or older who have committed an imprisonable offence. The supervision is for 1–3 years and the community service is 40–100 hours. The conditions for the order are the same as for a probation and community order. The offender should have a reasonable prospect of completing the order.

The various requirements which may go with a probation order may also be attached.

(4) Curfew orders: This requires the offender to remain at a specified place for 2–12 hours a day for up to six months. The court must consider information about the place and the effect on others of the enforced presence of the offender. The curfew may be reinforced by electronic monitoring (tagging) if the court has a scheme approved by the Home Secretary. The curfew must not interfere with religious beliefs or work or school. Someone must be responsible for monitoring the curfew. The offender must be willing to comply with the order.

Adults: custodial sentences

Custodial sentences are restricted to those cases in which nothing less than imprisonment will do – either because the offence is so serious or because it is needed to protect the public from serious harm (e.g. in the case of a violent or sexual offence). Reasons must be given in court as to why the sentence is being given. What is to be regarded as serious tends to come from Court of Appeal judgements. Serious harm is defined as 'death or serious personal injury, whether physical or psychological'. Seriousness should be balanced by any mitigating factors. In considering the seriousness of any offence the court may take into account any previous convictions of the offender or any failure to respond to previous sentences.

Having decided that a custodial sentence is required, the length of sentence will reflect the circumstances of the offence and the number of offences. In the case of violent or sexual offences, the length will reflect any need to protect the public.

(1) Determinate sentences. Custodial sentences which have a fixed length of time are known as determinate sentences. All prisoners serve at least half their sentence in custody, after that the rules controlling release reflect length of sentence. Misbehaviour in prison may lead to additional days being spent in prison before final automatic release.

    (a) Less-than-12 month sentence: half is spent in custody then automatic unconditional release in the community. Further offending in this period may lead the court to require the outstanding term to be served in prison in addition to any new sentence.

    (b) 12 month up to four years: Half in custody then automatic conditional release on licence (supervision by a probation officer) for the next quarter with the possibility of serving the outstanding term in prison for further offending in addition to any new sentence.

(c) Four years or more: Half in custody then the possibility of discretionary conditional release on parole between half and two-thirds of sentence. At two-thirds there will be automatic conditional release on licence (supervision by a probation officer) until three-quarters of the sentence.

Re-offending may lead to having to spend the outstanding term in prison as well as any new sentence.

In the case of sex offenders, the sentencing court may order that supervision be continued to the end of the sentence.

(2) Suspended sentence: In this case, the court sentences the offender to a period of imprisonment but chooses not to enact the sentence, rather the offender is permitted to go back to the community on condition that there are no further offences within a stated period of up to two years. Should there be a further offence in that period then the original sentence will be served plus further time for the new offence. The sentence would be used where the circumstances of the case justify it. It would usually be combined with a compensation order or fine.

(3) Suspended sentence supervision order: This combines a suspended sentence with supervision.

(4) Life sentences: This sentence means that the offender is held in prison for an 'indeterminate' length of time. There are two sorts of life sentences: (a) the mandatory life sentence where the sentence is mandatory for the offence (i.e. murder), and (b) the discretionary life sentence (one given for an offence other than murder where the court had discretion as to what sentence was passed).

The trial judge may recommend that, in the case of the mandatory life sentence, a minimum period be spent in custody to satisfy the requirements of retribution and deterrence (the tariff). The prisoner has a right to know what this is and the reasons for it so a representation can be made to the Home Secretary if it is felt to be unjust. The Home Secretary (after consultation) lays down a minimum tariff period to be served in each case which may be longer than that of the trial judge. The prisoner may obtain release some time after the tariff period has been served depending on the prisoner's behaviour and the nature of the case.

In the case of the mandatory life sentence, release is solely at the discretion of the Home Secretary following a favourable review by the Mandatory Life Panel of the Parole Board in consultation with the Lord Chief Justice and, if possible, the trial judge. The offender is then released to the community on licence to a probation officer. Recall to prison may occur at any time during this period of licence if the offender's behaviour is worrying. The condition of seeing a probation officer will continue for some years. However, even after that the offender remains eligible for recall for life.

In the case of the discretionary life sentence (for very serious offences such as rape, arson, etc.) the sentencing judge states in open court a tariff period. The European Court of Human Rights has ruled that the prisoner on a discretionary life sentence is entitled to have his detention reviewed by an independent body with the status of a court and not just left to the Home Secretary. In fact, under the Criminal Justice Act 1991 the Discretionary Life Panel (a judge, a psychiatrist and an independent member) of the Parole Board reviews the case at the prison in an open tribunal-like setting with the prisoner having legal representation. The Board can, when appropriate, direct the Home Secretary to release the offender.

The first review by the Parole Board of either type of lifer occurs three years before the tariff date and thereafter at regular intervals.

(5) Execution: Theoretically, an offender can still be sentenced to execution for the offences of treason or arson in Her Majesty's Dockyards.

Young adults (18 to 21 years): non-custodial sentences

The non-custodial sentences for young adults are the same as for adults with the addition of an attendance centre order for 16 to 20 year olds.

Attendance centre order: The offender is required to attend a senior attendance centre – for three hours at a time (usually Saturdays) to a maximum of 36 hours – as a punishment. The 'centre' may be based at a school or youth club where the offender is expected to take part in organized activities, e.g. physical exercise, carpentry etc.

Young adults (18 to 21 years): community sentences

The sentences are the same as for adults.

Young adults (18 to 21 years): custodial sentences

The law asks courts to avoid, if possible, the use of custody for this age group as well as for juveniles. Since the Criminal Justice Act 1988, custody must only be used for this group if (1) the offender is unable, unwilling or has repeatedly failed, to respond to non-custodial penalties, (2) it is necessary to protect the public from serious harm, or (3) the offence is of such seriousness that it would lead to imprisonment if the offender was over 21 years and a non-custodial sentence cannot be justified. The court must also specify what criteria they feel justify the sentence if custody is used.

Young adults (aged 18–20 years inclusive) can be sent to ordinary prison during this period of their life but as far as possible they are placed in a young offender institution where they can stay until 21 years when they must move to an adult prison. The custodial sentences are the same as those received by adults and follow the same rules. However, all young offenders are subject to at least three months supervision after a custodial sentence whatever the length.

(1) Determinate sentences: A determinate sentence generally begins in a young offender institution. These institutions are designed to provide an environment for young people with the emphasis on training and educational facilities. Some establishments specialize in young people with particular problems – e.g. Feltham Young Offender Institution specializes in inmates with psychological disturbances.
(2) Custody for life for those found guilty of murder aged 18, 19, 20. This is treated, in practice, as though it were a life sentence.

Offenders under 18 years

Offenders under 18 years ('young offenders') are divided into 'young persons' (aged 14–17) and 'children' (aged under 14 years). The powers of the courts are derived principally from the Children and Young Persons Acts 1933 and 1969 and The Criminal Justice Act 1991.

Young persons and children: non-custodial sentences

(1) Absolute discharge.
(2) Conditional discharge.
(3) Bound over to keep the peace: for 16 and 17-year-olds the court may order the parent or guardian to enter into recognisance (to be bound over) to take proper care and exercise control over the offender. The parent or guardian must agree to this but can be fined for unreasonable refusal. For those under 16 years the court must bind the parents over if it is satisfied that the exercise of these powers would be desirable to prevent further offending. Reasons must be given in court where the powers are not exercised.
(4) Fine: The parent(s) or guardian(s) must pay the fine if the child is under 16 years. The size of the fine can be based on the income of the parent(s) or guardian(s). If the offender is 16 or 17 the parents or guardians may be ordered to pay.
(5) Compensation order: This may be the only sentence for a crime or it may be in addition to others. The parents or guardians must pay the compensation order for offenders under 16 unless it is unreasonable to do so. The size of the compensation may reflect the income of the parents or guardians. The parents or guardians may be asked to pay if the offender is 16 or 17.

Young persons and children: community sentences

The court must consider the offence serious enough to require such a sentence and take into account any mitigating factors.

(1) Attendance centre orders: The offender is required to attend a junior attendance centre for young persons of 10–17 years for up to 24 hours (36 hours if 16 or over) on Saturdays and for up to three hours at a time. The centre is likely to be based at a school or youth club. The offender is expected to take part in organized activities, e.g. physical exercise; carpentry. Most centres are for boys, though some are mixed.

(2) Supervision order: The sentence may be made on an offender under 18 years. It empowers a social worker or probation officer to supervise an offender for up to three years. The court (or supervisor with the court's authority) may attach various requirements (if the offender consents) to the order some of which are limited in time. For example, to

(a) live in a particular place (for up to 90 days).

(b) attend a specified place (for up to 90 days).

(c) take part in various activities (for up to 90 days).

(d) remain at home from 6 pm to 6 am (for up to 30 days).

(e) refrain from taking part in various activities (for up to the whole of the order).

(f) receive psychiatric treatment (if medical evidence shows that the offender has a condition which requires and is susceptible to treatment). Consent is only required if the offender is 14 or over.

(g) attend school where the offender is of compulsory school age.

The court may make a 'residence requirement' for the offender to live in local authority-provided accommodation for up to six months if the offence was serious or if the offending was a significant consequence of the circumstances in which the offender had been living.

(3) Probation order: The court may make such an order (for six months to three years) on an offender aged 16 years or over. The offender must agree to comply with its requirements before the order can be made. It may be combined with another sentence for the same offence, e.g. a fine. Before making the order the court must be of the opinion that it is desirable in the interests of rehabilitation or protecting the public or preventing further offending.

The offender is required to be supervised by the probation officer. The court may attach other requirements provided the court is satisfied, after consultation, that it is feasible to get compliance with them. For example, to:

(a) have psychiatric treatment.

(b) live in a particular place (e.g. a probation hostel).

(c) attend, usually for up to 60 days, a probation centre (a day centre with a demanding regime aimed at making the offenders face up to their behaviour.

(d) attend, usually for up to 60 days, a specified probation scheme or activity.

(e) attend for treatment for drug or alcohol dependence.

(f) refrain from doing particular things during a period of time.

(4) Community service orders: This applies to 16-year-olds and above who have committed, in adult terms, an imprisonable offence. If the offender consents then the offender will be required to perform unpaid work for the community for 40–240 hours over 12 months. A report from a social worker or probation officer must be considered first. There are national rules about the nature of the work, which includes projects such as decorating old people's dwellings, making adventure playgrounds, helping at disabled clubs. The order may be combined with a fine for the same offence.

(5) Combination orders: This combines a probation order for 12 months to three years with a community service order for 40–100 hours. It applies to offenders of 16 years or more who have committed an imprisonable offence and who consent to the order. The conditions for community service apply to a combination order.

The court must be satisfied that it is desirable for rehabilitation or to protect the public or prevent further offending.

(6) Curfew orders: This requires the offender to remain in a specified place for a specified period (up to six months) for 2–12 hours per day. It applies to those of 16 years or more who consent. It is meant to keep the offender indoors and away from sites of trouble. Where the facilities are available it may be combined with electronic monitoring arrangements ('tagging').

Young persons (14 to 17 years): custodial sentences

A custodial sentence may be passed only where the offence was so serious that only such a sentence can be justified or where the offence was violent or sexual and only such a sentence would protect the public. Mitigating factors must be considered.

(1) Shorter sentences – 'Detention in a Young Offenders Institution': This applies to offenders of 15 years to 17 years inclusive. The sentence varies from two months to a maximum (at the time of writing) of 12 months. All sentences of 12 months or less are eligible for automatic release at six months.

(2) Longer sentences: Such sentences are dealt with under schedule 8 of the Criminal Justice Act 1991 and the Children and Young Person Act 1933. Section 53(1) of the latter Act deals with those under 18 years convicted of murder who are then detained 'during Her Majesty's

pleasure' (effectively a life sentence). Section 53(2) provides for the prolonged detention of juvenile offenders aged 14 or over who have been convicted in a crown court of an offence which, in adult terms, has a maximum penalty of 14 years or is a serious sexual offence. The juvenile may not be detained longer than an adult would have been. The sentence may begin in a local authority home or youth treatment centre (see Chapter 13) and go on to a penal institution (a young offenders institution and then later prison).

Children (10 up to 14 years): custodial sentences

(1) Children who are out of parental control or in need of care and protection might be placed (under the Children Act 1989) on a care order under civil proceedings started in a family proceedings court and detained in accommodation by the local authority (until, at the most, 18 years).
(2) A child on a supervision order may be required (a 'residence requirement') by the youth court, under the Criminal Justice Act 1991, to reside in accommodation provided by the local authority for up to six months if certain specified criteria are met. In certain cases this may be in secure accommodation.
(3) Persistent offenders aged 12–15 years: Persistent offenders who have not responded to any other measure may be subject to detention in a secure training facility (secure training order) for up to two years.
(4) Serious offences (murder, manslaughter) are dealt with under the Children and Young Person Act 1933, section 53 which allows the court to sentence the child to a determinate sentence or, in the case of murder, to be detained during Her Majesty's pleasure. This would begin in a local authority home or youth treatment centre. The scope of section 53 may be widened for 10–12 year olds, e.g. to include death by dangerous driving.

Young persons and children: remands in custody

Where bail for juveniles is refused, the rules vary by age:

(a) 17-year-olds may be remanded in a remand centre or prison,
(b) under 17 years, remands are to local authority accommodation. The court may add conditions, e.g. a curfew order. At present, however, until suitable alternatives are provided, the courts may, for very violent or serious offences or persistent absconding, remand 15- and 16-year-olds to a remand centre or prison if nothing else will do to protect the public from serious harm. The offender must be legally represented and there must be proper consultation.
    The arrangements for children depend on local authority observa-

tion and assessment centres being available. Some will need, because of the risk of dangerousness or persistent absconding, to be held in a secure unit within the centre. For this an order from the court is required for other than brief emergency admission.

Mentally abnormal offenders

Where the offender appears mentally disordered, the court will require a psychiatric report. If a custodial sentence is being considered then the court must consider its likely effect on the offender's mental condition. The court will be anxious not to send someone to prison whose mental state indicates that psychiatric care is needed. The court is assisted in this by diversion schemes (see Chapter 1). The sentences involving a psychiatric disposal include treatment in the community or treatment in hospital:

(1) Psychiatric treatment as a condition of probation: The powers of the Criminal Court Act 1973, section 3, and the Criminal Justice Act 1991 allow the court to attach to a probation order a requirement that the offender receives psychiatric treatment. This treatment may be as an outpatient, as an inpatient, or 'at the direction of' the psychiatrist. If the offender fails to attend the psychiatrist or refuses treatment then he can be taken back for the court to re-consider the case.
(2) Binding over to keep the peace: The condition attached to this can include accepting psychiatric treatment.
(3) Guardianship order: Attendance for treatment may be a condition of this order (see Chapter 3).
(4) Treatment in hospital using various orders under the Mental Health Act 1983 (see Chapter 3).

The probation service

Definition

The probation service was started to enable probation officers, who are servants of the court, to befriend and assist offenders. The service has now grown to a national service organized in England on a county basis. The activities of the probation service now cover many areas which include:

(1) Provision of pre-sentence reports to the courts on the backgrounds of offenders. In cases of offenders being considered for a custodial sentence, the report will help the court in reaching its decision as to whether custody is required. It will also provide detailed information about community alternatives for the court to consider.

(2) Provision of probation supervision to offenders placed on probation by a court. This may also include intensive probation programmes aimed at controlling offending behaviour.
(3) Secondment to penal institutions to offer resettlement plans as well as counselling, group work and welfare provision.
(4) The running and manning of probation hostels in which people on probation can be placed.
(5) The running and staffing of bail hostels in which accused persons can be given accommodation whilst on bail as an alternative to being remanded in custody.
(6) The provision and manning of probation centres for people on probation. This will include activities such as wood work, job training, social skills and job finding.
(7) The development of community service orders.
(8) The provision of statutory supervision for licensed and paroled prisoners, prisoners on life sentence, and some mentally disordered offenders on conditional discharge to the community under section 37/41 of the Mental Health Act 1983.
(9) The provision of aftercare to those prisoners who seek help.
(10) Running bail information services for the court.
(11) Playing a part in court diversion schemes.
(12) Supervision of juveniles in the community and playing a part in the juvenile justice bureau.
(13) The provision of reports to the divorce courts on the social background of divorcees and their children.

The forensic psychiatrist will find that probation officers will often provide invaluable information on the background of offenders on whom a psychiatric report is being prepared. The psychiatrist will often 'share' the care of offenders with the probation service, either seeing an offender as a condition of probation, or working with a probation officer to supervise a conditionally discharged restricted patient in the community. The probation service will value any help the forensic psychiatrist can give in the care of disturbed inmates in probation or bail hostels. The forensic psychiatrist is also likely to be involved in reporting to the court on any mentally abnormal offenders who find their way into a bail hostel.

References

(1) Criminal Justice Act 1991. *Sentencing: The New Framework*. NACRO, London.
(2) Criminal Justice Act 1991. *Defendants and Offenders Under 18*. NACRO, London.

Chapter 3

Legal Aspects: The Law and the Mentally Abnormal Offender

Introduction

This chapter deals with the way the mentally abnormal offender is helped by the Mental Health Act 1983, the Criminal Procedures (Insanity and Unfitness to Plead) Act 1991, and the Acts in relation to probation. The chapter goes on to show the various legal ways mental abnormality is used in court. It may be grounds for mitigation, reason to be excused trial, reason for diminished responsibility or to be excused guilt. The medico-legal problems of amnesia, intoxication, muteness, and false confessions are considered next. Mental abnormality and the civil law is dealt with in Chapter 18.

Definition of terms

It is imperative, in dealing with the legal profession, to realize that the various definitions referring to mental disorder used in the different Acts are technical terms. The careless use of such terms as 'mentally ill', 'psychiatrically disordered' leads to confusion and misunderstanding in the courts. The following terms occur in the Homicide Act 1957 and the Mental Health Act 1983. They must be used precisely in their proper context and not confused.

(1) Mental abnormality (used in the Homicide Act 1957)

This is a generic term meaning any abnormality of the mind and certainly encompassing illness, all mental impairment and psychopathic disorder.

(2) Mental disorder (used in the Mental Health Act 1983)

This is a generic term meant to encompass all mental disorder. It is divided into: 'mental illness, arrested or incomplete development of mind, psychopathic disorder and any other disorder or disability of mind'.

(a) Mental illness (Mental Health Act 1983)

The term is undefined in the Act and is a matter for clinical judgement. In practice it is used by psychiatrists to cover a range of psychiatric disorders, including psychosis, psychoneurosis and organic states. Whether the illness is of sufficient severity to warrant detention in hospital will be a matter of judgement depending on the severity of the illness, the dangerousness of the patient and the likelihood of co-operation with the doctor if not detained.

(b) Arrested or incomplete development of the mind (Mental Health Act 1983)

This may be grounds for detention only if associated with certain conditions which are laid down in the Act. It is then divided as follows:

(i) Severe mental impairment

This is 'a state of arrested or incomplete development of mind, which includes severe impairment of intelligence and social functioning, and is associated with abnormally aggressive or seriously irresponsible conduct on the part of the person concerned'. This definition clearly refers to people of very low intelligence (level undefined) but is not applied legally to people unless there is also impaired social functioning and associated abnormally aggressive or seriously irresponsible conduct. In practice, the IQ level tends to be below 50. There is no comment on what is meant by impaired social functioning, abnormally aggressive or seriously irresponsible conduct – this is left to the clinician to define. Clearly, a person (of low intelligence) whose behaviour was dangerous to others (e.g. fire-setting) or to himself (wandering in front of cars) would come within the definition. Persistent minor offending may well be classed as seriously irresponsible in this context.

(ii) Mental impairment

This is 'a state of arrested or incomplete development of mind (not amounting to severe mental impairment) which includes significant impairment of intelligence and social functioning and is associated with normally aggressive or seriously irresponsible conduct on the part of the person concerned'. This definition, again, does not give an IQ level, but, in practice, covers the IQ level between 50 and 70, although there will be variation on this according to local interpretations. Again, there has to be impairment of social functioning and associated abnormally aggressive or seriously irresponsible conduct to bring the person within this legal definition. Even if the person fits this part of the definition it will be seen later that orders for the detention of those with simple mental impairment (unlike severe mental impairment) cannot be made unless it is also the case that treatment would be likely to alleviate or prevent a deterioration in their condition.

(c) Psychopathic disorder (Mental Health Act 1983).
This definition is not identical with that of psychopathic personality or antisocial personality or any other personality disorder. It is a legal definition covering a group of disorders. The definition is: 'a persistent disorder or disability of the mind (whether or not including significant impairment of intelligence) which results in abnormally aggressive or seriously irresponsible conduct on the part of the person concerned'.

Section 1(3) of the Mental Health Act makes it clear that: 'a person may not be dealt with under the Act as suffering from a mental disorder by reason only of promiscuity or other immoral conduct, sexual deviancy or dependence on alcohol or drugs'. Again, 'abnormally aggressive or serious irresponsible' are not defined and neither is 'persistent'. It will be seen from further discussion that subjects within this definition cannot be detained in hospital on an order unless 'treatment is likely to alleviate or prevent a deterioration in their condition'.

(d) Any other disorder or disability of mind (Mental Health Act 1983)
As Jones[1] points out the conditions in this residual category will depend on how broad a view is taken of mental illness. However, it has been said to include some neuroses, personality disorders, sexual deviation, alcohol or drug dependence, the behaviour disorders of children, certain specific disorders of learning, disability after head injury or encephalitis, mental enfeeblement as an aftermath of mental illness, as well as other minor psychiatric disorders[2]. However, the common feature of the group, from a legal point of view, is that they cannot be the basis of an order for detention in hospital under the Mental Health Act. They may be considered in mitigation by the court, who may be happy to accept recommendations for the subject to receive treatment for them, perhaps as a condition of probation or on a voluntary basis.

Mentally disturbed offenders in court

Magistrates and crown courts have the power, in certain circumstances, to commit mentally disturbed people to a hospital before or during the trial, as well as after conviction. The power to do this lies principally in the Mental Health Act 1983 but also in the Criminal Procedures Act (Insanity and Unfitness to Plead) 1991. Disordered people may also be treated by a psychiatrist as a condition of probation, made possible by the Powers of the Court Act 1973 and the Criminal Justice Acts 1982 and 1991.

Details of the relevant sections of the Mental Health Act 1983

Part 3 of the Mental Health Act deals with mentally abnormal offenders. The relevant sections in Part 3 of the Act are described below. Useful annotations on these sections are provided by Jones[1] and Bluglass[3].

Section 35: remand to hospital for report on accused's mental condition
Before the 1983 Mental Health Act, psychiatric reports could be requested by the court only while the accused was on bail (which might be to a hospital), or after remand to prison. The court could not order (remand) a subject to hospital for assessment. As it was felt that some subjects might require observation in a psychiatric hospital before a report could be prepared[2], this section was included in the 1983 Mental Health Act. It is applicable for any offence punishable by imprisonment, except if the subject has been convicted of murder, in which case the assessment must be in prison. It should be noted that the section does not allow the patient to be treated against his will.

This section can be effected by:

(1) The crown court for people awaiting trial or during or after the trial but before sentence where the offence is punishable by imprisonment;
(2) A magistrates' court for defendants:
    (a) after conviction for an offence punishable by imprisonment but before sentence,
    (b) before conviction for such an offence if the court is satisfied the person did the act,
    (c) before conviction and the person agrees.

In order to effect this section there must also be:

(3) A report from a doctor approved under section 12 of the Mental Health Act 1983 to convince the court (oral or written evidence) that there is reason to suspect mental illness, severe mental impairment, mental impairment or psychopathic disorder;
(4) Recognition by the court that a report on bail is impractical;
(5) A hospital willing and able to provide a bed within seven days (there must be written or oral evidence from a doctor or manager of the hospital on this point.

The defendant must be held in a place of safety (usually the prison) until the hospital bed is available. The remand is for a 28-day period, renewable at the request of the doctor responsible for the report, up to a maximum of 12 weeks. The court can terminate the remands at any time, especially if the doctor requests it. The renewal up to 12 weeks can be done in the patient's absence if he is represented by his solicitor in court. The defendant can also arrange his own private psychiatric report or appeal against the remand. The Mental Health Review Tribunal has no power to discharge such a subject. The police will take the patient to the hospital in the first place but the hospital is responsible for taking the patient back to court (with police help if the patient is dangerous). If the patient absconds from the hospital he can be arrested and taken back to court for reconsideration. The court has to decide if the security in the hospital is appropriate for the case. The court cannot order the subject to a hospital in the absence of the hospital agreeing.

Treatment may be required during this period but consent refused. In these circumstances it seems the patient may[4] be placed under section 3 Mental Health Act 1983 and treated, if the criteria are met. The position, however, has never been tested in law.

Section 36: remand of an accused person to hospital for treatment – used for mental illness or severe mental impairment

The request that this new section be included in the 1983 Act followed the realization that a number of psychiatrically disordered defendants spent very long periods remanded in custody awaiting crown court appearances. The section is therefore restricted to those awaiting crown court. It was not felt necessary for those awaiting magistrates' court as their periods on remand are relatively short. It applies to any defendant whose offence is punishable by imprisonment except those charged with murder (they can be transferred under section 48 Mental Health Act 1983). The section can be effected by crown court only and is an alternative to prison remand. It may be done in the pre-trial period (in which case it may allow a defendant to become well enough to be tried) or during the trial.

The order requires

(1) Two doctors, one approved under section 12 of the Mental Health Act 1983, to say that the patient is suffering from mental illness or severe mental impairment of a degree requiring hospital treatment. (Both doctors may come from the same hospital.) Note that the order cannot be applied to those with psychopathic disorder or mental impairment alone – presumably because these disorders would never be thought to require emergency treatment in their own right.
(2) Evidence from the doctor who will be in charge of the patient or a hospital manager that a bed will be available within seven days.

The patient will then be remanded in prison for up to seven days until the bed becomes available. Once transferred to hospital, further remands of 28 days can be made by the court up to 12 weeks at the doctor's request, made by giving oral or written evidence. The remands can be made in the patient's absence if he is represented by counsel or solicitor. The patient is subject to 'consent to treatment regulations' and therefore may be treated against his will. The Mental Health Review Tribunal has no powers to discharge. The travel arrangements are as for section 35 patients.

Section 37: hospital order

This is the principal section within Part 3 of the Mental Health Act for it allows the magistrates' court and the crown court to order a convicted offender suffering from the appropriate mental disorder to go to hospital for treatment. Before making this order the court has to have certain conditions satisfied:

(1) The offence is one which can lead to imprisonment.
(2) Two doctors must offer reports and one of the doctors must be approved under section 12 of the Mental Health Act as having special experience. Both doctors may come from the same hospital.
(3) The two doctors must agree on the main diagnostic group, which must be mental illness, severe mental impairment, mental impairment or psychopathic disorder. Two doctors must also agree in the case of psychopathy or mental impairment that treatment is likely to alleviate or prevent a deterioration in his condition.
(4) The hospital must be willing and able to take the patient within 28 days of the order being made. The doctor who will be in charge of the treatment or a hospital manager must give oral or written evidence of this. Pending the move to hospital the court will direct the patient to a place of safety – in general this will be back to the remand prison. If, at the end of the 28 days, the arrangements for transfer break down, the subject must be released. To prevent this, the Secretary of State can direct the subject to another, more appropriate, hospital within the 28 days and the order will continue there, or, alternatively, the patient can be taken back to court and re-sentenced (section II(2) Crown Court Act 1971 and section 142 Magistrates' Court Act 1980). This new sentence can be a renewal of the hospital order to allow time for a bed to become available.
(5) Before making the order the court must be agreed that this is the most suitable way of dealing with the offender. If this disposal is used then other sentences cannot also be used for that offence, e.g. fine, probation. In some cases the court may feel that the suggestions by the doctor are not appropriate to the particular prisoner and the offender may be sent to prison instead. Sometimes a court may ask the doctors to find a place in a more secure hospital than the one suggested. The doctors may investigate this possibility but, at the end of the day, if a bed in a more secure hospital is unavailable, or if the doctors feel it entirely inappropriate, then the disagreement between the doctors and the court may be resolved by the court sending the offender to prison, rather than accepting what it regards as an unsatisfactory recommendation.

A hospital order has the following effects:

(1) It gives authority for the patient to be transferred to hospital for up to

six months in the first place. The order can then be renewed if necessary by the responsible medical officer applying to the hospital managers (see Chapter 4). The first renewal lasts six months and subsequent ones each last one year.
(2) The patient falls within the Consent to Treatment Rules.
(3) The nearest relatives have no power to order discharge.
(4) The patient or nearest relative can appeal to a Mental Health Tribunal only after six months.
(5) Should the patient abscond and stay away for more than 28 days then he will be discharged by law. However, during those 28 days he can be brought back to the hospital against his will, either by hospital workers, social workers, or the police. Should he abscond the doctors may choose to inform the police of his absence in order to have him brought back.
(6) When sufficiently well the patient may be released to the community on 'leave of absence' for a maximum of six months. This provision gives the responsible medical officer the power to both test the patient in the community and easily recall the patient to hospital if the doctor considers it necessary. Consideration is currently being given to extending this period to one year in order to have greater control over potentially dangerous patients.

The magistrates' courts can make a hospital order (section 37(3)) without convicting the accused if the accused is suffering from mental illness or severe mental impairment. The court has to be satisfied that the accused did the act. This is rarely used, but it is a way of dealing with a defendant when he is so ill as to be unable to take part in the proceedings and it seems to the court the best way of dealing with the matter. In a crown court, if the accused was that disturbed then the formal question of fitness to plead (see below) would have to be considered. The juvenile court has similar powers to make a hospital order in the case of mentally disturbed children.

The District Health Authority and local social services have a duty to provide after-care services to hospital order patients (section 117, Mental Health Act 1983). This will involve the 'care programme approach' in which Health and Local Authorities are required to draw up individual care programmes for discharged patients. A key worker is nominated to oversee the programme. Others involved include the general practitioner, relatives and the patient as discussed in the Code of Practice[4].

Section 37: guardianship order

The purpose of this order is to provide social worker control in the community for appropriate subjects. It is applied to those offenders who have attained 16 years (before that, control would probably be provided by a care order). The order can only be made if certain conditions are met. These are:

(1) Two doctors (one approved under section 12) must offer reports that the mental disorder is of a nature or degree which warrants reception into guardianship.
(2) The doctors must agree on the main category.
(3) The local social services, or any other person, have to be willing to receive the offender.

A guardianship order has the following effects:

(1) It can be used in cases where the offender does not consent (unlike a probation order, which is an agreement between the offender and the court).
(2) The subject may be required to live where directed.
(3) Access to the subject must be allowed for the approved social worker, registered medical practitioner, or other person specified.
(4) The subject must present himself for medical treatment, occupation, education or training if required to do so.

The disadvantage of the order is that there is no sanction available to the guardian if the subject refuses to co-operate, although he can be re-arrested if he fails to live where directed. The guardian has to rely on the moral position given to him by the order to gain the client's co-operation. The order tends to be used mostly to look after mentally impaired patients in the community, although it could be used for any diagnosis where supervision and control is desirable.

The lack of sanctions has led to the proposal that there should be some new order which would provide supervision with control for patients whose health, own safety or safety to others is deemed to be at serious risk. The most recent proposal is for a 'supervised discharge order'. This would involve:

(1) A negotiated agreement with the patient for a clear treatment plan.
(2) A named key worker, the patient being required to live in a specified place.
(3) The patient being required to attend for medical treatment, occupation, education, or training.
(4) The key worker being entitled to have access to the patient.

The order would be for six months initially but be extendable on application for initially a further six months then annually. Failure of the patient to comply with the order would lead to a review of the case by all the relevant workers with consideration to recall to hospital. The latter would be effected by the responsible medical officer and the approved social worker if the deterioration met the criteria for compulsory admission.

Section 38: interim hospital order

This new order, recommended by the Butler Committee[2], was designed to allow doctors to admit patients to hospital to have a trial of treatment. If it becomes clear that hospital placement is inappropriate then the patient could return to court for re-sentencing. The order was designed to facilitate trials for treatment with difficult-to-place patients, particularly those with psychopathic disorder or mental impairment. However, the Act does allow it to be used for mental illness and severe impairment as well.

In order to effect this section the following conditions must be satisfied:

(1) The offence must be an imprisonable one.
(2) Two doctors, including an approved one, must agree on the main diagnosis and make the recommendation. One of the doctors must be from the hospital accepting the patient.
(3) It can apply to mental illness, psychopathic disorder, severe mental impairment and mental impairment.
(4) There must be reason to suppose that the disorder may be appropriate for a hospital order.
(5) A hospital bed should be available within 28 days of the order being made and evidence of this must be given in to the court by the potential responsible medical officer or a manager of the hospital.

An interim hospital order has the following effect:

(1) The patient can be detained in a hospital for a trial of treatment for up to 12 weeks initially renewed every 28 days up to six months total.
(2) At the end of the trial of treatment the court converts the order into a hospital order or re-sentences the subject.
(3) Renewals and conversions to a hospital order can be done in the patient's absence if he is legally represented and medical evidence is available.
(4) If a patient absconds he can be arrested and taken back to court.
(5) The effect of the order in terms of treatment is the same as a hospital order.
(6) There is no appeal to the Mental Health Review Tribunal.

Section 39

This new section was introduced in response to courts complaining that they were often unable to get doctors to produce a bed for a mentally disordered patient. The section allows the court to require the Regional Health Authority to give information about hospital facilities in their region for such a patient. The court cannot order the patient to a hospital if the hospital is not willing to take him, but they hope, by this manoeuvre, to so embarrass the Regional Health Authority that a bed will be provided. The Regional Health Authority does have the power to order a hospital to accept a patient, although in practice they are very reluctant to do this. As Regional Authorities are abolished so District Authorities may be involved.

Section 41: restriction order

The purpose of this section is to protect the public by ordering that a patient detained on a hospital order will not be allowed to leave the hospital without the Home Secretary's permission. The order can be made for a stated period of time (several years) or unlimited in point of time (i.e. to last for the rest of the patient's life). This interference with the patient's liberty is so great that the order can only be made by a judge in a higher court. Judges are recommended only to make the order where there is a risk of the patient causing serious harm to others if set at large.

The requirements for a judge to make this order are:

(1) All the recommendations of section 37.
(2) That the restrictions are necessary to protect the public from serious harm.
(3) That the judge has heard oral evidence from one of the doctors writing the reports for the court about the patient. The doctor will be asked whether or not he feels the restriction order is required. The doctor will give his mind to the dangerousness of the patient, the chances of his absconding, responding to treatment, and complying with treatment when he has left hospital. However, whatever the doctor's opinion, the judge may impose the restriction order if it seems to him appropriate.

The effects of a restriction order under section 41 are:

(1) The patient comes directly under the Secretary of State for Home Affairs, although he would generally delegate this to a Minister under him. The freedom of the patient within the hospital grounds is left to the doctor's discretion. All questions of movement from the hospital and the management of the patient after discharge have to be referred to the Home Office. Thus, permission is required for:
    (a) The patient to have parole outside the hospital grounds with an escort (e.g. for a shopping trip);
    (b) The patient to have parole outside the hospital without an escort;
    (c) Leave of absence overnight from the hospital;
    (d) Transfer to another hospital;
    (e) Discharge or conditional discharge.
(2) Unlike a simple section 37, detention is continuous without renewals.
(3) When the patient is discharged the Home Secretary will generally impose conditions which the patient must fulfil otherwise the Home Secretary may issue a warrant for his recall to hospital (see below). The conditions are, usually, to be subject to social work supervision

and psychiatric care. These conditions will, in practice, generally last five years but may in certain circumstances be extended or shortened. The Home Secretary does have the power to absolutely discharge someone, which he will do when he is satisfied that the patient is no longer a danger to others. Recall by the Home Secretary may be exercised even without medical advice when the Home Secretary has reason to believe that the patient has a mental disorder such that he is liable to be detained and there is a risk to his own health or safety or a risk to others.

(4) The patient cannot obtain his discharge by absconding. No matter how long he stays away from the hospital he is liable to be recalled if found.

(5) The patient can apply to the Mental Health Review Tribunal after six months. The Tribunal does have the power to absolutely discharge or conditionally discharge the patient but other powers are limited (see below).

(6) Regular reports are requested by the Secretary of State.

Permission for increased freedom for the patient is obtained by writing letters to the Home Secretary's department describing the improvements in the patient's mental state, the reduction in his dangerousness, the new proposals and the lack of danger involved in the proposal (see Chapter 15).

It should be noted that a restriction order does not necessarily imply that a hospital must have security. The restriction order may be placed on the patient largely in order to enforce treatment after discharge. The initial treatment may, in appropriate cases, be carried out in open conditions. Similarly, the patient who needed secure conditions at the beginning of his treatment may improve sufficiently to move to open conditions for rehabilitation.

If the patient is conditionally discharged and has a relapse he can be readmitted to a hospital by the doctor without a formal Home Office recall simply by admitting informally or by admitting under Part II of the Mental Health Act. The hospital need not be the original hospital but any suitable to the case. The Home Office would become involved if recommended by the responsible medical officer or a dangerous situation had occurred.

A magistrates' court, wishing to make a hospital order on a mentally disordered offender, may have enough evidence before them to regard the offender as sufficiently dangerous to require a restriction order. In that case the court would have to refer the offender (see below) to a crown court, who would review the case before deciding whether or not to make a restriction order with the hospital order.

The 'problems' of a restriction order include:

(1) Interference in the clinical management of the case by legal controls. The clinician may find that he has to detain the patient in

hospital for much longer than he might consider necessary on clinical grounds in order to satisfy the Home Secretary's anxieties about dangerousness.

(2) The difficulty of deciding if someone is still dangerous. Patients, for example, with psychopathic disorder and sadistic offences, or psychotic patients not fully under control may be detained far longer in hospital than they would have been had they received a simple prison sentence for the same offence.

Section 42

This allows the Home Secretary to order a conditional or absolute discharge, or to withdraw the restriction order. It also allows the Home Secretary to recall a conditionally discharged patient. This is done by issuing a warrant, usually to the police, to arrest the patient and take him to an appropriate hospital. This would be prompted by a report from the patient's social worker, or responsible medical officer, that the patient was breaking the conditions of his conditional discharge or that his behaviour suggested that he was becoming dangerous again. Health Service Guidelines (HSG (93) 20) recommend that the patient has to be informed immediately that he is being recalled and given the reasons (orally and in writing) within 72 hours by the responsible medical officer, an approved social worker or administrator. The patient then has the right to appeal to the Mental Health Review Tribunal, within one month, against the recall. This protects the patient against arbitrary recall.

Section 43

This allows a magistrates' court to refer a case to a crown court if they believe a restriction order is required. It cannot be used for children under 14 years.

Section 44

This allows a magistrates' court to order a patient, on whom they want a restriction order placed, to be sent to hospital whilst awaiting for a section 43 to be enacted. Whilst the patient is in hospital, he is held as though a restriction order had been made until such time as the crown court can make the proper order. Before the order can be made, evidence from a manager or doctor from the hospital is required about the availability of a hospital bed.

Section 46

This allows the Home Secretary to detain indefinitely servicemen found Not Guilty by Reason of Insanity, or who have been found unfit to plead.

Mentally disturbed offenders in prison

The Mental Health Act allows for the transfer of mentally disordered people (remanded or convicted) from prison to hospital (sections 47 and 48). The doctors involved usually find the bed and then apply to the Home Office to make the recommendation for transfer. This is done without the courts being involved. If a bed has not been found then the Home Office pass on the prison doctor's recommendation to the appropriate health authority who has a duty to find a bed.

Section 47: transfer direction for convicted prisoners

This section allows movement of mentally disordered convicted prisoners from prison to a hospital. Once recovered in hospital the patient can be returned to the prison to finish sentence. However, if it is more appropriate to stay in hospital, then this may be allowed. If the illness is not relieved by the date the patient was due to be released from prison then the patient can still be detained in the hospital. The transfer direction is treated as though it were a section 37 from the date the patient was admitted to the hospital (see also section 49 below).

The requirements for section 47 are that:

(1) Two doctors (one approved) recommend to the Secretary of State that the patient is suffering from mental illness, psychopathy, mental impairment or severe mental impairment, which warrants attention in a psychiatric hospital. The doctors state what sort of hospital would be most appropriate.
(2) The Secretary of State judges it expedient to remove and direct the offender to a suitable hospital.
(3) That a hospital has accepted the patient.
(4) The transfer must be enacted within 14 days, otherwise a further transfer direction would have to be sought.

The effect of section 47 is that the patient is detained in hospital as though on a hospital order but without the same relationship to the Mental Health Review Tribunal. In practice, the section 47 is accompanied by a restriction direction under section 49 of the Mental Health Act (see below).

Section 48: a transfer direction for remanded criminal and sentenced civil prisoners

This section allows for the transfer to a hospital of men in prison who are on remand (or civil prisoners during their sentence) if they are suffering from mental illness or severe mental impairment only. It was used only for the most severely mentally ill or severely mentally impaired patients where urgent psychiatric treatment in hospital was required. It is now used more liberally as a way of getting the mentally ill into hospital quickly. This section requires that:

(1) Two doctors (one approved) recommend to the Home Secretary that such a transfer be effected on the basis of the severity of the mental illness or severe mental impairment of the prisoner.
(2) The Home Secretary considers that the transfer is expedient.
(3) A hospital is willing to accept the patient.
(4) The patient is moved within 14 days of the transfer direction having been provided.

The patient may stay in the hospital until he is well enough to return to prison to continue his remand. In the case of patients who have been remanded by a magistrates' court, they can only be detained for the length of that remand. However, that remand can be renewed by the magistrates' court to allow the patient to stay in hospital. In the case of patients remanded to await trial in a crown court, the date of appearance will be altered to suit the case. If the patient does not improve, the question of fitness to plead or a hospital order through section 51 may have to be considered (see below).

The use of section 48 is increasing as remand prisons and the NHS respond to the current policy of diversion of the mentally ill from the penal system.

Section 49

This section (known as a restriction direction) allows the Home Secretary to place restrictions (as in section 41) on a transferred convicted prisoner and makes mandatory that restrictions be placed on transferred remand prisoners. The restriction direction lasts, in the case of convicted men, until the earliest date of release from prison when the order effectively becomes a simple section 37. Should the doctor then continue the detention it would be without the restrictions. In the case of remanded men the restriction direction lasts until the court deals with the case, or until the man is returned to remand prison.

Sections 50–53

These sections deal with the management by the Home Secretary (or courts as well, in remand cases) of transferred prisoners once they are declared well again, or once it is found that no effective treatment can be given. This allows the transfer back to prison from hospital. Section 51(v) and 51(vi) allows the making of a hospital order on the mentally ill, or severely mentally impaired who are on a transfer direction whilst on remand, in their absence and without convicting them. This section is used when a prisoner has been moved from remand prison to hospital (section 48) and there is little likelihood of recovery sufficient to stand trial. Two doctors must give oral or written evidence about the mental state, and then the court can make a section 37 order in the patient's absence but without registering a conviction.

Mentally disordered people at home and in public places, and the role of the police

Section 135

Subsection 1 allows the police, with a magistrates' warrant, to enter the private premises of a person believed to be suffering from a mental disorder if it is suspected that they are either (1) being ill-treated, neglected or not kept under proper control, or, (2) unable to care for themselves if living alone. Subsection 2 similarly allows the police to remove from private premises a patient liable to be taken or recalled. For the warrant under subsection (1) the magistrate requires information received on oath from an approved social worker that there is reasonable cause to suspect the mentally disordered person of being ill-treated and neglected (either by himself or others), or not kept under proper control. For the warrant under subsection (2) the magistrate requires information on oath from a constable or a person authorized to retake the patient. Under subsection (1) the police constable should be accompanied by a medical practitioner and an approved social worker, and under subsection (2) a medical practitioner and a person authorized to take or retake the patient. The subject can be detained in a place of safety for up to 72 hours so that the person's condition can be assessed.

Section 136

This section allows the police to remove from a public place any person who appears to be suffering from a mental disorder and who is in need of immediate care and control. The constable may take the person to a place of safety (which may include a psychiatric hospital) where he can be detained for a period not exceeding 72 hours for his condition to be assessed by a doctor and an approved social worker. Such authority should only be used in the interest of the person or for the protection of others. In practice, it is likely to be used for patients who behave in a bizarre or dangerous way in a public place.

If further detention of the person was then required then an assessment or treatment order (section 2 or 3, Mental Health Act 1983) would be considered.

Mentally disordered offenders and probation

When a convicted man is mentally disordered, but not to such an extent that admission to hospital is necessary, it may be appropriate for him to receive psychiatric treatment as an outpatient as a condition of probation.

Probation can be a very useful disposal for patients for whom out-patient care is the most appropriate. It can also be applied to those mentally disordered people who fall outside the categories which permit detention, e.g. inadequate personalities with minor depressive swings, personality disorders accompanied by sexual deviations, alcoholics, etc. Treatment as a condition of probation can be required to last for up to three years and may be: (1) residential, (2) non-residential, (3) under the direction of a specified doctor.

To make such an order the court requires:

(1) Oral or written evidence from a doctor approved under section 12 that such treatment would be appropriate.
(2) Evidence that a named doctor is available to provide such treatment.
(3) The offender to be willing to comply with the order.
(4) A probation officer to have been consulted about the order.

The effects of the order:

(1) The patient is expected to accept the treatment as prescribed.
(2) The doctor can discharge the patient from treatment when the patient no longer needs it.
(3) If the patient breaches the conditions of the order (e.g. fails to attend) then the doctor should inform the probation officer who may choose to take the patient back to court for breach of probation. The court may then choose, depending on the circumstances, to leave the matter or to re-sentence the offender.

Under the same Act the court has the power to remand an offender in custody or on bail after conviction in order to obtain social and psychiatric reports to aid them in their sentencing. If the patient is remanded in custody the request for a psychiatric report from the court will be sent to the prison doctors. If the patient is remanded on bail then the request will be sent to a local psychiatrist.

Diversion from the legal system for mentally abnormal offenders

Systems for the diversion of the mentally abnormal offender from the legal system – have been discussed in Chapter 1.

The legal basis for diversion[5] of the seriously mentally ill depends on where the subject is when the diversion occurs, and also at what stage in the legal process (see also Chapter 3) the diversion occurs.

(1) After arrest: In the police station: admission may be arranged voluntarily or by using section 2, 3 or 4, Mental Health Act 1983.

(2) After arrest: police may bring the subject to the hospital for 72 hours' detention and observation, using section 136, Mental Health Act 1983.

(3) In the court:
  (a) before trial: if the subject is agreeable he may be bailed to the hospital (Bail Act 1976) by the court. Psychiatric reports may be requested. (Two reports (one by a doctor approved under section 12 of the Mental Health Act 1983) are mandatory under the Bail Act if the subject is charged with murder);
  (b) before, or during trial: section 35 of the Mental Health Act 1983 may be used to admit to hospital for reports; from a crown court, section 36 can be used for treatment.

(4) During remand in prison: A prison governors' order can be used to move someone to hospital in an emergency if immediate transfer is required. A section 48 (Mental Health Act 1983) transfer direction can also be arranged with the Home Office very quickly using fax and telephone.

(5) After conviction: A section 38 order (Mental Health Act 1983) can be used for a trial of treatment, or a section 37 treatment order (Mental Health Act 1983) can be made by the court in appropriate cases.

(6) After a custodial sentence: A transfer to hospital under section 47, Mental Health Act 1983 can be made.

Mental abnormality as a defence in court

In the majority of cases an accused person with a mental abnormality will stand his trial, and, normally it will only be after a plea of guilty or finding of guilt that medical evidence will be presented in order to mitigate the sentencing of the court. The offender is saying: 'At the time of the offence I was suffering from a mental disorder which I would like you to take into consideration in sentencing me and, if possible, send me for treatment rather than punishment'.

In certain uncommon cases, the accused is conveying to the court that:

(1) He is not fit enough to appear in court (not fit to stand trial);

or that:

(2) Although fit enough to appear in the courtroom he is not fit enough to take part in the trial. The phrases used to describe this are 'not fit to plead' or 'under disability in relation to the trial';

or that:

(3) Although he agrees that he did the act, he is claiming that he was not fully responsible at the time. He may claim that because of severe mental disorder he had
    (a) no responsibility for his acts and therefore should not be found guilty; or
    (b) (in the case of homicide) that he had diminished responsibility for his acts; or
    (c) that he was behaving automatically and therefore no crime was committed; or
    (d) that, in the case of a mother accused of killing her baby, the balance of mind was so disturbed that she should be found not-guilty of murder but guilty of the lesser offence, infanticide.

Thus, in these cases, the psychiatric evidence is heard before the trial or as part of the trial. These various pleas are described below.

Not fit to stand trial

An accused may not be fit to stand trial (to appear in court) on medical grounds, either because of severe physical illness or severe mental disorder, e.g. a state of mania. In such a case, if the man has been remanded in custody, it is quite likely that the prison doctor will already have initiated arrangements for a transfer direction under section 48 to have the offender treated in a local hospital. The consultant at the local hospital will then liaise with the clerk of the court over the weeks to keep the court acquainted with the offender's state of mind. When he is fit enough he can then be produced in court. In the case of the magistrates' court, the patient has to be remanded regularly. This can be done in the patient's absence if his solicitor is in court and there is a report from the doctor. In the case of a crown court the date of appearance in court can be simply put off until the patient is well enough to appear. If the offence is trivial and the patient is going to be treated anyway, the court or prosecution may choose not to proceed with the charge but allow the patient to stay in hospital to receive treatment. In a more serious case, on a transfer direction, section 51(vi) of the Mental Health Act 1983 allows a court to make a hospital order in the patient's absence (see above).

Not fit to plead (under disability)

It has been regarded as wrong, for centuries, to try a person who is unable to defend himself in court. This principle covers not only the mentally ill and the subnormal but also those who are unable to communicate, e.g. the deaf-mute with no ability to use sign- or written language. Both types of cases are dealt with by the new Criminal Procedure (Insanity and

Unfitness to Plead) Act 1991. If the accused is found to be under disability, the trial, as previously, shall not proceed. The court can now dispose of the case more appropriately. (Previously, under the 1964 Act, all cases were lumped together. A hospital order with restrictions had to be made which led to such anomalous situations as both the severely mentally ill and deaf-mutes being sent to psychiatric hospital.)

The question of the accused being unfit may be raised by the defence, the prosecution or the judge, and is a matter which has to be tried in a crown court. The question may be raised at the very start of the trial or the judge may allow it to be postponed until the prosecution case is heard – for if the case is weak then the accused may have no case to answer. The plea must be proven, on the balance of probabilities (if raised by the defence), or, beyond reasonable doubt (if raised by the prosecution). A new jury is empanelled just to decide the question. If the matter is not proven then the original trial goes on.

For a person to be found under disability it must be proven that the accused is unable to:

(1) Plead to the indictment.
(2) Comprehend the course of the proceedings of the trial so as to make a proper defence.
(3) Know that he might challenge a juror.
(4) Comprehend the details of the evidence.

Such a person, as a result of his disabilities, will be unable to instruct counsel or examine a witness. It is not enough simply that the accused might act against his own interests (e.g. in paranoia) or that he conducts his defence unwisely.

In order to 'prove' the disability in the case of mental illness, two psychiatrists (one approved under section 12, Mental Health Act 1983) are asked to give reports before a jury empanelled for the purpose. If the jury is convinced of the disability, then the court deals with the case under the Criminal Procedure (Insanity and Unfitness to Plead) Act 1991. A jury has then to hear the prosecution and defence case and decide whether or not the defendant committed the act. If not convinced then the defendant is acquitted; if convinced, a finding that the defendant did the act is recorded. The judge then has a number of possible disposals available under this new Act. These are:

(1) In a case of murder: an admission order to a hospital specified by the Secretary of State (effectively a hospital order with a restriction order unlimited in time).
(2) In other cases, the possibilities are:
    (a) an absolute discharge;
    (b) a guardianship order (under section 37 Mental Health Act 1983);
    (c) a supervision and treatment order. This is a new order leading to

supervision by a social worker for a period of up to two years with a requirement to submit to treatment by a registered medical practitioner. The order specifies whether the treatment be in a hospital, on an outpatient basis, or as the doctor directs. Medical advice must be given that compulsory detention for treatment is not needed, and the court must be satisfied that release into the community will not pose an unacceptable risk. The court has to be satisfied that social work supervision is available. Continuing care may be needed after the order is over. The order is designed for relatively minor offences where the offender is likely to co-operate. Failure to co-operate will lead to consideration for detention under Part II of the Mental Health Act 1983. If the person becomes dangerous it may be necessary to warn the police.

(d) an admission order to a hospital specified by the Secretary of State. This works like a section 37 from the date of the order. The court has the option of adding a restriction order.

If the jury is unconvinced of the disability then the accused is found fit to plead. The trial proper then begins and a new jury empanelled.

If the 'unfit' patient recovers, he can then be tried. If recovery does not take place within a reasonable time then it is unlikely there will be a trial. Under the old Act someone found guilty under disability was automatically detained as though under a hospital order with a restriction order unlimited in time. This dissuaded seriously ill people from this plea when the offence was a minor one. The present Act with its wide range of disposals will encourage more people to plead that they are under disability.

Not guilty by reason of insanity

In this case it is argued that the defendant cannot be held responsible for his actions because of the severity of the mental illness. The accused has to prove in a higher court on the balance of probabilities that at the time of the offence he laboured under such defect of the mind that he met the McNaughten Rules, i.e.

(1) That by reason of such defect from disease of the mind he did not know the nature or quality of his act (i.e. that he did not realize what he was physically doing at the time).

Or:

(2) By reason of such defect from disease of the mind that he did not know what he was doing was wrong (i.e. that he did not know that what he was doing was forbidden by law).

Or:

(3) Where a person is under an insane delusion which prevents the true appreciation of the nature and quality of his act, he is under the same degree of responsibility as if the facts were as he imagined them to be.

> A man had a delusional belief that he was in immediate mortal danger and he killed the person who 'threatened' him. His plea of 'not guilty by reason of insanity' was successful under the third rule.

A finding of not guilty by reason of insanity is known as the 'special verdict'. To prove the case, evidence must be presented by two or more medical practitioners one of whom is approved under the Mental Health Act 1983. The Criminal Procedure (Insanity and Unfitness to Plead) Act 1991 allows the judge to make use of a range of options for the care of the defendant. Under the previous 1964 Act the 'special verdict' was followed automatically by detention in hospital as though on section 37, Mental Health Act 1983 with a restriction order unlimited in time. In consequence the plea was used only by offenders who had committed serious offences. Offenders who met the McNaughten criteria but whose offence was minor lacked, at crown court level, a sensible disposal. The disposals now available are the same as for those defendants found to be under disability (see above).

This plea is of historical interest and has been discussed in detail by West and Walk[6]. For centuries, it has been a principle in English law that a gravely mentally ill person is not responsible for his actions. The Criminal Lunatics Act of 1800 allowed the acquittal of an accused if he was found not guilty on the grounds of insanity, though this finding was always followed by detention in custody pending His Majesty's pleasure. This custody came to mean incarceration in institutions for the psychiatrically ill.

> McNaughten was a Scotsman who in 1843 attempted to kill the Prime Minister, Sir John Peel, and in error killed the Prime Minister's secretary. McNaughten was under the delusion that his life was in danger from the Prime Minister's political party. He was found not guilty by reason of insanity. The finding was unpopular and there was a demand for clear guidelines to the court on such cases. In response to this the criteria known as the McNaughten Rules were laid down by the Law Lords.

The Rules became particularly important for mentally abnormal offenders charged with murder, because, until the abolition of the death sentence, a successful plea avoided execution. The Rules have, however, been subject to criticism. They are said to be based on a misunderstanding of mental illness and its effect on the patient. The Rules assume that mental illness is a disorder of reason only and do not recognize that mental illness may affect very severely aspects of mental life other than reason. The Rules are very strict and many severely mentally disordered people fall outside them, particularly those with disorders of emotion.

Diminished responsibility

The Homicide Act 1957 introduced, in the case of murder, the defence of 'diminished responsibility'. This Act allows a person charged with murder to plead that his mental abnormality, while not sufficiently severe to meet the strict criteria of the McNaughten Rules, is nevertheless sufficient to substantially diminish his responsibility. It has to be shown, on the balance of probabilities, that, at the time of the offence, the accused suffered from 'such abnormality of mind (whether arising from a condition of arrested or retarded development of mind or inherent causes or induced by disease or injury) as substantially impaired his mental responsibilities for his acts or omissions in doing or being party to the killing'. 'Abnormality of mind' has been ruled by the Court of Criminal Appeal (*R* v. *Byrne*) to mean:

> 'a state of mind so different from that of ordinary human beings that the reasonable man would term it abnormal. It appears to us to be wide enough to cover the mind's activities in all its aspects, not only the perception of physical acts and matters, and the ability to form a rational judgement as to whether the act was right or wrong, but also the ability to exercise willpower to control physical acts in accordance with that rational judgement'.

The meaning of 'mental responsibility' is unclear but is taken to refer to culpability. 'Substantially' is also undefined and is left for the jury to decide though the doctor will be asked his opinion. The effect of a successful plea is to reduce the charge from murder to manslaughter. Murder carried a statutory sentence of execution in the days of capital punishment; nowadays it carries the statutory sentence of life imprisonment. If the charge is reduced to manslaughter then the court is free to make any sentence, including hospital orders and probation.

The Homicide Act 1957 has been criticized because of the lack of definitions and the stretching of the meanings of the words which occur[7]. Nevertheless, because of its flexibility, the plea of diminished responsibility has largely replaced the plea of not-guilty by reason of insanity. In the case of the severely mentally ill the outcome of both pleas, if successful, is much the same – i.e. committal to a hospital for treatment with a restriction order attached. However, in the case of a successful plea of diminished responsibility, more choices are available to the judge, e.g. if the offender's mental state does not require admission to a psychiatric hospital, the judge is free to make treatment a condition of probation. If the psychiatric condition is such that treatment in a hospital is unlikely to be helpful (as in the case of psychopathic disorder, for example) then the judge may choose to sentence the offender to imprisonment – indeed to life imprisonment in appropriate cases.

It is important to note that the defence of diminished responsibility is specific to the Homicide Act 1957, and use of the term should be restricted to this defence against a charge of murder.

Automatism

This is a rare plea in which the defendant claims that at the time of the offence he was behaving 'automatically' and therefore is not guilty of a crime. In law, this term means a state where the mind is not ruling the body. Two forms are recognized.

Sane automatism
This is due to external causes, (e.g. behaviour in a state of concussion after a blow on the head or behaviour in a confusional state after an anaesthetic). The plea has even been successful with absent-minded behaviour at a time of stress or in a hypoglycaemic state from a large insulin injection. It is argued that in automatism there is no conscious capacity to control one's actions and therefore no possibility of *mens rea*. A successful plea of sane automatism leads therefore to a total acquittal.

Insane automatism
This is an automatism due to an 'internal' cause of behaviour without voluntary control, such as epilepsy, insulinoma, or degenerative brain disease. Such behaviour may, the law argues, recur until the illness is controlled. It is argued that the disease so affects the mind that the subject at the time of the incident does not know what he is doing. The subject thus falls into the McNaughten Rules. A successful plea of insane automatism leads to the subject being found not-guilty by reason of insanity. The defendant is then sentenced according to the Criminal Procedure (Insanity and Unfitness to Plead) Act 1991 (see **Not fit to plead** above). This new law allows considerable latitude in disposal which can be adjusted to the particular case.

Historically, people who have offended whilst their consciousness was affected by sleep (in sleep walking, night terrors or awaking from deep sleep) have been regarded as having sane automatism (despite the fact that sleep is an internal cause). They have been acquitted and advised to sleep alone with the bedroom door locked (see Chapter 9).

> A soldier dreaming of fighting, was woken from sleep. Before being fully awake he reflexly seized his bayonet and killed the person waking him. His plea of automatism was successful.

The illogicality of regarding all sleep disorders as having an external cause has been pointed out in court[8]. As a result, in the case of a man who behaved violently whilst sleepwalking, the court ruled (supported by the Court of Appeal) that a finding of insane automatism was appropriate just as it would have been if he were in fact in a hysterical fugue.

Infanticide

This is a plea which can be offered under the Infanticide Act 1938, as a defence when a woman is accused of the murder of her child. To be successful the child must have been less than 12 months old, and it must be shown that the balance of the mother's mind was disturbed by reason of her not having fully recovered from the effects of giving birth to the child, or by reason of the effects of lactation, consequent upon the birth of the child. The effect of a successful plea is to reduce the charge of murder to one of manslaughter – the same effect as a successful plea under diminished responsibility. It would clearly be the proper plea in a case occurring during puerperal psychosis but it is also used successfully where the degree of mental disturbance is less than would be required for a plea of diminished responsibility. It is not necessary to argue that the woman had a mental illness or abnormality; it is only necessary to show that the balance of the mother's mind was disturbed.

The problems of amnesia, drugs and alcohol, mute defendants and false confessions

Amnesia

Amnesia (loss of memory) may arise from organic causes (see Chapter 9) or psychological ones[9,10]. The latter occurs in the absence of detectable brain pathology. Psychological causes are suspected clinically when there is evidence of new information being retained normally or when there appears to be inability to retain any memory for even a few seconds. It may be caused by:

(1) A failure to lay down memory (in severe depression, extreme emotional arousal or severe psychotic arousal).
(2) The motivated forgetting of unpleasant memories.
(3) Impaired ability to recall due to a disturbed mood, e.g. in severe depression.

Amnesia for the offence has been found in 40% of men remanded for homicide and 10% overall in remanded men mostly due to psychogenic causes. Deciding whether an amnesia is feigned or a genuine psychogenic amnesia is extremely difficult, if not impossible.

Amnesia for the offence, or the period around it, is not in itself a defence: the trial will proceed regardless of whether the accused can remember the events or not. However, if it can be shown that the amnesia is due to a mental disorder, then, clearly, that mental disorder may be a defence – e.g. if an offence is committed whilst consciousness is disturbed following a fit, or during a state of extreme excitability during an acute psychotic breakdown, then it is those disturbed mental states that would form the basis of the defence, not the associated amnesia.

Drugs and alcohol

The relation of substance-induced disorders and the law is discussed in Chapter 9. In law, a person is held to be fully responsible for anything done after knowingly taking drugs or alcohol. The only possible exceptions to this are:

(1) Where substances have induced psychosis or a reaction which could not have been anticipated.
(2) Where the drugs and alcohol have removed the ability to form a specific intent.

There, there may be some defence (see Chapter 9).

Mute defendants

If a defendant is mute the court has to decide whether he is mute by 'malice or by visitation of God'. The doctor may be asked to assist in this. If the defendant is mute through some illness, whatever it is, then the question of fitness to plead is raised. The final outcome may then be a disposal under The Criminal Procedure (Insanity and Unfitness to Plead) Act 1991. If he is mute by malice then there is no bar to his trial.

False confessions

Attention has recently been drawn to the problem of people who come to deny the confession of guilt that they made to the police. Psychologists or psychiatrists may be asked to comment on the chances of a confession being false.

Clearly, when the original confession was truly false it may have been given because of undue pressure in interrogation or in an attempt to escape the pressures of custody which may include the effects of hunger, lack of sleep, fear, etc. It may also be due to suggestibility, undue compliance or acquiescence. Gudjonsson[11] reported on 100 cases of people who have retracted their confessions. He found they were characterized by lower intelligence and increased scores on a suggestibility and compliance test. However, this does not imply that such features necessarily indicate lack of guilt; they are the features of people who retract their confessions.

Three types of proven false confessions were described by Gudjonsson and McKeith[12]:

(1) Voluntary false confession: A person comes forward voluntarily to 'confess' (this may be due to a delusional state, a morbid depression, or perhaps for attention or notoriety).
(2) Coerced confession: The person confesses in the hope of stopping what is experienced as unbearable pressure from either style of questioning or the stress of the situation, perhaps exacerbated by hunger, fatigue or fear.
(3) Coerced – internalized: The person seems to become confused and appears temporarily convinced of his guilt during interrogation, perhaps due to the combination of the subject's suggestibility and tendency to compliance and methods of questioning.

Where the defendant is known to be vulnerable, then the Police and Criminal Evidence Act 1984 requires that an independent person be present in the interview to help protect the interviewee.

References

(1) Jones, R.M. (1991) *Mental Health Act Manual*. Sweet and Maxwell, London.
(2) Home Office and Department of Health and Society Security (1975) *Report of the Committee on Mentally Abnormal Offenders (Butler Committee)* Cmnd. 6244. HMSO, London.
(3) Bluglass, R. (1983) *A Guide to the Mental Health Act 1983*. Churchill Livingstone, Edinburgh.
(4) Department of Health (1993) *Code of Practice: Code of Practice: Mental Health Act 1983*. HMSO, London.
(5) Joseph, P.L. (1990) Mentally disordered offenders: Diversion from the criminal justice system. *Journal of Forensic Psychiatry* **1**, 133–8.
(6) West, D J & Walk, A. (1977) *Daniel McNaughten: His Trial and the Aftermath*. Gaskell Books (for The Royal College of Psychiatrists), Ashford, Kent
(7) Cordess, C. (1985) The Homicide Act: Origins, anomalies and proposals for change. *Bulletin of the Royal College of Psychiatrists* **9**, 245–6.
(8) Fenwick, P. (1990) Automatism, medicine and the law. *Psychological Medicine, Monograph Supplement* **17**.
(9) Stone, J.H. (1992) Memory disorder in offenders and victims. *Criminal Behaviour and Mental Health* **2**, 342–56.
(10) Lishman, W.A. (1987) *Organic Psychiatry*. Blackwell Scientific Publications, Oxford.
(11) Gudjonsson, G.H. (1990) One hundred alleged false confession cases: some normative data. *British Journal of Clinical Psychology* **29**, 249–50.
(12) Gudjonsson, G.H. & McKeith, J.A.C. (1990) A proven case of false confession: psychological aspects of the coerced compliant type. *Medicine, Science and the Law* **30**, 329–35.

Chapter 4

Legal Aspects: Appeals and Protection

Introduction

Patients have a protection against the activities of courts, doctors, the Home Secretary (responsible for restricted patients), and the managers of the hospital (responsible for detaining them). This protection comes from appeal courts, the Mental Health Act Commission, the Mental Health Review Tribunal, and the duties placed on the managers. Each of these will be considered in turn. The duties are described of the Home Office Advisory Board which is responsible for assessing certain dangerous restricted patients in order to protect the public. This is followed by a note on the role of the European Commission on Human Rights.

Appealing against court decisions

The appeal system

Appeals are made to the court above the one which gave the sentence. Thus, an appeal about the verdict or sentence of a magistrates' court is made to the crown court, and appeals about the crown court go to the Courts of Appeal. The latter are situated in the Royal Courts of Justice in London and consist of a Criminal Division and a Civil Division. The president of the Criminal Division is the Lord Chief Justice and he is assisted by 21 full-time 'Lord Justices of Appeal'. The court consists of one Lord Justice and two other judges.

On points of law one can then appeal to the Lords of Appeal in the House of Lords. It is also possible to appeal to the European Court of Justice if it is felt that the English Law conflicts with the European Treaties, e.g. the European Court of Human Rights agreed with an appellant that it was wrong that the Home Secretary should have sole right to discharge restricted patients under the Mental Health Act 1959. As a result, in the 1983 Act, the Mental Health Review Tribunal was given the power to override the Home Secretary's decision in restricted cases.

Whenever someone wishes to appeal he has to obtain permission from the court for the appeal to be considered. This permission will be given on the basis of there being good grounds for appeal.

Who may appeal?
Those who may appeal are:

(1) The Home Secretary – if requested, on behalf of someone found not fit to plead or someone found not-guilty by reason of insanity.
(2) The convicted offender.
(3) The Attorney General – against too small a sentence in certain serious cases (Criminal Justice Act 1988), and a new sentence may be set. The Attorney General, after an acquittal, may refer the case on points of law to the Court of Appeal but the effects of this appeal will not affect the acquitted defendant though the court's advice may affect future practice.

Subjects of appeal
The convicted offender may appeal against:

(1) Conviction.
(2) Sentence.
(3) Conviction and sentence.
(4) A verdict of not guilty by reasons of insanity.
(5) A finding of being unfit to be tried.

Grounds for appeal
These may be that:

(1) The verdict of the jury was unsafe or unsatisfactory, because:
    (a) inadmissible evidence was used;
    (b) proper evidence was excluded;
    (c) uncorroborated evidence was used;
    (d) there was misdirection of the jury by the judge on technical matters.
(2) The judgement of the court was wrong on a question of law.
(3) There were irregularities in the course of the trial.
(4) The sentence did not fall within the normal tariff for the offence – either it was too severe or too lenient.

The effect of the appeal

(1) At the crown court level: The crown court hears appeals against the judgement of the magistrates' court. The court may grant the appeal and change the finding or sentence of the magistrates' court. However, they may also increase the sentence if they believe the magistrate has been too lenient, though they have to keep within the limits of the magistrates' court's sentencing powers.

(2) At the court of appeal level, criminal division: The Court of Appeal deals with cases which come from the crown court. The Court of Appeal may quash the conviction or reduce, change, or increase the sentence if they feel that it is not within the normal tariff.

(3) At the House of Lords: this deals only with points of law.

Appeals and the forensic psychiatrist

A forensic psychiatrist may have to convince a court that a sentence was inappropriate or that a treatment should or should not have been made.

> A schizophrenic patient was convicted of breaking into a house and assaulting a sleeping girl. Psychiatrists recommended to the court that the man be sent to the local regional secure unit on a treatment order. The judge, however, felt that the security of the unit was not sufficient for the man and gave a life sentence. The defendant appealed and psychiatrists were called to the Appeal Court to give evidence about his mental state, the treatment and security available in the regional secure unit, and the safety of his being treated there. The appeal court re-sentenced the defendant to receive treatment on a hospital order at the regional secure unit.

Mental Health Review Tribunal

Definition

A tribunal is effectively a court under the Lord Chancellor's jurisdiction with the specialist function of dealing with disputes in which the weak are pitted against the powerful. The function of the Mental Health Review Tribunal is to deal with the dispute between the detained patient and his detainer.

Structure

There are 14 regional services (matching the regional health authorities) covering England and Wales. A regional chairman has responsibility for the tribunals which consist of a lawyer as president sitting with a psychiatrist and layman of appropriate experience. When the tribunal is dealing with a restricted case then the president must be a circuit judge or a recorder, otherwise the president is frequently a solicitor. Four administrative offices provide the support for the tribunals.

Legal aspects

Mental Health Review Tribunals are conducted with powers given to them under the Mental Health Act 1983[1] and their practice is governed by guidelines issued in association with that Act.

In all cases (except the restricted) even though illness may still be present, Mental Health Review Tribunals have the discretionary power to discharge the offender without any special conditions being met if they believe it appropriate. They must discharge under certain conditions (see below). In non-restricted (but *not* in restricted) cases the tribunal may recommend transfer or trial leave. Their decision may be deferred to allow further investigation or arrangements to be made. They may also direct that a patient's condition be reclassified, e.g. 'mental illness' to 'psychopathic disorder'.

Procedures of the tribunals

The tribunal is run in a relatively informal manner but with considerable attention to the rights of the patient to hear the case and be heard. It is now normal practice for the patient to be represented by a solicitor (for which legal aid is available). The patient and his legal representative, the responsible medical officer, the social worker and relatives will come together before the tribunal which will sit, usually, in a room provided by the hospital in which the patient is detained. The patient and his representative will give their case – possibly supported by their relatives – and then the doctor and social worker will give theirs. Other people who may have relevant information may be called, e.g. a nurse or psychologist.

The tribunals normally expect that the patient should hear the reasons for his detention, although the tribunal also recognizes that there may be instances where the responsible medical officer may wish to say something which would be damaging for the patient to hear. However, even in this case, the patient's representative will be present, though it is understood that he will not divulge the damaging material. Similarly, the patient's relatives may wish to see the tribunal without the patient being present, and they have an opportunity to write to the tribunal and ask for this before the tribunal sits. It may be that they feel unable at that time to support the patient's application but fear that if the knowledge came to the patient's ears it would permanently ruin their relationship with him. When all the evidence is heard the tribunal considers the case and conveys its decision to the patient and the responsible medical officer after a few days.

Tribunals are normally private and the proceedings may not be published unless the applicant applies for a public hearing (perhaps to publicize his case).

Preparation for a tribunal

Before the tribunal meets the responsible medical officer and social workers will be asked to supply a detailed account of the case including a view about the continued need for detention. The social worker should also obtain a description of the community resources in the patient's home area so that the tribunal has this information in case they wish to discharge the patient. In the case of a restricted patient, the Home Office will also be asked its view about the need for further detention. The patient will require a solicitor to represent him (a list of local solicitors able to provide this service is normally kept by the hospital or The Law Society). The solicitor must be given access to the patient and the opportunity to discuss the case with the responsible medical officer. The solicitor may instruct another psychiatrist to supply him with an independent report. It is proper to give this psychiatrist every facility to assess the case, including access to the patient's case notes. The psychiatrist on the tribunal will also visit the patient before the tribunal. He also must have every facility to investigate the case including the opportunity to see the medical notes and the chance to discuss the case with staff who look after the patient.

A patient's right to a tribunal

The Mental Health Act 1983 (sections 65–79) substantially increased the power of tribunals and the access of patients to them. The situation is complex, however, for the rights of the patient depend on this section as do the powers of the tribunal. They are discussed in detail by Jones[1]. The principal features are described below.

Patients detained under Part II of the Mental Health Act
Tribunals may be requested in the following situations:

(1) **After a patient has been detained for assessment (section 2):** The patient may apply for a tribunal in order to obtain his discharge within 14 days of the section being activated. The tribunal must discharge immediately or at a future date if:
   (a) the patient does not meet the criteria of any or sufficient mental disorder to merit assessment in hospital, or
   (b) the patient's detention is not justified in the interests of his health and safety or protection of others.

Leave of absence or transfer may also be recommended in appropriate cases.

(2) **After a patient has been detained for treatment (section 3):** The patient may apply within six months of the section being activated – as can his relatives. After six months, the managers of the hospital have a statutory duty to have a tribunal which, under Statute, must be repeated every three years. The tribunal must discharge the patient if they find that:
   (a) the patient is not suffering from any form of mental disorder needing treatment or detention in hospital, or

(b) it is not necessary to detain the patient in hospital in the interests of his own health and safety, or for the protection of others, or,
(c) in the case of psychopathic disorder, the disorder is no longer amenable to hospital treatment (*R* v. *Cannons Park Mental Health Review Tribunal, ex parte* A. *Times Law Report*, 24.8.93). This recent innovative ruling is to be challenged at Appeal Court.

If the patient is not fit for discharge he may be sufficiently well for the tribunal to recommend leave of absence or transfer. Such a recommendation, although not a mandatory order, does carry considerable weight. If this recommendation is not complied with, the tribunal may consider the case further, at a later date. When making these recommendations, or exercising discretionary discharge powers, the tribunal has to consider the likely effects of further treatment, and also the ability of the mentally ill and the severely impaired patients to care for themselves or guard themselves against serious exploitation. Tribunals must satisfy themselves on a balance of probabilities.

(3) After a patient has been subject to guardianship under section 3: The patient may apply, as may his relatives, within the first six months and thereafter as in the case of section 3 treatment orders. The tribunal must discharge if they find the patient is not mentally disordered or if they find it is unnecessary for him to be in guardianship.

In (4)–(7) below, the tribunal may order discharge or recommend transfer on trial leave.

(4) After a responsible medical officer has reclassified the patient under section 16 (changed the category of mental disorder): The patient or his nearest relative may apply for a tribunal in the first 18 days.
(5) After a renewal of detention: The patient or his relative may apply once during any new period of detention.
(6) After the issue of a certificate of dangerousness: If a responsible medical officer (under section 25) has issued a statement that the patient is dangerous to the managers in order to prevent relatives discharging a patient, then the nearest relative can apply to the Mental Health Review Tribunal within 28 days.
(7) After the county court directs someone to take over the function of the nearest relative: After a county court has directed (under section 29) that the function of the nearest relative (in terms of application or discharge) be taken over by another relative or social worker, then the nearest relative or social worker can apply to the Mental Health Review Tribunal within 12 months, and any subsequent period of 12 months.

Patients detained under Part III of the Mental Health Act
The rules for tribunals depend on the section:
(1) After a patient has been detained on a hospital order: The patient or

his relative may apply but only after six months have elapsed and then once during each time the section is renewed. The hospital managers, otherwise, have a duty to arrange a tribunal every three years. The powers of the tribunal are as for patients detained under section 3 (see above).

(2) **After the patient has been placed on a guardianship order by the court:** The patient may apply within 6 months and the nearest relative within 12 months. The powers of the tribunal are the same as for a section 3 guardianship order (see above).

(3) **After the renewal of a hospital order:** The patient or his nearest relative may apply after every renewal. The managers of the hospital have a statutory duty to arrange a tribunal for the patient every three years. The powers of the tribunal are the same as for patients detained under section 3 (see above).

(4) **After a patient has been detained on a hospital order with a restriction order:** The patient may apply to the tribunal after six months and then subsequently annually. The Secretary of State otherwise has a duty to arrange a tribunal every three years beginning from the day the order was made. In the case of restricted patients, the tribunal's powers are limited. However, the tribunal must discharge absolutely if they find that the patient is:

    (a) not now mentally disordered, or that the disorder is not such as to need detention in hospital, or that the patient is disordered but it is not necessary for the health and safety of the patient or for the protection of others that he should receive treatment, and

    (b) it is also not appropriate that he is liable to recall.

Or

    (c) in the case of psychopathic disorder, the disorder is no longer amenable to hospital treatment (*R v Cannons Park Mental Health Review Tribunal, ex parte* A. *Times Law Report*, 24.8.93). This recent and controversial Judicial Review ruling, if supported by the Appeal Court, will have considerable implications. Will refusal of a psychopath to co-operate with treatment mean release is inevitable? If so interpreted, then the use, already small, of section for psychopathic disorder will effectively cease. Before the ruling such patients were customarily detained despite being unamenable to treatment.

On the other hand, the tribunal must discharge conditionally if:

(a) it is felt that it is appropriate that he be liable to recall but now is
    (i)   not suffering from mental disorder, or
    (ii) his mental disorder is such as not to need detention in hospital for treatment, or

(iii) that it is no longer necessary for the health or safety of the patient or protection of others that he should receive treatment.

Thus, if the tribunal finds the patient completely well and not likely to require further psychiatric care or to be so mildly disordered that recall is inappropriate they must discharge absolutely.

> A patient was detained for a number of years in special hospital. At his tribunal it became clear that he had deliberately feigned mental illness in order to be detained in hospital so as to hide his shame for his offence. By the time of the tribunal he had repaired his relationships with his family and was therefore willing to admit his deception. The tribunal discharged him absolutely.

Conditional discharge would clearly apply to a psychotic patient who makes a very good recovery but for whom aftercare would be advisable.

> A schizophrenic patient was detained on section 37/41 after setting fire to his house. His illness came under control and the responsible medical officer recommended conditional discharge. The Home Office refused permission but the patient, supported by the responsible medical officer, successfully applied to the Mental Health Review Tribunal for this conditional discharge.

The tribunal can delay its final direction whilst arrangements are made for the conditional discharge so that the plans for aftercare can be approved by the tribunal.

In cases subject to a restriction order the tribunal has, however, no discretionary powers of discharge or powers to recommend transfer to another hospital or leave of absence from the hospital. They can merely offer these as suggestions to the Home Office.

(5) **After a conditionally discharged restricted patient has been recalled to hospital:** The Secretary of State has a statutory duty to arrange a tribunal within one month of the patient's return to hospital. This arrangement came about because there have been complaints to the European Court, under the old Act, that a man might be called without any form of appeal. Thus the tribunal now acts as an appeal against the Home Secretary's judgement that the patient should be recalled.

(6) **After a patient has been transferred from prison to hospital for treatment under sections 47 and 48:** The patient may apply for a tribunal within six months and there must be a statutory tribunal held every three years. The tribunal's powers are severely limited in these cases. The tribunal notifies the Home Secretary of their opinion about suitability for discharge, detention in hospital or return to prison. If the alternative to detention in hospital is only prison, the Mental Health Review Tribunal can suggest further detention in hospital. The Home Secretary then decides within 90 days whether he will accept the suggestion for discharge (absolute or conditional as the case may be). If he does not agree to discharge, then the patient returns to prison

or stays in hospital depending on the tribunal's suggestion. Life-sentenced prisoners, when well, are to be returned to prison to be considered by the parole board before release to the community.

(7) **After a restricted patient has been conditionally discharged:** The patient may apply to a tribunal for absolute discharge after 12 months and then every two years. The powers of the tribunal are the same as for restricted patients.

Patients detained under the Criminal Procedure (Insanity and Unfitness to Plead) Act 1991 (not guilty by reason of insanity or found not fit to plead)
The patient may apply within six months and thereafter in the next six months and then annually. The Secretary of State will otherwise refer the patient for a tribunal after the first six months and then every three years. The tribunal's powers are the same as for restricted patients.

Patients who have no right to a tribunal

Some patients detained in hospital have no right or access to a tribunal. These include patients who are detained:

- for 72 hours (sections 4, 135 and 136)
- under section 35 (remand to hospital for report)
- under section 36 (detained by the court for treatment before sentence)
- under section 38 (detained for a trial of treatment)
- under section 44 (detained in hospital awaiting sentence for a restriction order from a crown court having been found guilty in a magistrates' court)
- under section 5(ii) and 5(iv) (detentions of voluntary patients already in hospital).

Criticism of tribunals

Peay[2] studied the workings of tribunals in various settings and regions. A lack of consistency was the principal finding. Some regions discharge many more than others and different presidents vary in their 'results' – some seeming to have more discharges than others. On the whole, tribunals tend to be very cautious about discharging and are heavily influenced by the medical opinion and rarely disagree with the responsible medical officer. The tribunal system has also been criticized for being slow to respond to requests for a tribunal for people detained on the longer sections. It may take several weeks or months to set up such a tribunal, due in part to the pressure of work on the tribunals.

Managers of the hospital and detained patients

Definition

The Mental Health Act defines managers as members of the District Health Authority (DHA) or the Special Hospital Authority (SHA) responsible for the administration of the hospital. It also includes any person appointed by the DHA to any committee or subcommittee of the DHA. Managers may 'authorize' officers to act on their behalf.

Duties of the managers in relation to detained patients

These are to:

(1) Nominate officers to receive the reception papers (which are legal documents), to check the documents and their contents, and to ensure that all procedures are followed, as laid down in the Mental Health Act – including the duty to inform the patient and his relatives of their rights.

(2) Ensure that the patient's condition meets the criteria defined in the Mental Health Act (section 20) necessary for him to be detained. Managers have, in fact, the powers to review and discharge a patient at any time if these criteria are not met.

(3) Review the renewal (three managers are involved) when a detention order is being renewed. In the past this has been a procedure which tended to rubber-stamp the doctors' recommendations. However, the renewal should be a thorough affair[3] with the three managers reviewing the case thoroughly (with a full history before them) by interviewing the patient and considering the relatives' views.

(4) Review the case – apart from assessing the case when the order for detention is renewed – if (a) a patient requests it, (b) the doctor makes a report to the managers to over-ride – usually because of the patient's dangerousness – a nearest relative's application to discharge the patient detained under Part II of the Act.

Mental Health Act Commission

Definition

This body was set up as a result of the Mental Health (Amendment) Act 1982 with the express purpose of guarding the rights of detained patients following a general feeling that these rights may have been abused.

Functions of the Mental Health Act Commission

These are given in the Act and include:

(1) The appointment of medical practitioners and others for the purposes of supervising the consent to treatment procedures.
(2) To receive reports on treatment given under the consent to treatment procedures.
(3) To keep the Mental Health Act under review, to visit patients and investigate complaints. This is done by the commissioners making regular visits to hospital to see detained patients.
(4) To submit proposals for the Code of Practice[3] for the care of detained patients.

Rules in regard to consent to treatment and detained patients
Three categories of treatment for detained patients require special consideration (Mental Health Act sections 57 and 58). Other treatments for mental disorder outside these categories (e.g. occupational therapy) can be given without consent.

The three categories are:

(1) Those treatments which can be given without the patient's consent for three months from the date the treatment starts. If the patient, after three months, does consent after proper explanation, the consent is recorded on form 38 and the treatment continues. On the other hand, if the patient refuses to consent or withdraws consent, or is unable to give real consent because of the effects of mental disorder (see below), then a second opinion is required from a doctor appointed by the Commission for this purpose. This doctor will give consideration to the treatment plan put forward by the responsible medical officer after interviewing the patient, assessing the case, and discussing it with at least two members of the multidisciplinary team, only one of whom may be a nurse. He will also check that the legal documents are in order. The appointed doctor will record his agreement to the treatment on form 39. Such approval lasts until the section is renewed. The responsible medical officer then furnishes a report to the Commission who decide if the approval shall continue or if a further visit is required. Treatment which can be given under this category includes medication by oral or parenteral routes and includes any venesection needed for blood tests (as with lithium or clozapine therapy).
(2) The second group includes treatment which can only be given with the patient's consent or, failing this, after support has been obtained from an appointed doctor who will consider the case as above. This category of treatment includes only electroconvulsive therapy (ECT) at the present time (Mental Health Act 1983, section 58).

(3) The third category applies to informal as well as detained patients. It includes treatments which cause irreversible changes and for which the patients' consent is essential. The Commission must send a doctor (who must consult two persons professionally concerned with the patient) and two other commission members to review the case to confirm the patient's general understanding and consent and the appropriateness of the treatment. Without the Commission's agreement even an informal patient may not receive the treatment. At present this group includes only psychosurgical operations and hormonal implants (Mental Health Act 1983, section 57).

Who comes under the consent rules?
The 'consent rules' do not apply to every detained patient. Some sections do not allow patients to be treated against their will. These sections are the ones which hold people for 72 hours or less (sections 4, 5(ii), 5(iv), 135 and 136) and a remand to hospital for psychiatric reports (section 35). In the former cases, if treatment is required then the section should be re-graded. In the latter case, the Code of Practice[3] allows the use of section 3 (in conjunction with section 35) to detain the patient for treatment. This might occur in the case of a patient referred for a report who turns out to be so severely ill that treatment is required at once.

Conditionally discharged patients do not fall within the rules; they may refuse the medication though this may mean that recall has to be considered.

Consent and mental capacity
To give consent, a patient must have the capacity to do so[3]. The patient must understand what the treatment is, that someone says he needs it, and why it is he needs it. The nature, benefits and risks must be understood in general terms – as must the consequences of not receiving the treatment. The patient's capacity is a matter for clinical judgement subject to the above guidance and current professional practice. Clearly, the consent must be voluntary and can be withdrawn at any time. A record in the patient's case notes must be kept of the patient's capacity to consent.

Young people over 16 years are treated as adults (Family Law Reform Act 1969). Children under 16 are governed by a House of Lords decision (Gillick Case: *Gillick v West Norfolk and Wisbech Area Health Authority and Another,* 1985). Those with sufficient intelligence and understanding of the proposed treatment are treated like adults.

Treatment in an emergency
The Mental Health Act allows the doctor to treat without consent in an emergency under section 62 in order to:

● Save the patient's life
● Prevent a serious deterioration

- Alleviate serious suffering
- Prevent the patient from behaving violently or being a danger to himself or others.

The Aarvold Committee and the Advisory Board to the Home Office

Graham Young, with a history of poisoning others at the age of 14 years, was released from Broadmoor after 9 years and a short time later, in 1971, killed workmates by poisoning. The ensuing outcry led to the setting up of a working party in 1972 under the chairmanship of Judge Aarvold[4]. The purpose of the working party was to examine the way dangerous offenders were assessed before discharge from special hospitals. The recommendation for a three-man advisory board (a judge, a psychiatrist and a senior social worker or probation officer) was adopted (though it is now expanded). Patients in special hospital on restriction orders who are identified by the responsible medical officer as representing a special risk are referred to the Board by the Home Secretary for an opinion on dangerousness, as are any other patients causing concern to the Home Secretary. The Board's report to the Home Secretary is a further source of advice when the Home Secretary considers discharging or transferring a restricted patient.

The forensic psychiatrist will come across the work of the Board when looking after a patient who has been so identified. The Home Secretary may delay a decision about the psychiatrist's recommendations on such a patient in order to obtain the Board's advice. The Board makes its judgement by sending one of its members down to assess the case and interview the patient and staff. The Board then discusses the case in the light of the findings and all previous reports in order to prepare a report for the Home Office. Where there is a conflict between the advice from the responsible medical officer and the Board, the Home Secretary will necessarily have to choose between them. He does not automatically give precedence to the Board.

References

(1) Jones, R.M. (ed) (1991) *Mental Health Act Manual.* Sweet and Maxwell, London.
(2) Peay, J. (1989) *Tribunals on Trial: A study of Decision Making under the Mental Health Act 1983.* Clarendon Press, London.
(3) Department of Health and Welsh Office (1993). *Code of Practice. Mental Health Act 1983.* HMSO, London.
(4) Home Office and Department of Health and Social Security (1973) *Report on the Review of Procedures for the Discharge and Supervision of Psychiatric Patients subject to Special Restriction (Aarvold Report).* Cmnd. 5191. HMSO, London.

Chapter 5

Criminological Facts and Theories

Introduction

Studies show that the bulk of the population will break the law in some way at some time, though only a minority will be apprehended. A still smaller number will go on to become persistent serious offenders. This chapter touches on the facts and figures of offending, and goes on to discuss the factors which are believed to affect the chances of an individual behaving in a delinquent way. A disorder of personality is the commonest psychiatric condition associated with persistent offending, and it is not surprising therefore that the factors believed to be contributory to persistent delinquency are the same as those believed to lead to those personality disorders encompassed by the term 'psychopathic disorder'. The chapter finishes with a consideration of the effects of crime on the victim. Later chapters discuss the way mental disorder may lead to crime.

Definition

A crime has been defined as an 'act that is capable of being followed by criminal proceedings'. Some acts may be criminalized or decriminalized as the law changes, the classic example being homosexual acts between consenting adults in private which ceased to be a crime after the Sexual Offences Act 1967. Similarly, children used to be regarded as being criminally responsible from the age of 8 until the Children and Young Person's Act, 1963, changed the age of criminal responsibility to 10 years. Children under 10 who commit 'criminal acts' cannot be charged with an offence but are dealt with using civil procedures such as care proceedings. Between the ages of 10 and 14 children are presumed not to have responsibility unless the evidence rebuts this. Full criminal responsibility is reached at the age of 14 years.

The role of intent in the definition of crime and the nature of criminal responsibility are discussed in Chapter 2.

Crime rates

Introduction

A crime may be committed but not noticed by others, e.g. theft from a shop. The theft may be noticed but not reported to official bodies. If the theft is reported it may not be recorded by the police and therefore will not show up in police statistics. The offender, however, may or may not be detected and, if detected, he may or may not be arrested (if the offence is very minor there may be a simple warning). If arrested he may not be prosecuted but simply cautioned or prosecution may not proceed if the evidence is not strong enough. Prosecution may be unsuccessful. Clearly, therefore, there is an enormous gap between the number of crimes committed and the number of offenders found guilty. Indeed, there are gaps between all the levels in the above system. Crime which is not reported is known as 'hidden crime', other crime may be 'undetected crime', 'reported crime' or 'detected crime'.

Criminologists discuss at considerable length whether crime rates are truly rising. The increase in convictions which has accompanied an increase in reported crime, may reflect a decrease in tolerance of criminal behaviour by the population as well as an actual increase in crime. Historical studies indicate that the rate of crime does seem to swing from being at a peak in the eighteenth century, falling in parts in the nineteenth century, being fairly stable at the beginning of this century, steadily rising after the First World War until the 1930s when it remained stable again until the 1950s. Since the 1950s crime rates appear to have risen once more.

A guide to the total amount of certain sorts of crime can be obtained by house-to-house surveys to find out how much crime the householders have been subjected to. Four such surveys (in 1982; 1984; 1988; 1991) were completed by the British Crime Survey[1]. They showed the considerable gap between the crime experienced by householders and the amount appearing in police statistics – as well as the rise in crime over these years experienced by the public. Although the percentage of crimes reported to the police is rising year by year, many crimes are left unreported. They are felt to be too trivial or it is felt that the police has little chance of solving them, e.g. minor burglaries; minor thefts; minor assaults. It has been said that some crimes (e.g. rape; domestic violence) are not reported because of the embarrassment of the victim or fear of further violence.

Overall, comparing the British Crime Survey with official figures, it would seem as though only 30% of offences are reported. Another way of trying to estimate the amount of hidden crime is to do self-reporting surveys to find out how many offences have been committed by different groups of people. Such surveys[2] also show that there is considerably more crime committed than is recorded – though the biggest gap, naturally is in the minor offences.

It is apparent, therefore, that if the reporting behaviour of the public increased then the police statistics would also show an increase without there actually being a change in the real crime rate. Similarly, if the police record all offences reported to them then again there would be an apparent increase in the crime rate.

Criminal statistics for England and Wales record 50 000 indictable offences per year in the 1950s rising to 1 million in the 1960s, 2 million in the 1970s and 5.3 million in 1991[3]. Similarly, the total number of homicides has risen from 350 per year in 1946 to 675 in 1991, although this includes all forms of homicide including death by terrorism. The British Crime Survey estimates a total of 15 million crimes in 1991 against individuals and their property.

Rates of offending

Statistically speaking, delinquent acts are normal as West and Farrington have shown [2,4]. Some 80% or so of boys will have committed a delinquent act which could have taken them before the court by the time they were 17. However, it is also true that the majority of these acts will have been relatively trivial, e.g. minor thefts; minor damage. Only a tiny minority of delinquent acts lead to court appearance but the more substantial the offence, the more the likelihood of being caught. Thus, only 8% of shoplifters may be caught compared to 60% of those who break and enter. Offending is an activity of the young reaching its peak at around 17 years and declining rapidly by the late 20s. Some 30% of all males born in 1953, were convicted by age 31. A small group of men (6%) became severe recidivists accounting for 65% of all convictions.

Females offend much less than males. Self-report studies show that the difference is not as great as has seemed from official statistics but it may be that this is because the majority of female offending is very minor. However, there has been an enormous increase between the 1950s and 1970s in female offending. The male to female ratio for offences in 1957 was 11:1; in 1977 it was 5:1. Similarly, there has been a 379% increase in convictions of females under 17 in the same periods as the males increased by 148%. These ages and sex associations are reviewed in detail by Rutter and Giller[5]. Of women born in 1953, 7.1% were convicted by the age 31.

Patterns of crime

By far the commonest offence is simple theft. The British Crime Survey found that of 15 million crimes in 1991, 75% were acquisitive, 5% were violent offences (wounding and robbery), and 12% were common assaults. Sexual offences were not measured by the Survey but have been given as less than 1% from reporting figures.

The prognosis of offending

The majority of offenders are not re-convicted after the first offence, though the younger the offender the greater the likelihood he will be re-convicted. For children under 14, the re-conviction rate after the first offence is 60%[4], whereas for 17–19 years the rate is 35%, and for first offenders over 40 re-conviction is only 9%. Similarly, the chances of re-conviction are greater for those who have been previously convicted, e.g. amongst juvenile offenders with four previous convictions the re-conviction rate is nearly 80%. However, there appears to be a trend towards social conformity as the young offender matures. Only a minority of people are going to become persistent adult offenders. In Camberwell, a working class area of London, West and Farrington[2], showed that perhaps 80% of the boys would have committed an act which was criminal by the time they were 17, though only 20% would have been caught. Of those 20%, half went on to be convicted of a second crime and of these a small proportion would go on to become chronic recidivists. Each year after 17 years there would be some new first-time offenders but the number of first-time offenders and re-offenders fall with each year of life. There is a similar fall in the crime rate for females from the late teens – except in their case the fall is interrupted by a small increase in the rates around the late 40s and early 50s.

Factors associated with delinquency

Introduction

Why one person and not another should become persistently delinquent has promoted considerable theorizing and study. Historically, there was a desire to find 'the cause' of delinquency and, as a result, a number of rival 'monolithic' theories were developed from criminology, sociology and psychiatry to explain delinquency. Professor Lombroso (the 'father of criminology') in nineteenth century Italy proposed the idea that criminals were born and that they had a particular primitive constitution and physique associated with primitive impulsiveness, cruelty, etc. He believed, from his study of prisoners, that there were physical stigmata of criminality, e.g. absence of ear lobes, low foreheads, etc.

This theory held the forefront of thinking until it was toppled in 1913, by a careful statistically controlled study of criminals in Parkhurst Prison, when it was demonstrated that the so-called stigmata were, in fact, equally common in non-criminal populations. Attention after Lombroso moved to the idea of there being a deficiency of the 'moral faculty' in a similar way to there being a deficiency in some people of the intellectual faculty. The Mental Deficiency Acts of 1913 and 1927 encapsulated these concepts, covering both intellectual and moral deficiency. A moral defective was defined as: 'a person in whose case mental defectiveness was coupled with strongly vicious and criminal propensities and who required care and supervision and control for the protection of others'. This permitted the detention in hospital of people labelled as 'moral defective'.

Sociological theories developed in the 1920s and 1930s. These theories denied that criminality arose from some individual disturbance. Criminal behaviour was seen to be the result of social factors or pressure acting on normal people. Sutherland proposed that crime was learned, like everything else, and that the main factor leading someone into crime was due to the association and imitation of criminals. Merton saw criminal behaviour as one of the possible ways a disadvantaged person might obtain the goals of society (i.e. money and success), when unable to gain them by legitimate means or being unable to simply accept the status quo. Similar theories referring to social inequalities were developed to explain the phenomena of delinquent gangs.

However, the social theories, whilst adding to our understanding, failed to allay the clinical suspicion that individual personal experiences were of outstanding importance. Contemporaneous with the social theories was a growing body of evidence supporting the idea that there was a clear association between the individual's early family experience and crime. The main stream of this approach included the work of the Gluecks, the McCords, and Bowlby.

The more recent realization of the ubiquitousness of criminal behaviour has led to a different view. It now seems clear that delinquent behaviour is best understood on a multifactorial basis, the sum of many factors in a person's life. This view and the evidence has been reviewed in detail by Rutter and Giller[5]. The next section will discuss these factors which can be considered under the headings of inherited and acquired factors.

Inheritance and criminality

It has long been known that delinquency and antisocial behaviour often runs in families. The question arises about the extent that inherited traits contribute to these family histories. Twin studies have given rather conflicting results in the past. More recent studies of criminality in twins show a greater concordance for monozygotic than for dizygotic pairs (e.g. 35% to 13%) though the differences between them are reduced when the pairs are controlled for similarity in environment[5].

Further support for the idea of a genetic factor is derived from adoption studies. Mednick and Finello[6] studied in Denmark over 14 000 adoptees. They divided the biological and adoptive parents into criminal and non-criminal groups and looked at delinquency patterns in the adopted children. The rate of delinquency in children born to non-criminal biological parents and given to non-criminal adoptive parents was very similar (13.5%) to the delinquency rate for children as a whole in Denmark. Children of criminal biological parents given to criminal adoptive parents had a 24.5% official delinquency rate. The important finding, however, was that a higher rate of delinquency was found in the children of criminal biological parents given to non-criminal adoptive parents (20%) compared to the 14.7% in children of non-criminal biological parents given to criminal adoptive parents. Clearly from this study it would seem that both upbringing and inheritance contribute towards delinquency but that biological weighting seems more important. Other (though not all) adoptee studies have found similar results though there is evidence that part of the predisposition to crime arises from an inherited tendency to abuse alcohol[7].

Inherited and constitutional factors

What biological factors might be inherited is unclear. Current thought looks towards neurophysiological factors as well as intelligence. Chromosomal abnormalities are another factor which has attracted attention.

Neurophysiological factors

Disturbance of brain function

Electroencephalograph (EEG) studies
A number of workers have claimed to find abnormal EEG activity in particular types of offenders. These include:

(1) An excess of spikes and slow waves in the temporal lobes associated with pathological aggression in violent criminals[8];
(2) General slow wave activity observed to be more common in the EEGs of abnormal murderers[9], though there have been some conflicting findings since[10]. In ordinary clinical forensic psychiatry work, abnormal EEGs do not seem more common in violent men than in non-violent offenders.
(3) Slower recovery of the cortex from normal evoked potentials in schizophrenia and recidivist offenders of psychopathic personality compared to normal[11]. It has been argued that there is a reduced rate

of cortical excitability in psychopaths. This may, it is argued, lead the subject to search for excessive stimulation and excitement.

(4) A higher amplitude contingent negative variation demonstrated in primary psychopaths compared to normals[12]. Contingent negative variation is a slow negative potential change seen on the EEG recording when the subject is preparing to respond to a stimulus.

Absence of normal brain function

Cleckley[13] has argued, persuasively, that there is a: 'primary psychopath' (see Chapter 10) characterized by typical personality traits and an absence of psychologically damaging factors in the background. He has postulated that the primary psychopath has a defect in brain function so that there is no association between emotion and words, a semantic disorder. The psychopath learns to say: 'I am sorry' but cannot experience the emotions of regret or guilt normally associated with these words and therefore is not inhibited in the future by emotion. There is, however, no objective neurological evidence of this postulated disturbed brain function.

Disturbance of the autonomic nervous system and conditioning

It is argued that delinquency may be associated with an inability to condition normally due to abnormalities within the autonomic nervous system or to defects in cortical arousal. It has long been known in the animal world that some animals will condition easily and quickly and are therefore easily trainable whereas others are not. The evidence for an association of delinquency with poor conditioning or disturbed autonomic functioning arises from studies which, for example, show in 'psychopaths' that:

(1) Skin conductance was lower at rest and showed less spontaneous fluctuations than normal;
(2) psychopaths do not condition as quickly as normal to painful stimuli[14].

These experiments have methodological problems in defining psychopaths and in getting consistent findings. Nevertheless, this sort of observation underlies the hypothesis that delinquency may be a failure of 'passive avoidance learning'[15]. That is to say, the subject fails to learn to avoid certain behaviour (e.g. stealing) due to his inability to condition (learn) normally.

Attention-deficit disorder with hyperactivity

This condition of children is recognized in the ICD 10 as the hyperkinetic conduct disorder (ICD 10, F 90.1), and in the DSM IIIR as the attention deficit hyperactivity disorder (DSM IIIR, 314.01). It has been asserted that the condition is due to minimal brain damage and can persist into adult life and result in impulsive character disorders, irritability, lability, explosiveness and violence. A study of 94 subjects and 78 controls suggests that 32% with the disorder will develop antisocial disorders as young adults compared to 8% in the controls[16].

Raine *et al.*[17] have tried to bring these various findings together. Some 101 randomly selected English schoolboys were tested at 15 years for heart rate, skin conductance and EEG wave form. Their criminality was examined at 24 years, and 17 serious offenders were identified from criminal records. These 17 had lower heart rates, lower skin conductance and greater theta activity in the EEG at 15. These variables predicted 74% of the criminals in the group. Nevertheless, it is not clear if these features were the result of personality rather than the basis of it.

Abnormalities of brain chemistry
It has been postulated, based on levels in the cerebrospinal fluid, that habitually violent, alcohol-abusing men are deficient in the neurotransmitter, serotonin (see Chapter 7). It is not known whether this condition (if it proves to be a real one) is inherited or acquired.

Defect of intelligence

It seems likely from many studies that low intelligence is a factor in delinquency. West in his Camberwell study (see below) found that intelligence was one of the principal factors associated with persistent delinquency – a finding which is now generally supported. To the extent that this faculty is biologically based and inherited, it is an inherited factor which plays a significant part in behaviour.

Chromosome abnormalities

The chromosomal abnormalities which have been associated with antisocial behaviour include some of the disorders with an extra sex chromosome, i.e. the XYY, XXY (Klinefelter) and XXX (superfemale) karyotypes[18,19]. The incidence of XYY and XXY in the population is just over 1 per 1000 liveborn male infants, respectively. In the 1960s XYY men were found to make up 3% of patients at Carstairs, the Scottish State Hospital. A series of papers followed confirming a raised incidence of XYY and XXY males in special hospitals, though as the true national incidence became apparent it also became clear that only a small proportion of such cases were in institutions. Rates in subnormality hospitals and penal institutions for delinquent youths were normal. Are XYY youths easily identified and transferred to hospital?

The initial description of XYY males as tall, aggressive, impulsive and of dull intelligence has had to be modified. Only 50% are taller than 6 feet and behavioural disorder is probably not present in the majority and when present can take any form. The behaviourally disturbed cannot be distinguished on physical grounds. Their intelligence has been found to vary from the superior level to the subnormal, although the mean is said to be below normal.

XXY males are characterized by very poor testicular development, eunuchoid habits, tallness, feminine breast development, intellectual deficit, and small head. XXX females are characterized by tallness, long legs, intellectual defect and small head. Behavioural problems have been described in both XXY and XXX patients. The present view appears to be that these chromosomal abnormalities are not direct causes of criminal behaviour. Where they are associated with such behaviour they may exert their influence through the effects on intelligence or temperamental characteristics, the situation is unclear. Nevertheless it is calculated that an XYY male has a 1:100 chance of being sent to a special hospital[20].

Medicolegally, in England, (though not in all countries) chromosome abnormalities themselves are not regarded as relevant to the question of responsibility. When the patient also has a mental disorder (e.g. personality disorder) the knowledge that there is also a chromosomal defect may alter the perception of the court or professionals involved in the case who may be more ready to see it as a 'medical' problem.

Acquired factors associated with delinquency

There have been innumerable cross sectional studies concerning delinquents and non-delinquents to identify individual differences, but good longitudinal studies are rare. From a methodological point of view the best approach might be to study a random group of children from an early age and follow them through into adulthood.

Such a study was carried out by West[2] in Camberwell. Some 400 boys were identified at the age of 8 years from a working class neighbourhood in London and followed up at the age of 25, by which time a third of the group had acquired a criminal conviction record. The aim of the study was to assess: 'the relative importance of social pressures (such as low income), individual style of upbringing (manifest in parental attitude and discipline), personal attributes (such as intelligence, physique, and aggressiveness) and extraneous events (mischance of being found out)', i.e. to examine the influence of both acquired and inherited features. It was also hoped that it would be possible to identify criteria present at an early age which could be used to predict which individuals would be more likely to become persistent delinquents. The study was designed to encompass a wide range of items. Assessments were made by psychologists, experienced social workers and experienced research workers. Full assessments were made at the age of 8 and then every 2 years after that up to the age of 18. After that, specific groups were interviewed at 21 and 23 and 24. The persistence of the interviewers was such that 95% of the subjects were traced up to the age of 18.

The study was used to test many of the findings of previous workers and to try and assess the relative importance of the various associations which had previously been discovered. Nearly every one of the 200 items investigated proved to have some association with delinquency. However, the items could be grouped into five major factors. Perhaps one of the most important findings of the study was that no one of the five was predominant. The presence of any of the five factors had equal weight in its correlation with delinquency and the factors appeared to summate in their effects. Possession of one adverse factor significantly increased the likelihood of a boy becoming a delinquent compared to a boy who lacked these factors. The five factors were:

(1) Coming from a low income family.
(2) Coming from a large-sized family, defined as five or more children up to the subject's tenth birthday.
(3) Unsatisfactory parenting which includes marital conflict, the dominance of one parent over another, inconsistency between the parents, attitudes of indifference, rejection or neglect, overstrict or erratically varying discipline and harsh methods of enforcement. They also found that separations from parents were not in themselves important, only the cause for the separation. Separations due to illness or death had comparatively little relationship to offending, unlike separations caused by breakdown of parental marriage. It was also found that the timing of the disruption (early or later in life) had little importance on its effect.
(4) Having a parent with a criminal record (acquired before the boy's tenth birthday). Crime does seem part of a family tradition and it was found that 4.6% of the families accounted for half of all the convictions recorded by the boys. The risks of the subject becoming delinquent increased with the number of people in the family who were also delinquent. It was not clear how the parental delinquency was 'passed on' to the child, it might be due to attitude training or to hereditary factors.
(5) Having below-average intelligence on testing. Intelligence testing at 8 and 10 years showed that the future juvenile delinquents had a mean IQ of 95 compared with a mean IQ of 101 in the rest of the sample. The study looked at whether or not the lower IQ was a reflection of lower social class status but found that it was not.

Families of low IQ, however, do tend to be deprived in others ways. Furthermore, children of lower IQ do less well at school which will affect their perceptions of themselves. Failure at school can be associated with the development of antisocial attitudes and delinquent behaviour. There is clearly overlap between these adverse factors and it was found that the presence of one factor made the presence of another more likely. Some 63 boys had at least three of the five predictive factors and almost half of this group became juvenile delinquents compared with only a fifth among the sample as a whole.

Whilst these factors can be used to give a prediction score, the best single predictor of juvenile delinquency was found to be a measure of troublesomeness derived from teachers and classmates at primary school. This assessment covers things like application to work, scholastic performance, concentration, cleanliness, obedience, attendance and relations with other children. Of the 92 boys categorized as the most troublesome at primary school, half became juvenile delinquents, whereas only 3.5% of the 143 boys in the least troublesome group became a delinquent. West notes that this finding implies that deviant behaviour observable at an early age is likely to persist and to take a delinquent form as the boy grows older.

Other acquired factors contributing to delinquent behaviour

These are reviewed by Rutter and Giller[5] and include the following.

Racial background
In England the arrest rate amongst Asian juveniles has been lower than in the equivalent White groups, whereas, on the other hand, it was higher amongst West Indians. The difference may, to some extent, represent distortions due to differences in reporting rates, detection rate and policing methods. There have also been studies to indicate that the higher rate of crime amongst Black youths may be accounted for by greater socio-economic deprivations. The situation is unclear and further research is required.

Physical characteristics
Studies in the past have suggested that extreme physical characteristics are associated with delinquency, i.e. muscularity or being undersized. However, more recent evidence shows that these associations disappear once relevant social factors are taken into account. No connection between body build and delinquency was identified by West. Some workers have claimed an association between delinquency, ill health and multiple biological impairments such as those which might be obtained around the neonatal period due to bad maternal care, resulting perhaps in impaired growth or minimal brain damage. However, no such relationship occurred in West's study.

Living in large towns
Comparative studies indicate lower delinquency rates in rural areas,

compared to metropolitan areas. West found that the delinquent behaviour of his subjects dropped if they moved from London to rural areas.

Different crime rates also occur in different parts of the city. It has long been known that the crime rates are highest in the most run-down areas. Even within such areas there are high-risk communities and low-risk communities. The possible causes for this include the policy of local authorities to group problem families together and the drift of delinquent people into areas of high delinquency. The extent to which such areas influence the behaviour of people moving into them is unclear. Experimental initiatives which have tried to improve social cohesiveness and awareness, e.g. crime reduction schemes on large estates or community policing hold out hope of reducing delinquency.

The effect of 'bad' schools

Power[21] showed that different schools serving similar areas had enormous differences in delinquency rates. Most of the school variation could be explained in terms of differences in intake and in terms of behaviourally different children. Nevertheless, Rutter[5] was able to show that a school could influence, for good or bad, the development of the potentially delinquent boy. By giving a predictive score to children on factors similar to those found by West, he was able to show statistically that some schools persistently improved the chances of boys leaving their delinquent behaviour behind whilst other schools increase the chances of a boy becoming delinquent. The effect seemed due to the mix of pupils (the higher the intellectual ability and social status the less the delinquency) and the styles of management by the teacher which influenced the climate of the school. Styles which encouraged a positive atmosphere were the most successful.

Being labelled delinquent

There has long been a social theory that 'labelling' (i.e. identifying and processing) a child as a delinquent will increase his chances of continuing to be one. This labelling could alter the child's perception of himself and therefore his behaviour. West found evidence in support of this theory. He was able to match a small group of boys who had been caught by the police with a group of boys who were similar in all other respects except they had not been caught. The group who were caught were found to alter their view of the police from a positive to a negative one. Furthermore, the group who were caught went on to commit more offences (to judge by self-report and official records) than the group who were not caught. It remains possible that the group who were caught were in some way more incompetent as criminals or more antisocial than those who were not. West was unable to find evidence for this.

Exposure to violent films and television

There has been a great deal of debate, particularly in regard to violence, as to the effects of films and television on offending rates. There are many laboratory studies which show that children will play at violence and appear more aggressive immediately after seeing a violent film though such studies are criticized as being too artificial. A more realistic study examined delinquent boys living in cottages in a secure institution. Aggressive films were shown in one group of cottages and non-violent films were shown in another. The boys exposed to the violent films showed increased aggression compared to the controls for that week and to a lesser extent in the following period. There are no good experiments on the long-term effects of showing such films though some believe that frequent exposure to them desensitizes people to violence and makes violent behaviour more likely. However, aggressive people seem to favour aggressive films[22].

What factors protect a person against delinquency?

In West's study it was found that some people might have all the factors associated with delinquency and not show up as a recorded delinquent. When this was examined more closely it was found that many of the non-recorded delinquents had, in fact, avoided detection. Some boys, however, did not become delinquent but developed marked neurotic symptoms instead. Nevertheless, there were still some boys who seemed to survive, developing neither persistent delinquency nor neurotic symptoms.

Factors which may protect the child

Personality

Werner[23] studied the development of 689 infants born in 1955 in Hawaii. Children who survived adversity seemed to have, even as babies, more equable temperamental characteristics with greater competence socially, at school and at play. This may be the reverse of a disposition to criminality but may also be due to their being more advantaged as babies (more first born, less sibling pressure). Rutter[24] argues that inherited temperamental traits (emotionality, activity levels, sociability) influence interactions with parents and others (for good or bad) and thus contribute to the final personality and view of the world.

A good peer group

West's study showed that those who moved away from a delinquent career abandoned their delinquent friends. However, what is not clear is whether it is the change of associates which led to a change in the subject's behaviour or vice versa. The evidence from the effects of school, discussed above, does suggest that, in the right setting, peer group effects may have a protective influence. Similarly, the observation of the change in delinquency behaviour which occurs when the person moves from the city to a rural area supports this hypothesis.

Successful employment

It is clear that delinquency and unemployment are strongly associated. Whether the experience of unemployment increases the chances of a subject becoming delinquent is uncertain – though social studies have claimed that there is a rising crime rate in periods of high unemployment. Clinically, one sees delinquents who do seem to settle down when a job goes well, only to break down again when the job collapses. A recent study[25] showed that unemployment has most effect on the criminality of those who already have a delinquent history. The non-delinquent is not easily precipitated into offending by unemployment.

A good marriage

Clinically, subjects who have been delinquent may gradually reduce their delinquency in their early twenties, marry and largely cease their delinquent career. Against this it seems likely that the effect of the marriage will depend on the extent to which it improves the psychosocial situation of the individual. Undoubtedly some youths with a very marked antisocial lifestyle who marry before the age of 21 show no obvious benefit to their delinquency, though other aspects of their behaviour may improve. If the marriage is to a delinquent woman then the chance of delinquency may increase.

An improvement in life circumstances

Rutter[5] has shown that conduct disorders in children improve as family discord or stresses die down. Similarly, it was found that problem behaviour shown by children of divorcing parents improved if the divorce brought harmony to the family. Rutter concludes that major changes in environment in this way can lead to major effects in terms of children's social behaviour. In clinical practice similar relationships are seen amongst adults between life events and offending behaviour.

One good relationship

It has been found that a good relationship with one parent can protect children from adverse experiences around them. However, this relationship must be a particularly good one and with a parent living with the child. To what extent such a relationship would protect a child from all the influence leading to delinquency is uncertain.

Good life experience outside the home

Rutter[5] has shown that the rate of behavioural disorder among children from seriously deprived or disadvantaged homes is considerably less than expected if they did well at school. Whether this is because those particular children were more resilient or whether their teachers had been particularly successful in encouraging the children is unclear. There is also evidence to suggest that children from disturbed homes can only become successful either by dropping their contacts with their family or maintaining an emotional distance.

The effects of crime on the victims

In the last two decades there has been an increased awareness that the victim not only suffers from the immediate effect of the crime (loss, injury) but may also suffer psychological after effects (see Chapter 7). These range from immediate shock to short- and long-term symptoms, such as anxiety, depression, sleep disturbance, fear, anger, inability to perform ordinary tasks, nightmares, intrusive thoughts – the symptoms of post-traumatic stress disorder. People emotionally close to the victim or offender may also be affected, especially in the case of homicide. Black[26] has drawn attention to the effects of a murder in the family on children and the need they have for specialized help. Counselling for victims[27] may be helpful both for practical matters (insurance, security) and for psychological ones (see Chapter 18).

References

(1) Mayhew, P. & Maung, N.A. (1992) *Surveying Crime: Findings from the 1992 British Crime Survey.* Home Office Research and Statistics Department. *Research Findings* No. 2. HMSO, London.

(2) West, D.J. & Farrington, D.P (1977) *The Delinquent Way of Life.* Heinemann Educational, London.

(3) Home Office (1992) *Criminal Statistics. England and Wales 1991.* Cmnd. 2134. HMSO, London.

(4) West, D.J. (1982) *Delinquency: Its Roots, Careers and Prospects.* Heinemann, London.

(5) Rutter, M. & Giller, H. (1983) *Juvenile Delinquency: Trends and Perspectives.* Penguin, Harmondsworth.

(6) Mednick, S.A. & Finello, K.M. (1983) Biological factors and crime: implications for forensic psychiatry. *International Journal of Law and Psychiatry* **6**, 1–15.

(7) Bohman, M., Cloninger, C.R., Sigvardsson, S. & Van Knorring, A.L. (1983) Gene-environment interaction in the psychopathology of adoptees: some recent studies in the origin of alcoholism and criminality. In Magnusson, D. and Allen, V. (ed.) *Human Development: An Interactional Perspective.* Academic Press, New York and London.

(8) Williams, D. (1969) Neural factors related to habitual aggression. *Brain* **92**, 503–20.

(9) Hill, J.D.N. & Pond, D.A. (1952) Reflection on one hundred capital cases submitted for electroencephalography. *Journal of Mental Science* **98**, 23–43.

(10) Driver, M.V., West, C.R. & Faulk, M. (1974) Clinical and EEG studies of prisoners charged with murder. *British Journal of Psychiatry* **124**, 583–7.

(11) Shagass, C. & Schwartz, M. (1962) Observations on somatosensory critical reactivity in personality disorders. *Journal of Nervous and Mental Disease* **135**, 44–51.

(12) Howard, R.C., Fenton, G.W. & Fenwick, P.B.C. (1984) Contingent negative variation, personality and antisocial behaviour. *British Journal of Psychiatry* **144**, 463–74.

(13) Cleckley, H. (1976) *The Mask of Sanity* (5th edition). The C.V. Mosby Co., St Louis, Missouri.

(14) Hare, R.D. (1970) *Psychopathy, Theory and Research*. Wiley, New York.

(15) Trasler, G.B. (1973) Criminal behaviour. In Eysenk, H.J. (ed.). *Handbook of Abnormal Psychology* (2nd edition). Pitman Medical, London.

(16) Mannuzza, S., Klein, R.G., Bonagura, N., Malloy, P., Giampino, T. & Addalli, K.A. (1991) Hyperactive children almost grown up. *Archives of General Psychiatry* **48**, 77–83.

(17) Raine, A., Venables, P.H. & Williams, M. (1990) Relationship between central and autonomic measures of arousal at age 15 years and criminality at age 24 years. *Archives of General Psychiatry* **47**, 1003–7.

(18) Pitcher, D.C.R. (1971) Criminological implications of chromosome abnormalities. *New Law Journal* **121**, 1078–9.

(19) Pitcher, D.C.R. (1982) Sex chromosome disorders. In Granville-Grossman, K. (ed.) *Recent Advances in Clinical Psychiatry*. (Number Four). Churchill-Livingstone, Edinburgh.

(20) Editorial (1974) What becomes of the XYY male? *Lancet* **ii**, 1297–8.

(21) Power, M.J., Benn, R.T. & Morris, J.N. (1972) Neighbourhood, school and juveniles before the courts. *British Journal of Criminology* **12**, 111–32.

(22) Heath, L., Bresolin, L.B., Rinaldi, R.C., 1989 The effects of media violence on children: A review of the literature. *Archives of General Psychiatry* **46**, 376–9.

(23) Werner, E.E. (1989) High risk children in young adulthood. *American Journal of Orthopsychiatry* **59**, 72–81.

(24) Rutter, M. (1987) Temperament, personality and personality disorder. *British Journal of Psychiatry* **150**, 443–68.

(25) Farrington, D.P., Gallagher, B., Marley, L., Ledger, R.J. & West, D.J. (1986) Unemployment, school leaving and crime. *British Journal of Criminology* **26**, 335–55.

(26) Black, D. & Caplan, T. (1988) Father kill mother. *British Journal of Psychiatry* **153**, 624–30.

(27) Shepherd, J. (1988) Supporting victims of violent crime. *British Medical Journal* **297**, 1353.

Chapter 6

Offences Against Property and Forensic Psychiatry

Introduction

This chapter defines property offences (acquisitive and destructive). The different 'motives' (including psychiatric disorder) for acquisitive offending are discussed using shoplifting as an example. Similarly, the motivations for destructive offending are discussed with particular attention to arson as an example of a destructive offence.

The normal human motives for property offences (greed, envy, anger, jealousy, resentment, etc.) occur also as motives in the mentally disordered. The presence of a mental disorder does not preclude the patient from experiencing such feelings. The disorder, by intensifying emotional reactions or distorting perception, may engender similar feelings which precipitate an offence.

Definition

The term 'property offence' covers a variety of offences including:

(1) Theft: Dishonesty appropriating property belonging to another with the intention of permanently depriving the other of it.
(2) Taking a conveyance without authority: Taking and driving away a conveyance without the consent of the owner or other lawful authority (but without the intention to permanently deprive the owner of it). If the act is associated with injury, dangerous driving or damage to property then it makes the offender liable to a charge of aggravated vehicle taking.
(3) Robbery: Using force or seeking to put a person in fear of being subjected to force at the same time or immediately before stealing.
(4) Blackmail: Making unwarranted demands with menaces with intent to gain for oneself and to cause loss to another.
(5) Burglary: Entering a building as a trespasser with intent to steal. The charge may also be with intent to inflict grievous bodily harm, rape or to do unlawful damage to the building.

(6) Going equipped: Having an article for use for stealing, cheating or committing a burglary.

(7) Fraud: Dishonestly obtaining by deception; there are several varieties:
   (a) obtaining property by deception;
   (b) obtaining pecuniary advantage by deception;
   (c) false accounting and false statements by company directors;
   (d) obtaining services by deception;
   (e) evasion of liability by deception.

(8) Handling stolen goods: The receiving of goods or assisting in their retention, removal or disposal, knowing or believing the goods to be stolen goods.

(9) Forgery: Making of a false document in order that it may be used as genuine.

(10) Criminal damage to property: The destruction or damaging of property without lawful excuse. The offender must have intended the effect or have been reckless as to the effects of his action. A more serious charge is criminal damage with intent to endanger life or being reckless as to whether life was endangered.

(11) Arson: The destruction or damaging of property by fire (without lawful excuse). A more serious charge is arson with intent to endanger life or being reckless as to whether life was endangered. For arson to have occurred the arsonist must have intended to set the fire and intended its effects, or to have been careless of its effects.

It will be seen that there are two forms of property offences: (1) the *acquisitive offences* which cover the various forms of theft, robberies, burglaries and fraud, and (2) *destructive offences* which include arson and malicious damage to property. From a psychiatric point of view the acquisitive often have a different psychopathology from destructive offences.

Acquisitive offences

In these offences the question of specific intent has to be examined as its presence is legally necessary for an offence to have been committed. The absence of the intent will form a defence to the charge, e.g. if a person absent-mindedly carried goods out of a shop, it would not be a crime as there would be no intent to permanently deprive.

An understanding of the variety of patterns and motives for theft has been derived both from clinical practice and from various studies – the principal English study being on shoplifting[1]. The findings from that study have application to other acquisitive offences. A classification of 'motives' can be divided into a group without and a group with psychiatric abnormality. The latter, of course, will form the basis of medicolegal defences.

Patterns of offending not associated with psychiatric disorder

Avarice

The bulk of theft is carried out by psychiatrically 'normal' people. Examples include stealing from places of work where such thefts are accepted as normal 'perks' by the workmen, and from shops where studies of 'wastage' have shown that a substantial proportion of the goods are taken by the people who work in the shop.

Poverty

The shoplifting study identified a very small group of offenders who were stealing through poverty. The motives included a need to provide for the family or to maintain appearances.

Excitement

Excitement appears to be the principal motivation in certain groups, e.g. children or adolescents in groups. Amongst young, foreign women in London caught shoplifting excitement appeared to be an important factor in the motivation. Excitement may be part of the motive when groups of youths urge each other on to stealing, taking and driving cars, or even breaking and entering.

Antisocial families

A group of shoplifters from antisocial families was identified where the whole family took part in the shoplifting, accepting it as normal behaviour. Such families tended to be involved in other forms of acquisitive offence.

Professional theft

In the shoplifting study a gang drove from one town to another where they systematically deceived the shop assistants and took the goods back to the first town for distribution. The desire for gain often appeared associated with resentment and bitterness towards the society and was part of the cultural lifestyle adopted by this group. Similar groups may organize themselves to take part in other property offences.

Acquisitive offending and psychiatric disorder

The incidence of psychiatric disorder among adult acquisitive offenders is unknown, though serious disorder must only occur in a small proportion. In 1959 Gibbens[2] thought that 10–15% of shoplifters fell into the disordered group, though in 1981[3] he thought it might be only 5% – an expression of the increase in shoplifting among those without disorder. Gibbens and Prince[1] analysed the psychiatric disorders among shoplifters and these give an insight into the types of disorder one might see among other acquisitive offenders. The following expansion of their findings is based on clinical practice and relates offending to different disorders.

Acquisitive offending and neurosis

Depression
Depression is perhaps the commonest symptom among mentally ill offenders convicted of theft. It is often appropriately treated on an out-patient basis, perhaps as a condition of probation. Four groups can be identified based on the study of shoplifters:

(1) Isolated young adults under stress
In the shoplifting study a group of young women with children was identified. Characteristically they lived in multi-storey blocks of flats, separated from parents, looking after children on their own with a husband out at work and without support from neighbours. Depressive symptoms appeared and then after some months an offence occurred. The theft could be understood as a cry for help and the acquisition may have been comforting.

(2) Older people with a chronic depression
The study identified a group of women in late middle-age with chronic depression isolated within their families with children having left home, and the husband having become rather neglectful. This depression occurred at the menopausal period which, of course, coincides with these other losses. Characteristically, the woman would have attended her doctor for some weeks with vague symptoms. After a time she would sense his loss of interest and would stop going. A month or so later she would be convicted of shoplifting. The motivation was similar to that in group (1) above.

(3) Subjects with depression associated with acute loss such as a death in the family, etc.
Sometimes the subject will claim to have been so distracted as to have

been unaware or only have a hazy recollection of the act. There may be, therefore, a genuine lack of intent and certainly mitigating factors.

> A very respectable woman became very sad on hearing of the sudden death of a life-long friend. She was arrested the next day for taking a small packet of food. She denied any conscious awareness of the act.

4 Personality disordered subjects experiencing a depressive swing

Such people often have aggressive feelings of resentment. The offending can be understood as: a sudden impulse to give themselves a treat; an attempt to embarrass and therefore punish their family by bringing disgrace on themselves; an attempt to gain the family's sympathy by drawing attention to their plight.

Anxiety

Anxiety states may cause a state of distraction and in this state it is possible that a subject may 'absent-mindedly' take goods from a shop without paying. In such a case there would be a defence of 'no intent'.

> A professional woman under considerable stress at work had become very anxious and distracted. She was arrested outside a shop and accused of taking goods without paying for them. She successfully pleaded in court that her state had been such that she had behaved automatically and taken the goods without thinking. She was found not guilty.

Compulsive states and 'kleptomania'

Phobias and obsessional states with unwanted intrusive thoughts are rarely associated with theft. However, some persistent offenders appear or claim to experience a compulsion to steal and fit the DSM IIIR and ICD 10 description of kleptomania. The compulsion is characterized by a feeling of tension associated with a particular urge to steal, excitement during the theft (which in a minority of occasions may be sexual) and relief after committing the act. At the same time the urge is recognized as senseless and wrong and the act is followed by guilt. The stealing is not an expression of anger or vengeance nor part of a conduct disorder or antisocial personality. The goods are usually worth little and often not required. They may be hidden, hoarded or given away. Such a compulsion seems associated with other neurotic symptoms such as:

- Depression
- Anxiety perhaps associated with other compulsive behaviours (hand-washing, compulsive checking)
- Bulimia nervosa
- Sexual dysfunction (promiscuity or frigidity).

The literature suggests that the condition occurs at any age and is commoner (77%) in females[4]. Behavioural therapy, psychotherapy and antidepressants have all been used with clinical evidence of success in relieving the compulsion in some cases. Overlapping with this disorder are those with chronic feelings of sadness, tension and depression whose dysphoria is relieved by theft[5].

Another example of compulsive behaviour is that of youths who, at times of despondency, persistently drive and take away vehicles. Once behind the wheel they feel a sense of well-being and a return of self-esteem. After driving around they then abandon the car. They become very skilled at taking cars and carry keys for this purpose. It is basically a neurotic behaviour said to occur particularly in association with dominating mothers.

Such offenders have to be distinguished from people with antisocial personalities who show opportunistic and impulsive behaviour in many areas but without a neurotic cause. They must also be distinguished from those where psychosis or brain damage underlies the repetitive behaviour.

Subjects with depression using shoplifting to manipulate
These subjects find themselves in very unhappy situations (e.g. the newly immigrated young woman who hates the new country) and consciously or unconsciously use shoplifting to draw attention to their plight or force a change of circumstances.

Acquisitive offending and psychosis

Schizophrenia

Delusional states may lead directly to theft

> A subject with schizophrenia suffered from the delusion that God had given him permission to take the things he required. He helped himself from Woolworths and was arrested for stealing. The court, after receiving the appropriate reports, made a hospital order for treatment.

Schizophrenia may lead to a deteriorated vagrant state leading to theft. Without sustenance or money and handicapped by severe mental illness the subject may well steal in order to obtain food. The theft may be a simple one from a shop or a doorstep, or may be more complicated involving a burglary.

> A schizophrenic man of excellent previous personality deteriorated under the influence of his illness until he became a vagrant. He held strongly paranoid views about the world and communicated with no one. One morning he attempted to steal from a milk cart. The milkman tried to stop him and the subject responded violently. He was found guilty of theft and violence but the court accepted a medical recommendation for treatment in hospital on a hospital order.

Affective psychosis
Offending may occur in association with mania, either due to an expansive grandiose mood or due to associated delusions. When a manic person offends in this way, it typically might be by writing cheques which could not be met, ordering goods which can not be paid for, or taking articles believing that 'all is in order'. These offences all arise from an exaggerated grandiosity and elevation of mood, possibly associated with delusional beliefs. In severe depression the 'theft' may be due to an absent-minded state, a desire to comfort, an attempt to draw attention to the subject's plight or arising from an associated delusion.

Acquisitive offences and organic states

Dementia
Stealing might occur because of (1) a state of confusion where a person might walk out with goods without paying, or (2) because the dementia undermines the subject's resistance to temptation. A careful examination and history from the subject and relatives will reveal the diagnosis.

Brain damage
Some subjects following brain damage show a marked deterioration in personality and develop antisocial behaviour which may well include theft.

> A young man, who had shown some delinquency, sustained a severe brain injury followed by epilepsy as a result of a road traffic accident. His character deteriorated and his antisocial behaviour increased. He offended in a number of ways including impulsively taking and driving away cars, and minor stealing. It was felt that much of his behaviour was due to his resentment and his failure to come to terms with the handicap caused by the brain damage. Initially he was placed on probation with a condition of treatment (support and counselling), but this failed to modify his attitude or his behaviour and eventually he was imprisoned.

Epilepsy

Associated with an epileptic attack
The epileptic attack may be followed by a state of confusion in which, theoretically at least, a person might leave a shop with goods without remembering to pay, though this must be extremely rare.

Associated with an antisocial personality and epilepsy
The offending will almost always be unrelated to actual fits though an experienced criminal may try and claim such an association. Such a claim should be examined sceptically.

Substance abuse
Alcohol or drugs may be associated with theft in a number of ways, though substance abuse is not a defence (see Chapter 9).

(i)   the impoverished subject may steal drugs or drink to maintain the habit,
(ii) food may be stolen due to poverty,
(iii) the substance abuse may disinhibit the subject sufficiently for him to take part in a burglary or other offence either by himself or with others.

Acquisitive offending and mental impairment

Stealing may occur in subjects with mental retardation due to there being:

(1) Less resistance to temptation;
(2) An associated personality disturbance;
(3) Resentments which are due in part to recent or chronic difficulties and frustrations experienced by the handicapped person as a result of the effect of low intelligence.

Acquisitive offending and psychopathic disorder

The shoplifting study revealed a group of young people who stole impulsively and who also had other offences. Their backgrounds were likely to be severely disordered, their adjustment to life unsuccessful, and they led lifelong chaotic, disturbed lives. Their ability to sustain relationships, maintain themselves in work and manage their own affairs was also poor.

Acquisitive offending and other 'disorders'

'Absent-minded' taking of goods
Patients may taking things from shops in an 'absent-minded' state[5] without intent to deprive, in which case they should be found not guilty. Absent-minded behaviour may occur in a number of conditions including depression, anxiety, dementia and post-epileptic confusion.

Preoccupation, distraction or harassment
This may be a common cause of absent minded behaviour.

> The author entered a shop to purchase a postcard. He selected one and became distracted by a book. Suddenly remembering his need to post the card he rushed from the shop and sent it off. He then recalled that he had failed to pay for it. The shop told him afterwards 'Not to worry, lots of people do that.'

Similar distraction is said to have occurred in association with painful or severe physical illnesses such as painful arthritic conditions[5].

Impaired concentration due to medication
This has been described[5] in association with excessive night sedation, antidepressants, anti-epileptic medication, steroids. Typically, such people are honest people who have offended whilst taking medication. In such cases, there should, obviously, be no history from observers (e.g. the store detective) of stealth or attempts to conceal the goods. It is most common in the elderly.

Confusion
States of confusion may be induced by mental disorders – e.g. panic induced by claustrophobia in a shop followed by a desire to leave the shop as rapidly as possible. In these cases the confusion would probably be obvious to the store detective and shop assistant.

Impaired concentration due to endocrine disorders
Endocrine states may affect concentration or mood (e.g. hypothyroidism, thyrotoxicosis, hypoglycaemia).

> A middle-aged woman of previously excellent personality was charged with shoplifting. On examination she claimed to have no memory of taking the goods. She was found to be suffering from thyrotoxicosis, though in this case the court would not accept her defence of 'no intent' and she was found guilty.

Clinical assessment of the case

A full history should give an indication of any psychiatric disturbance. Subjects may claim to be unable to recall the actual offence. Possible causes of such failure to remember include:

- Malingering
- Hysterical denial
- Poor retention due to being:
  distracted
  ill
  under the influence of medication
  under the influence of alcohol or drugs
- Dementia with poor memory
- Rare disturbances of consciousness, e.g. hypoglycaemia, postictal phenomena, etc.

In clinical practice malingering and hysterical denial appear to be by far the commonest cause of failing to remember. It is very important to check as much of the history as possible from other sources. Relatives should be seen, if possible, or information obtained second-hand through a social report (probably prepared by the probation service). A detailed history of past offences should be obtained from the patient (and checked with the probation or police record). Ideally, an objective account of the present offence should be obtained from statements or the police. This becomes particularly important where it is being asserted that there was no intent. The observations of others are essentially to make a balanced appraisal of the case.

> A middle aged woman, who had had a very unhappy life, developed panic attacks after her first divorce. Her second husband gave a very clear description of the panic attacks occurring in shops when he was there as well as in other situations. After an argument at home she went into a shop alone and was accused of theft on leaving it. She assented that she had developed a panic attack in the shop and had left it hurriedly. She denied any intent to deprive. However, the store detective's account was of a woman deliberately stealing. The psychiatric report referred to both accounts of the events and attempted to show where there was compatibility and incompatibility. The court was left to decide which account was the correct one.

If, of course, one feels certain on psychiatric grounds that there was no intent then this opinion should be given to the court. On the other hand, some subjects will not proceed with such a defence fearing that it will increase the chances of their case being publicized in the newspaper. They hope, by pleading guilty, to dispose of the matter quickly and anonymously.

Management and treatment of mentally disordered property offenders

The appropriate treatment is that of the underlying mental disorder. Whether or not this will require admission to hospital will depend on the severity of the disorder and the likelihood of the patient co-operating with treatment. Generally it will be the psychotic or severely organically disturbed who will need hospital treatment on a hospital order. The neurotic disorders (minor depressions; anxiety states) may be managed on an outpatient basis, often as a condition of probation. All patients will benefit not just from medication, but also from supportive counselling and sound advice, e.g. leaving bags outside shops, shopping with others, getting rid of car keys, etc.

The most difficult patients include those with severe personality disorders (who may not be amenable to treatment) and the 'compulsive' groups. Various attempts have been made with behavioural techniques in the latter group including[6] aversive conditioning, covert sensitization, re-directed activities, and mass practice. Of primary relevance is the motivation which may be dependent on mood (frustration, low self-esteem, depression).

Prosecution and the courts

There have been cases where a prosecution for shoplifting has led to the suicide of a vulnerable person. The Code for Crown Prosecutors gives guidelines to the prosecution indicating that sympathetic consideration should be given to those with some form of psychiatric illness or impairment. The subjects may be cautioned or not prosecuted, or the prosecution abandoned – particularly where the adverse effects on the defendant's mental health from prosecution outweigh the interests of justice.

However, where there is a successful prosecution, and psychiatric disorder is also present, then the disorder may be put forward in mitigation on behalf of the subject. The courts are usually very anxious to assist those who are clearly psychiatrically disordered and usually willing to go along with a psychiatric recommendation. It is the case, however, in shoplifting particularly, that the courts had become so disillusioned with the frequent plea that the shoplifter must have been depressed that there are signs of the courts having less sympathy when this plea is put forward. Nevertheless, they usually accept recommendations for outpatient treatment as a condition of probation, or inpatient hospital care on a hospital order in appropriate cases.

> A housewife of previously good personality, became depressed and began to abuse alcohol following the breakup of her marriage. She was caught shoplifting and charged. A psychiatric report explained her illness and its possible relation to the offence. The recommendation for a probation order with a condition of outpatient treatment was accepted by the court.

Destructive offences

Introduction

The literature in this area has principally been about arson which seems to have been of a particular interest to psychiatrists, though many of the findings apply to other destructive offences. It has always been recognized that arson could be due to mental illness as well as common motivations like jealousy, revenge or anger. The first descriptions go back to Esquirol in 1835[7] who described arsonists suffering from psychotic illness, dementia and subnormality etc. At that time repeated arson without other psychiatric disorder led to a diagnosis of pyromania (in keeping with the then fashionable diagnosis of monomania), though now repeated fire raising is seen as the end-result of a number of disorders.

Scientific surveys of arsonists began in the 1950s with the classical study by Lewis and Yarnell[8] of 1100 arson cases which threw further light on the motives behind fire raising and resulted in a classification of fire raisers. Whilst that study gave a view of a representative sample, other studies have been on very selected groups, e.g. arsonists in special hospital and arsonists in prison. These latter studies[9], although lacking the overall view obtained by Lewis and Yarnell's study, have, nevertheless, added to our understanding and expand the classification.

Prins, Tennant and Trick[10] attempted to test a simplified version on 113 arsonists. Inter-rater reliability was obtained in two out of three cases but often multiple motivations were seen. The present classification below is modified from that of Lewis and Yarnell. The classification might equally well be applied to other destructive behaviour, such as malicious damage. Psychiatric abnormality can be associated with any of the sub-groups.

Fire as a means to an end

In this heterogenous group the fire is used to achieve an end – such as the collection of insurance money, revenge, or self-protection.

Insurance fraud
In this group the fire is set in order to claim insurance money. It is unlikely that a psychiatrist will be asked to see such a case except where the accused has a history of mental illness or there is a suspicion of illness.

Desire to earn money
Cases have been described where part-time firemen have deliberately created work for themselves by setting fire in order that they will be called out and thus earn extra money. Such cases are unlikely to come the way of the psychiatrist and are usually dealt with by prison or other penal sentences.

Covering up the evidence of a crime
Here, a fire is set to hide a crime or destroy clues. Such cases are unlikely to be referred for a psychiatric report but may be if the situation is sufficiently bizarre. The psychiatrist must ensure that he has seen all the relevant statements which were made to the court. These may throw light on what appears to be an otherwise perplexing event. Sometimes the excuse of covering up a crime may be offered by a defendant who wishes to hide more pathological motives, such as a repetitive urge to set fires, and sometimes the original crime may spring from a mental illness.

Political motives
A fire is set to achieve a political goal. It is unlikely that a psychiatrist will

be asked to see a person who has set fire for this purpose (except for the rare psychotic subject) for such persons usually take great pains to point out that their actions are those of a sane and responsible man. Some may have a history of personality instability but generally a hospital disposal is inappropriate.

Gang activities for excitement

Immature people, particularly adolescents, may work themselves up into a state of excitement during which time they may commit various offences, including arson (for which there seems to be a very good prognosis from the re-offending point of view). One sometimes sees cases where there is one very disturbed member influencing a group of relatively normal boys to indulge in wild behaviour, or one sees a disturbed youth attempt to gain attention or status with other youths by behaving in a dangerous way. The relatively normal youths are unlikely to set other fires once the dominating or disturbed youth is separated from them.

Revenge, self-protection, anger etc.

In this group the fire is the result of intense emotions of fear or anger often arising out of interactions with others:

> A man with a history of schizophrenia came to feel that the articles in his parents' home were persecuting him so he set fire to the home to destroy them. Assessment showed that he had been an uncooperative patient in the past who, whilst easy to stabilize, would quickly become unstable once released to the community through his failure to cooperate with his doctor. A recommendation for treatment under a hospital order was accepted by the court who also took up the suggestion of a restriction order so that obligatory supervision and treatment would be a part of the man's care when he re-entered the community.

> A plausible, superficial, but mistrustful and hypersensitive young man was employed in a large store. After an altercation with his manager he set fire to a pile of cardboard boxes in the storeroom out of anger and resentment. He had set several previous fires of a similar nature and had been dangerous and aggressive in other spheres. He was found to fall within the definition of psychopathic disorder. However, a prison sentence was thought more appropriate than a hospital order as it was considered unlikely that he would benefit from psychiatric treatment in hospital.

A cry for help state

In this group the fire is a way of drawing attention to the plight of the subject:

> A chronic schizophrenic, after years in hospital, was rehabilitated to the community. After an argument in his lodgings he wandered the countryside becoming increasingly despondent. In such a state he set fire to a barn one night. Assessment showed that he was actively psychotic believing that his

landlord was hostile to him. His act could be understood as an attempt to draw attention to his plight (as well as discharging tension). He was very willing to accept further hospital care. The judge, believing him to be dangerous, made a restriction order with the hospital order.

A conscientious man in his late twenties ran into occupational and domestic difficulties. He became depressed and following another rejection for a job he set fire to his house. Initially he was suspected of setting the fire in order to obtain insurance money. Assessment revealed his depressive state and his predicament to which he could see no solution. His fire raising could be understood largely as a cry for help. The incident exposed his difficulties to his family who rushed to his aid. From the psychiatric point of view, the chance of setting further fires seemed remote. The offer of outpatient treatment was put to the court.

Desire to feel powerful

This group obtain satisfaction from the sense of power they feel by setting something alight, watching the fire and commotion, and reading about it the next day – whilst enjoying the feeling of being the cause of it. They are usually inadequate people of low self-esteem:

A middle-aged recidivist thief and fireraiser had spent most of his adult life in prison and had no roots in the community. Whilst in the community, he became increasingly despondent and knew that he would feel better if he set fire to something. After doing so, he stood back and watched the consequences, and read about it the next day.

Desire to be seen as a hero

This group tends to be of subjects of rather inadequate personality with low self-esteem who construct a situation in which they appear to be heroes. They set a fire, call the Fire Brigade and rush to the rescue of people caught in the blaze in the hope of capturing the limelight. Long-term follow-up studies do not clarify whether this motivation necessarily means a bad prognosis. One might expect supportive therapy to be helpful in such cases.

A fire as a thing of interest

This consists of a heterogenous group in which there is fascination with the fire itself.

Irresistible impulse

People in this group are aware of a repeated urge to set fires which they do not fully understand and when questioned about it are very inarticulate. They are often isolated, inadequate people. They overlap with the tension-reducing group. They usually have a history of setting several fires and of being caught. The fires may escalate in severity.

A subnormal man aged 30 was charged with breaking into a garage and setting fire to it. At first he said that he had set the fire because he was angry that he had been unable to find anything to steal. Information from his probation officer, however, made it clear that the man was in fact more disturbed than this and had set fires which he could not explain. The offender feared that the fireraising would continue. In view of the offender's mental retardation and his dangerousness an application was made to a special hospital. The court made a hospital order on the grounds of mental impairment and placed a restriction order on him as well.

Sexual excitement

Although fire as a fetish was thought in the nineteenth century to be a common cause of fire raising in practice men who are directly sexually stimulated by fire seem to be rare (though there has been considerable psychiatric interest in the sexual symbolism in fireraising[5]). The surveys of arsonists have described people who are sexually aroused by the fire which they have set though this is a very small proportion of all fire-raisers. Some receive prison sentences where they may receive psychotherapy, others find themselves admitted to special hospital. The motivation seems so bizarre in these cases that a psychiatric report is usually requested. It is usually believed (without much evidence) that the prognosis must be bad. Certainly the subject should be regarded as dangerous as long as the fantasies of sexual arousal by fire raising persist.

Tension- or depression-reducing

In this group the principal motivation arises from the discovery by the subject that the act relieves feelings of despondency or tension. This group overlaps with the 'irresistible impulse' group and the 'cry for help' group. Such fireraising may be associated with other tension-reducing activity such as self-mutilation and suicide. In women, there are clinical grounds for suspecting an association with early sexual abuse. Virkkunen[11] found evidence of reduced levels of cerebrospinal fluid serotonin in this group (see Chapter 4) and an impaired glucose tolerance curve.

Management depends on how easily their depression and anxiety can be reduced, perhaps by offering asylum in hospital or supportive therapy as an outpatient (with or without medication), or whether it is necessary to contain the patient in a more secure establishment until, through time and treatment, there is maturation and greater self-control.

A 19-year-old boy (of dull intelligence) from an apparently stable home had grown into a shy, isolated youth. He was arrested for setting fire to a shed but it became clear that he had set fires to various objects for a number of years. He was very inadequate in social relationships and had a fetish for female underclothes. The combination of his personality difficulties (which brought him within the definition of psychopathic disorder) and low intelligence led to the view that it would be appropriate to offer psychiatric treatment. In view of his recurrent fireraising it was thought necessary to begin treatment in a special hospital. This case illustrates not only how fireraising can be used to relieve tension states but how fireraising may be related to sexual difficulties.

Dangerousness of fireraisers

Lewis and Yarnell painted a picture of arsonists being a very handi-capped group of people of whom 30% were likely to repeat fireraising. However, prediction in individual cases is often difficult[12]. A recent study showed an overall recidivism rate of only 4% for arson amongst convicted arsonists, although many commit other types of offences[13]. Offenders on short sentences have a very low re-offending rate for arson over a five-year period (2%) but 20% of arsonists who have served long terms of imprisonment committed further arson[14]. 25% of the short-termers and 50% of the long-termers were found to commit a destructive offence (arson, sex, property damage or violence) in the follow-up period. If all offences are taken into account then 43% of the short-termers were re-convicted of some offence (including theft) and 80% of the long termers reoffended overall. As with other crimes, the best predictors were the number of previous convictions, the parole score (see Chapter 14) and the time served in prison for the last sentence (a reflection of the offender's previous criminality and the severity of his last offence).

In summary, whilst it may be difficult to tell whether a particular person may commit arson again, the statistical chances of a repeat after serving a period in prison or other institutions appear to be low overall.

Clinical assessment of arsonists and other destructive offenders

As with all potentially dangerous offenders, the best chance of making a good assessment depends on getting the best objective information as well as taking a careful detailed history. Nothing can replace a pains-takingly detailed examination of previous psychiatric records, social reports, lists of previous convictions (with details if possible) and state-ments relating to the current offence. There should be current information from people about his background, obtained best of all by interviewing the relatives, and certainly by discussing the case with a social worker, or probation officer who knows the case.

The assessment will be aimed at elucidating whether there was a psychiatric abnormality – either at the time of the offence or since – and the motivation for the offence. The relationship with a psychiatric abnormality may be direct (e.g. acting on a delusion), or indirect (e.g. reflecting the stresses which occurred secondarily to the illness). The assessment will also be aimed at estimating dangerousness. This will be based on the history of previous fireraising and offending, understanding the precipitant to the fireraising and the likelihood of the precipitant recurring, and listening to the subject's own account and assessment of his potential for further fireraising together with his account of his fantasies and impulses. Clearly, previous fireraising (precipitated by minor stress) and an awareness of persistent impulses to set fire, must be given a high dangerousness rating.

The psychiatric report

The psychiatrist preparing the report will deal with the presence of psychiatric abnormality and what treatment can be offered and where. The subject of dangerousness, as already discussed, can be addressed but always with some diffidence, in view of the studies (see Chapter 14) which tend to show how unsatisfactory is a doctor's ability to gauge dangerousness successfully in any individual's case. The question of intent rarely seems a medicolegal problem for the psychiatrist in cases of fireraising though it may be for the court. Intent will be assumed from the nature of the fireraising, e.g. evidence of paper being piled up, etc.

Outcome in court

In cases of arson, the court is, as usual, generally very anxious to help those with psychiatric disorder. The court will also be anxious to keep the protection of the public in mind. Recommendations for treatment should therefore take cognisance of this and be seen to be realistic in terms of safety. Whilst it is not necessary to recommend everyone for a special hospital or regional secure unit, recommendations for outpatient care for an actively psychotic person who has just set a fire would also clearly be inappropriate. Recommendations for a restriction order may be appropriate when it is advisable to have obligatory after-care in the community or where absconding from hospital (with a risk to others) is likely.

References

(1) Gibbens, T.C.N. & Prince, J. (1962) *Shoplifting.* Institute for the Study and Treatment of Delinquency, London.
(2) Gibbens, T.C.N., Palmer, C. & Prince, J. (1971) Mental health aspects of shoplifting. *British Medical Journal* **3**, 612–15.
(3) Gibbens, T.C.N. (1981) Shoplifting. *British Journal of Psychiatry* **138**, 346–7.
(4) McElroy, S.L., Hudson, J.I., Pope, H.G. & Keck, P.E. (1991) Kleptomania: clinical characteristics and associated psychopathology. *Psychological Medicine* **21**, 93–108.

(5) Editorial (1976) The absent-minded shoplifter. *British Medical Journal* **1**, 675–6.
(6) Gudjonsson, G.H. (1990) Psychological and psychiatric aspects of shoplifting. *Medicine, Science and the Law* **30**, 45–51.
(7) Esquirol, J.E.D. (1965) *Mental Maladies, Treatise on Insanity.* Hafner, London.
(8) Lewis, N.D.C. & Yarnell, H. (1951) Pathological firesetting. *Nervous and Mental Disease Monograph.* No. 82. New York.
(9) Faulk, M. (1979) Arsonists and the psychiatrist. In Gaind, R.N. and Hudson, B.L. (eds) *Current Themes in Psychiatry.* Macmillan Press Ltd, London and Basingstoke.
(10) Prins, H., Tennant, G. & Trick, K. (1985) Motives for arson (fire raising). *Medical Science Law* **25**, 275–8.
(11) Virkkunen, M., De Jong, J., Barto, J., Goodwin, F.K. & Linnoila, M. (1989) Relationship of psychobiological variables to recidivism in violent offenders and impulsive fire setters. *Archives of General Psychiatry* **46**, 600–3.
(12) Faulk, M. (1982) Assessing dangerousness in arsonists. In Hamilton, J.R. and Freeman, H. (eds) *Dangerousness: Psychiatric Assessment and Management.* Gaskell (for the Royal College of Psychiatrists), London.
(13) Soothill, K.L. & Pople, P.J. (1973) Arson: a twenty-year cohort study. *Medical Science and the Law* **13**, 127–38.
(14) Sapsford, R.J., Banks, C. & Smith, D.D. (1978) Arsonists in prison. *Medical Science and the Law* **18**, 247–54.

Chapter 7

Offences Against the Person and Forensic Psychiatry

Introduction

This chapter defines offences against the person, including sexual offending. Basic criminological data, theories of violence, the relationship of mental abnormality to violence, and the forensic aspects are all discussed. This is followed by a description of the psychiatric assessment of violent offenders. Finally, sex offences and poisoning are covered.

As in all offending, violence may be the end-result of several different chains of events of which mental abnormality is but one. The task of the psychiatrist in any particular case must be to detect the presence, and demonstrate the influence of, any mental abnormality. The motive (anger, jealousy, etc.) that drives the 'normal' person to a violent offence may well be the final motive in the mentally abnormal. In the latter case, however, the motive will often be exaggerated by, or the result of, mental abnormality.

Definition

An 'offence against the person' is a legal term and includes:

(1) Homicide

This is the killing of a human being by another. It is subdivided into lawful and unlawful homicide.

(a) Lawful homicide
This includes justifiable killing (e.g. on behalf of the state) and excusable homicide (e.g. death resulting from pure accident or as a result of honest and reasonable mistake).

(b) Unlawful homicide
This is defined as the unlawful killing of any reasonable creature in being

and under the Queen's peace, the death following within a year and a day of the deed. It is subdivided into murder and manslaughter.

(i) Murder
The offender must be of sound mind and discretion (i.e. sane, and over 10 years of age). It must be proven that there was malice aforethought (i.e. intent to cause death or grievous bodily harm), or that the death follows unlawful and voluntary intent to do serious injury. Courts have varied in their rulings but currently it seems that intent may be assumed if there was recklessness as to the effect of an action either when the offender appreciated that death or serious harm was a virtual certainty or had given no thought to an obvious risk. This is known as the subjective test. Previously (the objective test) it had been ruled that intent was assumed if an ordinary person (not necessarily the offender) would have realized that the death or serious harm was the natural result of the act. A person found guilty of murder is automatically sentenced to life imprisonment. The court has no discretion in this sentence.

(ii) Manslaughter
In this case the homicide follows an unlawful act or omission but the circumstances do not meet the full criteria of murder, or there are mitigating factors, i.e. there is:

(a) an absence of intent to kill or cause grievous bodily harm,
(b) negligent behaviour without intent to kill (e.g. a drunken surgeon),
(c) an immediate reaction to severe provocation, e.g. finding a spouse in bed with a lover,
(d) having a mental abnormality of such severity as to substantially diminish the responsibility of the accused,
(e) homicide as part of a suicide pact.

In the case of manslaughter the court has discretion to give any sentence ranging from life sentence to conditional discharge including, in appropriate cases, hospital orders.

(iii) Infanticide
This crime is defined under the Infanticide Act 1938. A woman may be found guilty of infanticide instead of murder after she has killed her child if the child is under 12 months and, at the time of the act or omission, the balance of her mind was disturbed by reason of her not being fully recovered from the effects of giving birth to the child or the effects of lactation. If she is found guilty of infanticide and not murder then she is dealt with as in the case of manslaughter.

(2) Death of infants

There are three offences connected with the death of infants:

(i) *Child destruction*
The killing of a child capable of being born alive before it has an existence independent of its mother. The Abortion Act 1967 protects doctors from being charged with child destruction.

(ii) *Concealment of birth*
It is an offence to dispose of the dead body of a recently born child whether or not it was born alive.

(iii) *An attempt to procure an abortion*
It is an offence to attempt to procure an abortion except in the situation defined by the Abortion Act 1967. If a woman died as a consequence of an illegal abortion then the person attempting to procure the abortion would be indicted for manslaughter.

(3) Assaults

An assault occurs when a person strikes another or does an action which makes the other fear immediate personal violence. 'Battery' is the actual application of unlawful force, though 'assault' is frequently used to cover both. In certain situations an assault or battery is justifiable, e.g. in the furtherance of public authority, self-defence, or by consent. Relevant offences in this group include:

(i) *Wounding*
Here the skin must be broken. Wounding is subdivided into:

(a) 'wounding with intent to cause grievous bodily harm' (i.e. serious bodily harm). The prosecution must prove intent;
(b) 'Unlawful wounding', where there is no intent to cause grievous bodily harm even though grievous bodily harm may be caused.

(ii) *Assaults*
Here there may be little or severe damage but the form of it is not that of wounding. It includes:

(a) assault causing grievous bodily harm,
(b) assault occasioning actual bodily harm (a hurt or injury which interferes with the health or comfort of the injured but not such as to amount to grievous bodily harm),
(c) common assault in which there is an attempt to offer violence or do harm but without wounding or actual bodily harm.

(4) Poisoning

Poisoning is the deliberate administering of a noxious substance intending to cause harm or death. It has been discussed by Cordess[1]. Four situations can be recognized:

(a) Poisoning of children
Some parents poison their children

(i) as a form of non-accidental injury to punish, control or sedate them
(ii) as a form of Munchausen's syndrome by proxy presenting themselves as caring, worried parents with a mysteriously ill child and enjoying the attention of, and intimacy with, the hospital staff.
(iii) in order to claim the life insurance.

(b) Poisoning of sick parents by their carers
Often altruistic motives are professed ('to put them out of their misery') though sadistic motives or financial gain may be suspected.

(c) Poisoning to kill or get rid of people
This may be:

(i) within relationships as in other forms of homicide,
(ii) for financial gain,
(iii) for sadistic reasons – as in the case of Graham Young[2] who was fascinated by poisons and their effects and enjoyed observing the effects of poisons and the power poisons brought him.

(d) Threats and acts of mass poisoning:
This may be:

(i) to secure a ransom,
(ii) to achieve a political or terrorist goal: 'Do what we want or we will poison your products',
(iii) because of some unknown motivation – manifested by the discovery of the poisoned foods, the offender perhaps enjoying the feeling of power accompanying the widespread concern and panic caused by the action.

(5) Driving offences

The driving offences in this section are those which are dangerous to others and include:

(a) Careless driving
Driving without due care or reasonable consideration.

(b) Driving or attempting to drive when unfit
Whether this is through drink or drugs or with excess alcohol in the blood.

(c) Being in charge of a motor vehicle when unfit
Again, whether unfit through drink or drugs or with excess alcohol in the blood.

(d) Causing death by careless driving while under the influence
Under the influence of alcohol or drugs.

(e) Reckless driving
Driving recklessly at speed or in a manner dangerous to the public (automatism, e.g. sudden unconsciousness, would be a defence).

(f) Causing injury or death by reckless driving.

(g) Dangerous driving and causing death by dangerous driving

(h) Failure to provide a specimen
This would be a specimen of urine or blood needed for laboratory tests (a medical certificate to say that it would make the offender ill might be a defence).

(6) Sexual offences

These are listed and described below.

Criminological details of offences against the person

There are two principal sources of data. The best source is derived from the British Crime Survey in which over 10 000 people were questioned about their experience as victims. The traditional police statistics of reported crime are now known to be unreliable by comparison, as they are an underestimate as people do not always report crime and the police do not always record it; also, they distort the true figures because people report some crimes more than others.

The number of recorded crimes of violence has risen in the last few decades[3]. Total recorded crimes of personal violence (severe and trivial) rose from 89 599 in 1974 to 265 000 in 1992[4]. Crimes of violence reported to the police in 1991 amounted to just over 5% of all reported offences.

The British Crime Survey[5] found that violent offending is rising, although not at the high rate suggested by the police figures, and at a lower rate than property offences. The survey showed that only one in five woundings and robbery were reported. The relatively greater increase in the police figures suggests that people are perhaps more willing to report violent offences.

Violence known to the police seems to be committed by a very small proportion of the population. Of the 31 436 males born in Denmark between the years 1944–47, 2.3% of them accounted for all the convictions of violence by the time they were 30 years. Some 43% of the violent convictions were committed by 0.6% of the cohort[6].

The type of offence affects whether it is reported. Trivial assaults may not be worth reporting. Rape may be under-reported, on the other hand, because of the embarrassment of the victim. Serious violent assaults in the home may also be under-reported, in part, due to the fear of the victim that reporting the offence will anger or alienate the attacker and provoke further violence.

Over 90% of violent offenders are male, and over 50% are aged between 17 and 24 years. The principal victim outside the home is another young male. The offences are often carried out in association with the abuse of alcohol. In serious woundings, male victims are six times more frequent than female but only three times for less serious wounding. Two-thirds of the victims of robberies are male though older victims tend to be female. Violence is commoner in areas of social deprivation.

The amount of unreported homicide is unknown; there are a large number of missing people each year some of whom may be homicide victims. The reported homicide rate in England and Wales per million has varied throughout the century with peaks in the first, third and present decades. Currently, the rate has risen to 13 per million per annum (675 homicides in 1991) having been around 10 per million for a number of years. The equivalent rate in the United States of America is in excess of 140 per million, whereas in Denmark, in the 1970s, it was 5 per million.

In cases of homicide the victim is acquainted with the offender in three-quarters of the cases. In half of the cases the victim is a family member or lover. The offence usually arises as the result of quarrel, jealousy or an outburst of temper. A sharp instrument is the commonest method of killing in the UK.

Within the family, children under the age of 1 year are most at risk (32 babies/million/year) with males at slightly greater risk than females. These deaths commonly arise as baby battering but also from psychosis and the killing of unwanted babies.

Parricide (killing of parents) is rare (4% of homicides) and is committed by sons more often than daughters with the father more at risk. Schizophrenia is said to be common in the offending adult sons (75%). In childhood or adolescence, non-psychotic children who commit parricide do so as an explosive reaction to prolonged provocation or abuse – sometimes to the relief of the entire family.

Female parricide is rare (4% of female homicides) and is usually matricide[7]. The matricide arises in a setting of chronic discord, social isolation with a widowed daughter who has become mentally ill or alcoholic. Patricides by younger women (c. 18 years) occur in relation to long-term abuse and violence.

To give proportion to the figures it should be remembered that the number of people killed on the roads in the United Kingdom is around 5000 per year – one-fifth of which are due to dangerous driving.

Causes of violence

There have been many attempts to find, as in delinquency, a single 'monolithic' theory of violence. These attempts have each been criticized as failing to explain the whole range of aggression and violence[8,9]. Violence, like delinquency, has to be understood in a multifactorial way. It is useful, however, to be aware of these 'monolithic' hypotheses as each contributes to our understanding. The main hypotheses include (1) the instinct hypothesis, (2) the frustrated-drive hypothesis, and (3) the learned-response hypothesis.

The instinct hypothesis

Lorenz[10] from his studies on lower vertebrates came to the conclusion that aggression is a spontaneously generated force, a natural instinct, which has the biological functions of ensuring proper spacing of the animals, the maintenance of dominance hierarchies and therefore group stability and aiding natural selection. He observed that the release of aggression on members of the same species occurred when there were specific threats in these biological situations. He postulated that, despite our complex social situation, there is such a spontaneous, aggressive force in man. Normally, he argued, it is expressed and released in socially approved, aggressive activities, e.g. sport. Failure to find such expression leads to undesirable, aggressive acts. He linked this force to the instinctual forces postulated by Freud of Eros, the basic life instinct and Thanatos, the death instinct. The hypothesis has been criticized because of the failure to find support for the idea in man that aggression (as in lower animals) is released by specific aggression-releasing stimuli and inhibited by other behaviour (e.g. gestures of submission), and also because the theory is extrapolated from lower forms to man.

The frustrated-drive hypothesis

Dollard *et al.*[11] postulated that aggression arises as a result of the frustration of goal-directed behaviour. Thus, it is argued, that frustration always leads to some form of aggression, and the occurrence of aggression always presupposes some form of frustration. The degree of frustration reflects both the importance of the behaviour which has been frustrated and the number of times it occurs. It is argued that frustration may not immediately give way to aggression if inhibiting forces are present, such as an awareness of anticipated consequences of aggression.

It is also noted that the aggression, when it occurs, can be displaced onto objects other than the frustrating agent.

Although the frustration hypothesis may explain some aggression it cannot account for the whole picture. It has been pointed out that frustration may be followed by a variety of responses from dejection and resignation to positive, active effort. But it fails to explain various sorts of violence including sadistic acts or that done in defence of a reputation.

Learned-response hypothesis

Bandura[12] is a leading proponent of the hypothesis that aggressive responses are largely learned, though they may be motivated by emotional arousal resulting from any aversive stimuli. Aversive stimuli lead to a variety of responses, from withdrawal, to escape and aggression. The learning to be aggressive (and learning to inhibit aggression) occurs in two principal ways. These are:

(1) By learning from experience – aggressive behaviour being encouraged or not by others, rewarded or not by success or a rise in self-esteem, followed or not by unpleasant consequences. The pleasurable feelings achieved by the violent behaviour may come to have the features of an addictive experience[13].

(2) By observation of the behaviour of others, particularly adults by children (i.e. by modelling). A 20-year follow-up of children of violent parents, in fact, found an increased risk of violence in the children, although the majority were not violent[14].

Thus, the occurrence of aggression depends both on conditioned responses (by shaping or by classical conditioning) and on cognitive elements based on modelling and experience – as for example[15] goal-directed violence intended to sustain a subject's reputation and self-image, e.g. 'no-one walks over me'.

Modifying factors on aggressive or violent responses

Whether or not any individual is aggressive or violent in any particular situation is modified by many factors. These include:

- Personality
- The immediate social group
- The behaviour of the victim
- The presence of disinhibiting factors, such as alcohol or drugs
- Environmental factors
- Physiological and biological factors
- The presence of mental abnormality.

Personality

Megargee[16] related the presence and extent of aggressive behaviour to the presence of either an overcontrolled or undercontrolled personality. Blackburn[17] extended this hypothesis by the cluster analysis of personality test data obtained from violent offenders. He identified four major groups using two factors. The two factors are:

(A) Antisocial aggression (impulsivity, aggression, hostility, low denial of anger), distinguished between the undercontrolled (psychopathic) and the overcontrolled group.
(B) Sociability (social anxiety and proneness to mood disorder). This second factor divided them into groups:
    (1) undercontrolled, low social anxiety (primary psychopath),
    (2) undercontrolled, high social anxiety (secondary psychopath),
    (3) overcontrolled, low social anxiety ('controlled' group),
    (4) overcontrolled, high social anxiety ('inhibited' group).

He had previously found that being undercontrolled was associated with more frequent aggression whilst being overcontrolled was associated with infrequent but extreme aggression. It seemed as though the undercontrolled, used to aggressive outbursts following relatively little provocation, had learned, with practice, to control the extent of it. The overcontrolled person, being unused to aggressive feeling and reactions, becomes overcome and loses control once the aggressive outburst begins, with excessive violence as the result. Comparison with other studies shows that group (3) is most like the general population in personality and may, therefore, be best called 'controlled' and not, 'overcontrolled'. This group contained the largest proportion of mentally ill. Group (4) contained men with considerable interpersonal and emotional difficulties, and included a high proportion of sex offenders.

The immediate social group

The influence of the immediate social group can obviously be a big factor – as seen in football hooliganism, groups of adolescents, angry crowds, etc. Care has to be taken to distinguish between true aggressive behaviour in terms of actual violence and mere aggressive posturing, the latter being more common than the former. Aggression exhibited by certain minority groups is perceived to be the result of the social frustrations and prejudices experienced by the group. Nevertheless, the individual's behaviour in the group may owe more to the effect of group pressure than to his own experience.

The behaviour of the victim

Victims of aggressive attacks are often well known to the aggressor. There has been considerable interest in the role the victim plays in provoking and precipitating the violence. Wolfgang[18] concluded that the victim played a substantial part in precipitating the violence by provoking the aggressor in a quarter of the homicides he studied. Bluglass[19] found half of spouse murder victims were alcoholic, psychotic or disabled, and had played a significant part in their own death. Studies of battered wives have revealed a subgroup who were repeatedly provocative to their explosive husbands[20]. A study of victims of assault found a correlation between the severity of the injury and the alcohol intake of the victims[21].

Disinhibiting factors, such as alcohol and drugs

There seems, clinically, to be a clear link between the abuse of alcohol and aggressive behaviour in individual cases. Certainly alcohol plays a significant part in dangerous driving and in association with serious offending[3]. Drugs seem related to aggression by the pattern of life of the user rather than the disinhibiting effect as in alcohol. The need to obtain drugs or money leads to violent crime, though in England drug abuse does not, as yet, contribute significantly to violent offending.

Environmental factors

The extent of the violence may be influenced by such simple matters as the availability of weapons and the attitudes of the group towards them. Other features in the environment may influence the level of arousal or instability of the subject. Overcrowding, temperature, noise, environmental or social pressures may all play a part at the time of the aggression. The influence of the social mores is much debated but presumably is extremely important. How much the general social standards influence behaviour and how much specific experiences do, such as exposure to violent films and television, is still debated. The latter may be merely a symptom of the former and not harmful in itself.

Physiological and biochemical factors

A disturbance of the physiology of the body may alter the subject's irritability or self-control. The more common influences are likely to be such things as fatigue, hunger, and lack of sleep. Rarer medical conditions may occasionally be seen, such as endocrine disorders (e.g. thyrotoxicosis, hypoglycaemia, and brain disorders (e.g. brain tumours, brain injury).

Impulsiveness and aggression may be linked to a decrease in brain serotonin turnover in the limbic system and cortex. Serotonin is thought to be a possible inhibitor of impulsiveness and aggression. Virkkunen[22] followed up impulsive fire raisers and violent, alcohol-abusing offenders after imprisonment and found a correlation between recidivism for violence and arson and lowered cerebrospinal fluid levels of 5-hydroxyindoleacetic acid (a metabolite of serotonin), homovanillic acid and a flattened glucose tolerance curve.

A raised testosterone level has also been associated with aggression though this may be a secondary effect, not a primary one (see Chapter 12).

The presence of mental abnormality

It is the relationship of mental disorder to violence that is of particular interest to the forensic psychiatrist and will therefore be described in more detail.

(i) *The incidence of violence in the mentally disordered*

The question may be asked: 'Are the mentally disturbed more dangerous than normal?' The question, stated so baldly, is almost meaningless. Does the question apply to those in hospital under treatment, or to those in the community treated or untreated? Clearly, the potential for violence will be decreased by effective treatment in those whose illness predisposes them to violence. Similarly, detention in hospital will reduce the possibility, however remote, of the patient attacking a member of the public. The subject has been usefully reviewed by Berger and Gulevitch[23] and Taylor[24]. Up to the 1960s it had been asserted that the rate of offending, including violent offences, was less amongst discharged psychiatric patients than amongst the general population, with the patients having offending rates fourteen times lower than normal.

More recent work, however, presents a different picture and a number of studies suggest that discharged patients have rates of offending (including violence) which is the same or higher than in the normal population[25,26]. Sosowsky[27], for example, demonstrated that in a three-year follow-up of discharged patients from 1972–1975 the rate of offending for violence and property offenders was higher in the discharged patients than in the general population. He did show, what others had claimed, that the rate of re-offending amongst the patients was, as is true of all criminal activity, related to the number of previous offences. Nevertheless, even the group with no previous offences had higher rates of offending after discharge than the normal population. His own explanation for the change is that in modern settings dangerous patients are released more quickly than they used to be as part of the de-institutional programme. Other possibilities for the phenomena include:

(1) A failure in the earlier studies to identify all the criminality of ex-patients – some may have been returned to hospital instead of being arrested.
(2) A greater tendency in modern times to send mentally abnormal offenders to hospital and not to prison.
(3) An increase in hospital admission for drug addicts and alcoholics – groups notorious for associated criminal activity.

If the psychiatrically abnormal are more likely to be dangerous then the diagnosis of psychiatric abnormality should be made more frequently in populations of violent offenders than in the community. Care must be taken, however, to be clear what the 'psychiatric abnormalities' are and which population is examined. In a study of 'felons' Guze[28] did not find raised prevalence of schizophrenia, manic depressive psychosis or organic brain damage. What was raised was the prevalence of sociopathy, alcoholism and drug dependence. Similar results were found in a study of female felons[29]. What is not clear is whether or not the seriously mentally ill had been removed from the sample by transfer, at some stage, to the hospital system.

Taylor and Gunn[30,31] studied remanded prisoners charged with violent offences and found a higher prevalence of schizophrenia among men subsequently convicted of homicide (11%) than would be expected from the prevalence in the local population (0.1–0.4%). They also found an excess of schizophrenia among men on a variety of criminal charges which supported the belief that criminal behaviour is commoner in schizophrenia than in the general population. It is possible that the figures were distorted by schizophrenia increasing the chances of detection or of being remanded in custody – nevertheless there does seem to be an association. This offending, although greater than normal, represented the activity of only a small percentage of schizophrenics. It was assumed, therefore, that only a small proportion of schizophrenics were violent. Humphreys *et al.*[32] in a study of new schizophrenics found that 20% had exhibited life-threatening behaviour to others, though only a fraction were arrested (or admitted to hospital). Violent behaviour seemed to be a function of the length of time the illness had been untreated.

It may be that a careful study of the behaviour of schizophrenics, rather than counting official offences, would reveal, at least in the untreated, unexpectedly high levels of violence – though the same may be true of the general population!

Hafner and Boker[33] reviewed all serious violent offenders over a 10-year-period in West Germany. Whereas the seriously mentally disordered, as a group, appeared no more frequently than expected (approximately 3%), schizophrenia appeared more often than would be expected, and depressives, the mentally handicapped and brain damaged appeared less. Support for these findings came from a study by Teplin[34] in which a psychiatric assessment of a severe mental disorder (psychosis) was made in a sample of police call-outs in an American town: severely mentally disordered subjects were identified in about 5% of cases; the normally expected rate would be around 1.7%. However, a note of caution has to be entered because the study did occur in a part of the town in which there were many after-care hostels, and this may have artificially raised the incidence. Lindquist and Allebeck[35] in a 15-year-follow-up of 790 schizophrenics discharged from Stockholm hospitals found that the overall crime rate was normal in males, though increased twice in females. Nevertheless, males had a four times increase in violent crime though most of it was minor. Coid *et al.*[36] reviewed 280 twin pairs where one was psychotic. Criminality did increase in the psychotic individual compared to the non-psychotic twin, with schizophrenia having the greatest effect, especially for violence (approximately 7% of ill compared to 0.5% of well). The illness seemed to precede the criminality.

These studies do support the assertion that violence is commoner in some untreated mental disorders than normal, particularly sociopathy, alcoholism, hysteria and schizophrenia.

(ii) *The connection between the violence and the mental abnormality*

The relationship between the violent behaviour and the psychiatric abnormality may be: (a) direct, (b) indirect or (c) coincidental.

A direct relationship may be said to occur when the phenomena of illness directly relates to the offence. Such would be the case in schizophrenia when the subject's behaviour is directed by hallucinations, the effects of delusions or thought disorder induced by the illness. Taylor[37] found such a relationship in 80% of schizophrenic offenders, though at first sight it might not be obvious. It is not uncommon for a subject to attempt to rationalize behaviour and hide the 'true' motive. In schizophrenia, delusions are the commonest cause for violence:

> A man accused of beating his children refused to talk to anyone, having first intimated that his action was based on biblical interpretation. It later emerged that he held the delusion that God was giving him special thoughts and special abilities to understand the Bible. It was this special understanding that prompted him to beat the children.

In some subjects the offences may follow ordinary motivations but be directly affected by the disorder because the intensity of the motivation is heightened by the disorder.

> A young man of egocentric and explosive personality was angered at work by a mildly abrasive interaction with a foreman. Because of his particular personality disorder he over-reacted to the sleight and violently attacked the foreman.

An indirect relationship may be said to occur when the illness causes a change in the social circumstances of the subject which then leads to offending. This is seen in severely ill people who may offend because the social decline they have experienced results in their being without money or social contacts. The case may be complicated by an excessive emotional reaction due to the effects of the mental disorder.

> A schizophrenic man had declined in social position and adopted a vagrant existence. He was without insight and resented being taken into hospital. He stole a hospital knife, with the intention of robbing a shop, to help him to escape.

Similar situations may be associated with the social and psychological deteriorations caused by alcoholism or drug abuse.

A coincidental relationship may be said to occur when a person, with a violent history, develops a mental disorder but continues to be violent. The disorder may increase the violent behaviour and may also be associated with a deterioration of functioning in other areas. Such a picture is seen particularly in violent men who sustain brain damage from a head injury and become more impulsive and violent.

(ii) *The medicolegal aspects of mental abnormality and violence*

The mental abnormality, if severe enough, may be a reason for being unfit to plead, for being regarded as not responsible (or, in the case of a charge of murder, for having diminished responsibility). Finally, it may be used in mitigation. Such defences are available even if the link between the offence and the abnormality is indirect or coincidental. It will be seen that the nature of the abnormality, its severity and (in the case of psychopathic disorder and mental impairment) its treatability, are the important factors. Subsequent chapters will deal with particular disorders and their relationship to the law.

Special cases of violence and the psychiatrist

The charge of murder

Murder has been of particular interest because of its association (in the past) with the death penalty and the dramatic effect psychiatric testimony could have on the outcome. It remains of special interest not only because of the serious nature of the charge and the mandatory sentence of life imprisonment but because of the special defences available and also as a paradigm for other violent offences.

Defences to murder

There are a number of possible defences to the charge of murder including a number of medical defences. The defences include:

(1) Self-defence.
(2) Lack of intent to kill or cause grievous bodily harm.
(3) Provocation: In this case the jury must decide if the provocation was sufficient to provoke a reasonable man. The provocation must be immediately followed by the killing, there can be no time for reflection. Such a defence applies only to the charge of murder and if successful may reduce it to a finding of manslaughter.
(4) That the death was in pursuance of a suicide pact between the offender and the victim. A successful plea would bring in a finding of manslaughter. It would be for the offender to prove that he was acting in pursuance of such an act.
(5) Diminished responsibility: Here the offender asserts that he was suffering from such an abnormality of mind at the time that his responsibility was substantially impaired. A successful plea will, under the Homicide Act 1967, lead to a finding of manslaughter.
(6) Insanity: Here the offender asserts that he was so mentally ill at the time of the offence that he was not responsible for his acts and therefore has not committed a crime.
(7) Automatism: Here the offender asserts that his state of consciousness was so disturbed at the time that he was behaving automatically and therefore has not committed any crime.
(8) Infanticide: Here a mother is claiming that at the time of the death of the child (which must be under the age of 12 months), the balance of her mind was disturbed because she had not fully recovered from the effects of giving birth or the effects of lactation consequent upon the birth of the child. If her plea is successful she will be treated as though guilty of manslaughter.
(9) Not fit to plead: Here the offender is not really putting up a defence against the charge but simply saying that he is too mentally ill to be tried. If the plea is successful then the offender is dealt with under the Criminal Procedure (Insanity and Unfitness to Plead) Act 1991 (see Chapter 3).

Incidence of psychiatric abnormality in homicide

Figures vary from year to year, but, in 1991 there were 675 people suspected or charged with homicide in England and Wales of which almost 20% (a typical figure) were found guilty of manslaughter due to diminished responsibility. Of the 471 dealt with, there were only two cases of infanticide and two cases of insanity. A number of people (45 in

1991) who commit homicide also commit suicide and it may be assumed that some will have had a mental abnormality. A classic pattern, for example, is a man in a state of severe depression who feels that there is no future for himself or his family. He may kill his family and then himself. It is usually said, therefore, that up to 30% of those who commit homicide are found (in England and Wales) to have some form of judicially determined mental abnormality ('abnormal' homicide) covered by insanity, diminished responsibility, infanticide, being unfit to plead or having committed suicide. The incidence of abnormal homicide expressed as a percentage of the normal population seems remarkably constant in different countries[38], with the rate between 0.1–0.2 per 100 000 population. The difference in homicide rates between different countries seems to be accounted for by differences in 'normal' homicide which may reflect social norms and conditions, and the availability of weapons.

Assessment of the offender

The assessment described below acts as a pattern for the assessment of any violent offender. A useful description of the assessment in homicide is given by Bluglass[19].

Where is the assessment done?

The bulk of offenders charged with homicide will be remanded in custody because of the nature of the offence. There are a few, where the circumstances are appropriate, who remain on bail and may be seen as outpatients. The majority will therefore be assessed in prison where they are detained, usually in the prison hospital for observation. In due course the court or prosecution will formally request a report from the prison doctors but the assessment begins from the day the man enters the prison. Of the cases remanded on bail, the request for a report will be sent usually to a local psychiatrist.

Who makes the assessment?

The prison medical service begins the assessment on those in custody. Should they suspect a psychiatric disorder they may choose to call in a psychiatrist from outside the prison medical service for an independent opinion. If it is thought there is a psychiatric disorder which will require hospital treatment then a psychiatrist will be called in from an appropriate hospital (depending on the security needs of the offender) in order to consider whether treatment can be offered. The defendant, through his solicitor, may request a report from a psychiatrist of his choosing. When a report is being prepared on behalf of the defence it is sometimes helpful to communicate with the prison medical service or the independent psychiatrist (with the permission of the defence), especially where it is likely that all the doctors are going to agree in order that a well-organized recommendation can be put to the court.

What is required in order to make an examination?

The doctor making the examination must take a full history from the offender and must obtain copies of prosecution statements, and forensic reports relevant to the case so that he can get a full account of what is said to have happened. It is always helpful to see relatives or have an account from them of the offender to try and get a clearer idea of his mental state at the time of his offence. It will also be helpful to find out from the prison staff how the offender has behaved while under observation. It has become traditional to obtain an electroencephalogram (EEG), although in the writer's experience this rarely produces useful results. In cases of suspected subnormality there should be a psychological assessment of intelligence. This can be done either by the prison psychologist or by an outside psychologist. Other relevant documents which should be obtained include previous psychiatric records, a list of previous offences and a copy of any reports on the social background (probation or social worker).

What are the questions the psychiatrist is addressing himself to?

The psychiatrist will have in his mind the following questions for his report:

Question 1: Is the client fit to plead?
See Chapter 3.

The illness which makes the person unfit to plead may have been present at the time of the offence or may have developed whilst in custody. Should the subject be considered unfit to plead then it is sensible to find out what the other doctors involved in the case think. If they are of like mind then the doctors can present their views to the lawyers and the case be put before the jury. If there is disagreement between doctors then the court or solicitors may choose to obtain a further psychiatric opinion. Where the defendant is thought to be unfit to plead the psychiatric report might conclude:

Opinion:

X is suffering from the severe mental illness of schizophrenia, an illness, which in his case, was not only present at the time of the offence but is also affecting him now. In this case the illness severely disrupts the defendant's ability to think logically or converse comprehensibly. So severe is the disruption that the defendant is unable to understand what is going on in court or give instruction to his legal advisers. He is therefore under disability within the meaning of the Criminal Procedure (Insanity and Unfitness to Plead) Act 1991. He requires treatment in a psychiatric hospital.

Whether or not someone is fit to plead is a decision made by a special jury. The prosecution or the defence advise the court that they consider the accused unfit to plead, and they do this before the plea, or after the prosecutor's case is heard. A special jury is empanelled and evidence about the offender's fitness is put before them. Sometimes there is disagreement between the doctors and both opinions must be put to the jury. If the jury finds the accused unfit to plead then the court deals with the case under the Criminal Procedure (Insanity and Unfitness to Plead) Act 1991.

Recovery in hospital may be followed by a trial (see Chapter 3).

Question 2: Was the patient mentally disordered at the time of the offence to the extent that he was without responsibility within the meaning of the McNaughten Rules? (See Chapter 3.)

In this case the disorder must have been present at the time of the offence.

A middle-aged man developed a paranoid illness from which he came to believe that his life was in immediate danger from his father and relatives. In a state of considerable agitation he killed his father in the night, immediately informing the neighbours of the deed and the 'reasons' for it. On remand in prison he accepted antipsychotic medication. By the time of the trial he had lost his delusion. Nevertheless he was able to successfully plead 'not guilty by reason of insanity'.

A typical wording at the end of a report of which the man is insane would read as follows:

Opinion:

(1) The defendant is fit to plead and stand trial.
(2) At the time of the alleged offence the defendant knew what he was doing and whether or not it was wrong. However, at the time he was suffering from the severe mental illness of schizophrenia, and he was under the delusion that the victim was about to kill him. He was therefore insane at the time of the offence within the terms of the third limb of the McNaughten Rules.
(3) Although he is much improved following treatment on remand, he will continue to require psychiatric treatment in hospital until his condition is stabilized.

If the plea is successful then the judge informs the Home Secretary of the finding and a hospital place is sought, via the Department of Health, under the powers of the Criminal Procedure (Insanity and Unfitness to Plead) Act 1991. In hospital, the patient (in a case of murder) is detained as though on a hospital order (section 37) with a restriction order unlimited in time (section 41).

Question 3: Was the defendant suffering from a mental abnormality which substantially diminished his responsibility at the time of the offence? (See Chapter 3.)

This can present the most difficulty to the psychiatrist: it is easy if there was a psychosis at the time; less easy are cases with a past history of psychosis who become obviously psychotic shortly after the offence. It is possible that, in these cases, the offenders have been suffering from a pre-psychotic mental disturbance sufficient to substantially diminish their responsibility. Much more difficult are the cases of severe personality disorder, complicated by a neurotic disturbance at the time, such as a depressive reaction. Examples of mental states which have been found to be grounds for diminished responsibility include psychoses, endogenous depression, severe neurotic depression, severe psychopathy coupled with neurotic depressive episodes (psychopathy alone is usually insufficient), organic brain damage and subnormality. The finding of diminished responsibility does not rule out the possibility of the offender receiving a life sentence particularly where the main diagnosis is psychopathy.

In the cases where treatment in hospital would be appropriate, the psychiatrist may reasonably contact the other doctors seeing the case. If they are all in agreement then one of the doctors can take responsibility for obtaining a place in an appropriate hospital. That doctor should also be sure that two reports will also go to the court recommending a hospital order. If the case is such that treatment as an outpatient is appropriate the arrangements should be made beforehand so that the court can be informed of what would be available if the court wished to make use of it. Typical reports might conclude:

Opinion:

(1) The defendant is fit to plead and stand trial.
(2) At the time of the alleged offence the defendant was not insane within the McNaughten Rules. He knew what he was doing and whether or not it was wrong.
(3) At the time of the offence the defendant was suffering from the mental illness of depression. The illness developed over the preceding three months and was characterized by excessive sadness, disturbed sleep, loss of weight, suicidal feelings and increased irritability. This illness constitutes a mental disorder which substantially diminished the defendant's responsibility within the meaning of the Homicide Act 1967.
(4) The defendant is still suffering from this mental illness and requires treat-

ment in hospital. The court may feel that an order for treatment under section 37 of the Mental Health Act 1983 would be appropriate in his case. A bed will be available at Barchester Hospital within 28 days of the order being made should the court feel that this would be an appropriate disposal.

(5) In this case, in view of the need to supervise the patient in the community once well enough to return, the court may feel that a restriction order, unlimited in time, would be appropriate.

A supplementary report to the court on form F1303 recommending an offender's admission to hospital under section 37 is expected and convenient, although this is not strictly necessary legally if sufficient data is included in the original report. The psychiatrist may well be expected to attend court to give his opinion as to whether or not a restriction order would be appropriate, though the court may make the restriction order whether or not the doctor recommends it. The court may also be interested in the degree of security the hospital can offer and may wish to assure itself that the security offered is sufficient for the case. If the court feels it is not, the court may request the psychiatrist to try and obtain a bed in a more secure institution, or refuse to send the offender to hospital.

Question 4: Was the defendant so disordered at the time as to be able to plead the defence of automatism? (See Chapter 3.)

This defence is very rarely put forward. It has been successfully used in cases of homicide committed in association with epilepsy (see Chapter 9) for people in stage 4 sleep (sleepwalking, night terrors, confused waking from stage 4 sleep) and rapid eye movement (REM) sleep (waking from a dream)[39]. It has also been successfully associated with degenerative brain disorder and might be successful after a head injury. The courts have accepted, in a lesser case, the mental confusion arising from hypoglycaemia as a basis for automatism (*R* v. *Quick*, (1973) Ct. of App. R. 722).

> A man was knocked unconscious by a blow to the head. He appeared to recover and sought out and killed his assailant. However, he had no memory of this act and in retrospect appears to have had a period of disturbed consciousness which lasted from the head injury until some hours later. It was during this period of disturbed consciousness, when he appeared to outsiders to be behaving normally, that he committed the offences. His plea of automatism was unsuccessful though he was successful with the alternative plea of diminished responsibility on the grounds that the head injury had caused a mental disorder (a disturbance of consciousness) which substantially diminished his responsibility. He received a seven-year prison sentence.

Question 5: Is the woman, charged with the murder of her baby, sufficiently disturbed to be brought within the Infanticide Act? (See Chapter 3.)

The psychiatrist has to decide whether the balance of her mind was disturbed and, if so, whether it was related to birth or lactation. Clearly, this would be simple enough in the case of a puerperal illness but becomes less so afterwards. The problem is nowadays somewhat reduced because the alternative defence of diminished responsibility is available to cover cases where an illness supervenes with a less definite relationship to the birth or lactation.

> A woman who had been suffering from schizophrenia for some years became pregnant. She feared, understandably, that her medication would be present in her own breast milk and therefore refused to accept it in the last month of her pregnancy. Within days of the child being born she became grossly psychotic and she came to believe the child was in terrible danger and, as a result, she killed it. In her case the choice of a defence under the Infanticide Act or the Homicide Act was available to her. She could have claimed that the balance of her mind had been disturbed from the effect of giving birth to the child as it could be argued that it led to an exacerbation of her illness. On the other hand she could have claimed that she had diminished responsibility under the Homicide Act because of the mental abnormality (her mental illness) which substantially diminished her responsibility. Her plea of diminished responsibility was accepted and a hospital order was made.

A report putting forward an infanticide plea in this case might conclude:

> Opinion:
>
> (1) The defendant is fit to plead and stand trial.
> (2) Although mentally ill at the time of the offence the defendant was not insane within the McNaughten Rules.
> (3) At the time of the offence the balance of the defendant's mind was disturbed (as described above) within the meaning of the Infanticide Act. The disturbance results from the effect of giving birth to the child.
> (4) At the present time the defendant suffers from the mental illness of schizophrenia characterized in her case by delusional ideas. She requires treatment within a psychiatric hospital. The court may feel that a hospital order (under section 37, Mental Health Act 1983) would be appropriate with a restriction order unlimited in time. A bed will be available at Barchester Hospital within 28 days of the order being made should the court feel this to be an appropriate disposal.

Multiple homicide

There have been a number of cases recently which have focused attention on murderers who have several victims. The newspaper reports of such dramatic cases suggests that the incidence may be increasing. Multiple 'murderers' may be classified into those with:

(1) Multiple victims from one event, as in:

(a) atrocities of war;
(b) terrorist activities;
(c) organized crime activities;
(d) 'mass murderers' in which (typically) a non-psychotic white male, aged 20–30 years, creates a dramatic scenario by going berserk with a firearm killing a number of strangers and often ending by being killed or taking his own life. The act is believed to represent a boiling up at deeply felt resentments and anger at life's frustrations and personal difficulties. Sometimes the offence seems a 'copycat' of a similar dramatic offence committed elsewhere in the world;
(e) the killing of a specific group, e.g. the killing of the offender's family during a depressive or psychotic illness.
(2) A number of single victims killed separately over a period of time, as in:
(a) criminal or terrorist assassination;
(b) 'serial killers' – people who kill repeatedly motivated by psychological needs. Three main types can be recognized:
    (i) psychotically motivated killings, e.g. the repetitive killing of prostitutes in response to hallucinatory voices and delusional beliefs. The killings then are usually (in the UK) by strangulation or battering,
    (ii) sexually motivated, sadistic killings. The victims may be tortured or bizarrely mutilated. The offenders – (typically) white, male aged 25–35 years – are normally reserved, quiet and conforming in appearance. They pick strangers as victims and plan the offence (see Chapter 9). Persistent escalating, violent, sexual fantasies underlie the behaviour[40]. They may be associated with deviant sexual behaviour (e.g. fetishism, cross-dressing, voyeurism),
    (iii) the killing of consecutive babies by psychopathic mothers as an expression of an unwillingness or inability to cope (see Chapter 13),
    (iv) psychopathic offenders preoccupied and enjoying thoughts of killing or experimenting on others, e.g. by poisoning.

Aftermath of homicide and other serious offences

The psychological shock waves caused by the offence pass not only to the surviving victims (and offender) but also to the relatives of the victim, especially to any children of the victim or the offender (see Chapter 5).

Children

Black[41] has drawn attention to the disturbances which occur in the children of men who kill their wives. They may develop in reaction to the violence and double loss (death of mother, imprisonment of father) both a pathological grief reaction (repressed or extended) and a post-traumatic syndrome with intrusive thoughts, nightmares, fears, anxiety and increased arousal and sensitivity. Black recommends referring the child to a special child psychiatric team with experience in this field. The children should give, within 24 hours, a comprehensive account of the offence and their feelings. The child should be taken into social work care or wardship and great care taken with placement and future access. It is asserted that it should be generally assumed that contact with the father will be therapeutic.

The offender

The offender who has killed a friend or relative not only has to come to terms with his own behaviour, to understand it and digest it, he must also come to terms with his feelings of guilt and loss and feelings of ambivalence towards the victim. In those who were mentally ill at the time of the offence the process has to be integrated with knowledge of the illness.

After a psychotic killing, counselling will help the patient understand his illness and its effect on reducing his responsibility or even absolving him from responsibility for the act and give the patient an understanding of the need to monitor his illness in the future. A depressive illness may be exacerbated by the offence or mistaken for a grief reaction. On the other hand a grief reaction may be suppressed by enthusiastic treatment for a supposed depression[42].

The victim

Some 90% of victims who survive a serious crime will have psychological after-effects up to 2.5 years later to a greater or lesser extent[43]. Sexual assault victims are likely to be the most disturbed. Voluntary victim support agencies have sprung up to assist in such cases, both with material advice (insurance and security, etc.) but also offering psychological support. Specialist support has been developed for rape victims (see later), battered wives (see later), and sexually assaulted females. The Criminal Injuries Compensation Scheme also gives (on application) financial compensation to injured victims.

Lesser (non-sexual) offences against the person and psychiatric assessment

The principles of the assessment are the same as for those accused of murder. The psychiatrist will require a full history from the defendant, a copy of the prosecution statements, a copy of previous convictions, social reports, and an interview with relatives. Information must be obtained of any previous psychiatric care, and contact should be made with the probation officer or social worker involved.

Where will the assessment be done?

The more serious the case the more likely the offender will be remanded in custody. A number of cases will be remanded on bail and can be assessed in outpatients.

Who will do the assessment?

A report will be requested only on a fraction of those charged with assault. Factors which will lead to the request of a report include any known mental disorder, bizarre behaviour in court, bizarreness of the offence, a recommendation of the probation officer, and the request of a solicitor. If the defendant is in custody, and the court requests the report, then the prison medical officers will be the doctors principally involved. A solicitor, on the other hand, may instruct a psychiatrist to go to the prison to prepare a report independently whether or not the court has requested a report. If needed, a request for a remand to hospital (section 35, Mental Health Act 1983) can be requested (see Chapter 4). When a psychiatric disorder requiring treatment is discovered then whoever is seeing the case will have to ensure that a second medical report is available if a recommendation for a hospital order or trial of treatment is required. It will also be necessary to ensure that a hospital bed can be made available in case the court wants to take up the recommendation to place the offender in a hospital. Offenders on bail may be assessed at the request of the court or the solicitors. Identical arrangements must be made as above if an order under the Mental Health Act is to be made.

What questions does the psychiatrist consider?

The defence of diminished responsibility and infanticide are limited to the charge of murder. The 'defences' of being unfit to plead or insanity are available to any offender though both are used rarely, particularly the latter. The insanity defence under the new Criminal Procedures (Insanity and Unfitness to Plead) Act 1991 may be used more than it was now that courts have wider powers (see Chapter 3). While automatism is a possible plea, it is also very rare. Psychiatrists' reports, therefore, are used principally in mitigating the sentence. A psychiatrist will ask the following questions of the case.

(1) Is the defendant fit to plead or insane within the Insanity and Unfitness to Plead Act 1991?
(2) Is the defendant suffering from a mental abnormality?
(3) Is enough known about the case to reach a diagnosis or is it necessary to recommend admission to hospital for observation under section 35?
(4) Does the defendant suffer from a psychiatric disorder for which it would be appropriate to recommend a hospital order under section 37 of the Mental Health Act? If so, should one also recommend a restriction order under section 41?
(5) Is the disorder such that a trial of treatment would be indicated under section 38 rather than making a recommendation immediately for a hospital order under section 37? This might be most appropriate in cases of psychopathic disorder or mental impairment where it is unclear how the subject will respond to psychiatric treatment.
(6) Where should the treatment be given? (taking the dangerousness of the patient and the safety of the public into account); the options are:
    (a) ordinary psychiatric hospital,
    (b) medium secure unit
    (c) special hospital.
(7) Does the defendant suffer from a lesser degree of psychiatric disorder such that he does not fall within mental health act definitions, or does not require to be in hospital for treatment? In this case treatment might be offered as a condition of probation or on a voluntary basis. The court may prefer to place the defendant on probation. If the patient then refused to co-operate with treatment, or if his behaviour gave cause for anxiety in other ways, then the probation officer would be able to bring the defendant before the court again for the case to be reconsidered. This approach can be very useful in the care of personality-disordered people who benefit from support, and also some psychotic people who would benefit from support and continued medication whilst in the community. Guardianship orders, though a possibility, are rarely used.

> A man of an over-controlled schizoid nature developed an idea with almost delusional intensity that his affections for a girl were reciprocated. When she refused to have anything more to do with him he became increasingly distraught, took to following her about, and eventually, in frustration, attacked her. He was brought to court for this assault and dealt with by receiving outpatient treatment as a condition of probation. He benefited from medication and the support of the clinic and probation, and returned to a normal life pattern.

(8) If the defendant has no disorder requiring psychiatric intervention, are there psychological or social problems which may be assisted in other ways? The psychiatrist may feel, after discussion with the probation officer, that the defendant would benefit from a simple probation order or probation combined with placement in a probation hostel, or a placement in a specialized hostel, such as a therapeutic community run by a voluntary body.

(9) What is the prognosis of the case, what are the chances of assaultive behaviour continuing or getting worse? The psychiatrist will need to have a clear idea of the pattern of violence in the defendant's life, how easily violence occurs and the situations in which it does occur, in order to give his mind to this question. The court will want an estimate of the likelihood of the interventions proposed by the psychiatrist altering the chances of assaultive behaviour continuing.

Battered wives and spouse abuse

Over the last three decades, there has been an increased appreciation of the extent and severity of violence within the home – much of which has been and still is, hidden away. Domestic violence encompasses the violence between man and wife (or cohabitee) – and perhaps should also include violence to children within the home. The literature has been extensively reviewed by Smith[44].

Definitions

'Battered wife' is a loose term covering the situation where the wife or cohabitee is being physically attacked by her husband in order to oppress or control her. Sometimes it is used to refer to any violence; other times it is used to refer to repetitive, severe violence. Psychological abuse and severe intimidation may also be used to the same ends. All these behaviours are often coupled with excessive jealousy, restraints on movements and control of money.

Incidence

Few of the violent incidents are reported to the police. The victims are too afraid or ashamed to report the violence or they hope that matters will somehow improve spontaneously. In studying the incidence there are problems in deciding how violent the act should be to count as 'battering'. In the USA it was found that: in 25% of marriages, one partner would push, shove or grab the other, at some point; there was severe violence (punch, bite, kick, hit with an object, beat up, threaten with a weapon) at some point in 13% of marriages; and the most severe violence (beating up or using a weapon) would occur at some point in 5% of marriages. Such surveys have also revealed that wives attack the husbands only slightly less frequently but it seems that this is less violent and generally a defence response to the husband's violence.

Aetiology

This is best considered as the end-product of a number of factors. First the background includes maleness and the sociocultural background with its history of patriarchy with the wife seen as a possession subject to the husband's will. Background factors in individual cases may then include the offender being exposed to domestic violence as a child (this occurs in approximately 50% of wife-abusers) and belonging to a family or culture in which dominance of the wife and the use of violence in family discord are implicitly accepted. Additional factors will include stresses such as unemployment, poverty (the majority of wife abusing occurs in lower socioeconomic groups) work problems and frustrations and the effects of alcohol (50% of assaults occur at times of drinking). The attack may arise due to the disinhibiting effects of alcohol on the angry fulminating husband or the precipitating effects of minor or imagined slights, jealousy or 'insubordination'. Studies of the individuals who have killed or attacked their spouse reveal patterns of repetitive violence, alcohol abuse, neurotic and personality difficulties; actual mental illness seemed to be rare. How much the victim precipitates the violence, encourages it or accepts it, is unresolved.

Management

In general terms attempts to reduce the violence include:

(1) Offering refuge to the battered spouse
This provision began on a voluntary basis and is now widespread.

(2) Providing counselling and group work for the battering husbands
This may be with or without their wives. This has been offered extensively but the recruitment rate of husbands is low and the drop-out from counselling high. There is, therefore, very little evidence of overall success.

(3) Encouraging the police to arrest and hold the offender in the police cells
This is usually after a call to the home. Studies from Canada and the USA suggest that this approach may be the most effective way of inhibiting the violence. Whether a court appearance and a heavy sentence would increase the inhibition is not known. There is some evidence to suggest that a court order for mandatory attendance at the counselling group

increases effectiveness but the work awaits confirmation by other studies[44].

(4) Rehabilitating the victim and the children
This is also something of a problem. Anecdotal accounts suggest that a great deal seems to be gained by the victim from the support received by other victims, either in the refuge or from groups. Attention has to be given to the children too, to help put their experience into perspective and break the cycle transmitted from one generation to another. The emotional disturbance and feelings that follow domestic violence (nervousness, distress, guilt feelings) must also be dealt with in children.

Non-accidental injury to children

Non-accidental injury covers those injuries sustained by children through violence and is a concept that has developed from the battered baby syndrome.

Examination of the defendant

The conclusion that the child has suffered an injury will rest on medical findings; the decision to prosecute will rest with the police. In order to assess the defendant it is necessary to have available (1) descriptions of the injuries, (2) interviews with, or statements from, people who can give a description of the children and their relationship with the defendants, and (3) interviews with the defendants. Oliver[45] has described how easy it is to be deceived and overlook child abuse in those chaotic families where abuse is transmitted through the generations. Abuse is associated with bigger, more mobile, poorer families; unemployment, criminality, young motherhood and substitute fathers are other features associated with abuse.

Classification by motive

Scott[46] proposed the following classification of motives:

(1) Desire to rid the defendant of an encumbrance
(2) Desire to relieve suffering (mercy killing)
(3) Motives arising directly from frank mental illness
(4) Displacing onto the child of anger, frustration or retaliation arising from elsewhere ('He is not going to get away with it – if I cannot have the children then neither shall he')
(5) Desire to stop the immediate infuriating and frustrating behaviour of the child, e.g. persistent crying, screaming, soiling.

As in most offences, the motives can be seen to be numerous and to reflect all aspects of human emotion – anger, pity, jealousy and resentment – as well as possibly being due to mental disturbance.

Management of the situation

The prevention of the offence must be the first priority. In the special case of non-accidental injury, recommendations for the early recognition of children at-risk include an effective at-risk register, more health visitors, better nursery facilities, more links between school and primary care services, and greater public and professional awareness. The legal aspects (Children Act 1989) involve steps to protect the child and promote its welfare through the use of various orders (emergency protection, child assessment, care orders). There may also be prosecution of the offenders.

Sexual offences

Whereas all civilized and most primitive legal codes prohibit unjustifiable personal violence, including some sexual behaviour, other sexual behaviours are criminal in one country, a civil wrong in another, and simply a matter of private morals in others. In some American states extramarital intercourse is still a crime on the statute book, though seldom prosecuted. Homosexual acts between males is still an offence in most states in America, and was in Britain until, in 1967, the recommendations of the Wolfenden Committee were accepted that sexual acts in private between consenting males over the age of 21 should no longer be criminal. Prostitution in some states in America is a crime which could be prosecuted, though in England prostitution itself is not. Incest was not deemed a criminal act until 1908 though it was strongly discouraged by social pressure and was punishable under ecclesiastical law.

Definition

The sexual offences are legally classified as offences against the person and include:

(1) Buggery.
(2) Indecency between males.
(3) Indecent assault on a male.
(4) Rape.
(5) Indecent assault on a female.
(6) Unlawful sexual intercourse with a girl under 13.
(7) Unlawful sexual intercourse with a girl under 16.
(8) Incest.

(9) Procuration of women and girls.
(10) Abduction of a woman or girl.
(11) Bigamy.
(12) Soliciting by a man.
(13) Gross indecency with a child.
(14) Offences against mentally defectives.
(15) Offences against women receiving treatment for mental disorder.
(16) Indecent exposure.

Incidence of sexual offences

West[47] has described the difficulties in estimating the incidence of sexual offences from the police statistics. First, the reporting rate is less than the actual rate; secondly, whether a particular offence (e.g. an attempt at rape) is classified as rape, attempted rape, or indecent assault, may vary with police practice; third, only a proportion of reported cases end in a conviction. In bald terms the figures for reported rape show rape to be increasing (1100 cases in 1974 to 4000 in 1991), as well as indecent assault on a female (12 400 in 1974 to 15 000 in 1991).

Classification of sexual offenders and their motives

The sexual offences themselves may be considered to be of two main types:

(1) Those in which the 'victim' is a consenting partner, e.g. in homosexual acts between an adolescent and an adult homosexual, some sexual acts between adults and children who have acquiesced in (or even initiated) the activity. In this group the offender may have a genuine feeling and affection for the victim or at least no wish to harm, though some offenders will callously take advantage of their victims. Where there is affection the sexual behaviour may arise as a consequence of this.

(2) Those in which the 'victim' is a non-consenting partner. In such a case the offender is more likely to experience motives such as anger, or a desire for power as well as any sexual feelings.

There is no good classification of sex offenders. The following is an amalgam of other classifications, modified by clinical experience. The main purpose of the classification is to make the psychiatrist aware of the range of motives for a sexual offence; sexual deviancy is only one of the motives.

(1) 'Normal' men in abnormal circumstances
In this case the offending arises out of a combination of circumstances, e.g.

(a) A lonely old man in lodgings befriends the neglected child of the busy landlady, friendship blossoms, and from affectionate contact, mutually acceptable sexual behaviour springs.
(b) A young man identified with riotous group gets caught up in the group excitement and takes part in a gang rape.
(c) A father becomes sexually aroused by his daughter and gives way to temptation during his wife's illness, his daughter becoming a willing partner.

(2) People with suppressed sexual desires
Cases are seen of men who, when under stress which threatens their status or self-image, experience anger, depression or tension which they cannot manage. In such a state, the man may give way to his suppressed forbidden desires and become sexually involved, perhaps with another man or a child, either by force or seduction. In some cases the anger is dispersed by an aggressive attack; in other cases, depressive feelings are relieved by the offender 'giving' himself the pleasure of indulging in the forbidden sexual activity. There may be no previous episodes of sexual offending.

(3) The sexually deviant person
The deviations (see Chapter 12) may lead to a sex offence when the deviation involves children, young men, animals, sadistic thoughts, exhibitionism or frotteurism. The deviant person may be a persistent offender or he may be a person who contains his behaviour, giving way only at times of stress or great temptation. The offence may well be one in which the victim is a ready partner (e.g. homosexual acts) or it may be one in which there is extreme violence (e.g. associated with sadistic fantasies) with mutilation, rape, and a need to dominate the victim.

(4) Mentally ill subjects
Sexual offending of all types may be secondary to any mental illness, including organic illness, e.g. brain damage with disinhibited sexual behaviour. A man suffering from schizophrenia believed he was being persecuted. He believed that women were being used as part of the persecution against him so he attacked one and raped her in revenge. A man with frontal lobe damage had developed into a fatuous, irresponsible person who committed numerous petty offences. He got pleasure and excitement by touching women whilst they were shopping or in public places. He was charged with indecent assault.

(5) Mentally retarded subjects
Some mentally retarded subjects will make clumsy sexual approaches which will lead to a sex offence, e.g. indecent assault. Others, through frustration, in conjunction with poor life experiences (unsatisfactory

parenting, delinquent models), may give way to aggressive sexual assaults of all degrees as an expression of their anger as much as of their frustrated sexuality.

(6) Psychopathic disorder

There are egocentric men who see people as objects to be used. As a result, depending on the situation, there may be a sexual offence, including rape or incest. The intensity of the assault depends on the man's aggression or seductive powers and the ease with which he attains his ends. In such a case there is usually a long history of egocentric behaviour though sexual offences may not have occurred previously. The offence may be precipitated by some minor psychological setback such as an argument at work.

(7) Severely inhibited personalities

Cases are seen of men who may desire to form sexual relationships with others but are too inhibited. They may become aware of desires to touch, caress, seize or rape. The urge may be resisted and an awareness of it may lead the subject to seek psychiatric help rather than give way to it. The desire may be towards adults or children. The actual offence committed depends on the strength of the urge and its direction.

The above classification can only be a guide. Clearly, offenders may have characteristics of more than one group, e.g. the mentally retarded may also have developed a sexual deviation, the 'normal' man is likely to have some degree of egocentricity.

Role of pornography

Although pornography is sexually arousing, some assert that it can actually reduce offending by offering the potential offender another outlet for his fantasies. Others assert that it provides a stimulation and model for imitation. Despite this latter 'common-sense' view it is very difficult to prove that pornography 'causes' sexual deviation or offending[48]. Certainly many people with sexual deviations (some of whom will offend) enjoy pornography which reflects their fantasies and predilections. Thus pornography, at the very least, must help sustain and develop fantasies, but also further an unrealistic and egocentric view of women and children.

Particular sexual offences, mental states and their management

These have been discussed by Chiswick[49].

Buggery

This is anal intercourse in humans (or anal or vaginal intercourse with animals). The participants may be prosecuted unless they are consenting males in private, older than 21 years. This behaviour may occur in all male societies due to absence of 'normal' outlets, (e.g. normal men in abnormal circumstances).

It may be committed by sexually aroused aggressive psychopaths as a way of displacing aggressive feelings onto a hapless victim as a form of rape. It may occur among young males prostituting themselves for money, or for affection and attention (e.g. among drug addicts or very deprived children). Mental illness or mental stress may underlie sporadic homosexual behaviour in people who might otherwise resist the impulse. However, persistent homosexual inclinations must be the commonest cause. Where there is a mental disorder requiring treatment the usual channels can be used. Lesser degrees of psychiatric disorder where the offender wants assistance may be helped by treatment on probation, depending on the underlying problem.

Male victims of forcible buggery have similar adverse reactions as occur in rape (see below) with increased sense of vulnerability, impaired sexuality (with doubts as to whether it may mean they are homosexual), loss of self-respect, depression, and anxiety[50]. They should receive help similar to that offered to rape victims (see below).

Rape

This is defined as sexual (vaginal) intercourse with a woman without her consent and knowing that she did not consent, or being reckless as to whether or not she had consented. It is only necessary that the penis enters the vagina, for intercourse to be said to have taken place. Consent is invalid if obtained by fear, fraud or deliberately making the woman insensible with drugs or drink.

In the past, husbands enjoyed legal protection from a charge of rape unless the couple were legally separated. This protection was removed by the Court of Appeal in 1990.

Under recent legislation boys younger than 14 years can now be charged with rape whereas previously they could not.

In about 30% of cases the victim and offender are strangers; in 30% brief acquaintances; in the rest, long-term acquaintances or relatives.

Psychopathology of rape
Rape is a very aggressive act which includes not only sexual inter-course but often deliberate defiling of the woman, e.g. by forced oral sexual contact, masturbating over the victim, or attempting to degrade her in other ways. In such a situation the victim is being subject to

displaced aggression – possibly a rejecting mother or rejecting society. The anger may have been precipitated by recent threat to self-esteem (from work, home or elsewhere). This may be exacerbated by intoxication or overarousal during the execution of other crimes. The final triggering may be the presence of the woman in the situation which makes rape possible.

Grubin and Gunn[51] interviewed 136 rapists serving a prison sentence. They found the following: 50% had a chaotic family background (violence, delinquency, parental promiscuity, changes of care-giver); a similar number had experienced physical or sexual abuse; some 60% had been drinking or used drugs in the 24 hours before the rape; and 37% were alcohol dependant; nearly half had been convicted of an offence before they were 16 years; and nearly one-third gave a history of disordered sexual behaviour (voyeurism, frotteurism, fetishism, bondage). Although this is not a sample representative of all rapists, the disturbances in background throw some light on the psychopatholoy. The majority of rapes were unplanned and occurred impulsively, e.g. during the course of a burglary.

Classification of rape
The following classification is an amalgam of other classifications[52,53,54] modified by clinical experience.

(1) Circumstantial rape:
This occurs when normal social sanctions are removed and new group pressures are substituted, e.g. invading armies and gang rapes. It is asserted, perhaps with little evidence, that normal people will not take part in these activities and men who do have some of the features seen in other rapists. Certainly in Grubin and Gunn's study, many (not all) such offenders although younger, had a history of criminality and a disturbed background.

(2) Aggressive personalities:
Rape may be one aspect of a generalized egocentric, impulsive, aggressive, psychopathic behaviour. People are seen by such a rapist as objects to be used or defiled and put aside. It may be that in such a case the cause of the personality disorder is linked to disturbed parenting – particularly a disturbed relationship with the mother which may underlie the rapist's attitudes to women.

(3) Inhibited personalities:
Some men are isolated, and because of their timidity and anxiety, unable to relate normally to adult women. A few become aware of (but may dislike) their increasing drive to rape. As the drive becomes stronger they may follow women and the drive escalates from simple assault, to touching, to grabbing, and then to rape.

(4) Reaction to stress:
In this case an inadequate man responds with displaced aggression to considerable personal strain which is threatening his status and self-image. There will be no history of a build-up in terms of previous fantasies and escalating attacks. The rape simply corrects the balance of dominance or power.

(5) The sexually disordered paedophilic rapist:
Rapes occur in paedophiles: first, where paedophilia is associated with aggressive personalities and an inability to form warm relationships with children; second, in very inhibited frustrated men who have paedophilic fantasies and who feel guilty, inhibited, and unable to relate to children (or indeed to adults). When under some psychological stress their tension may be displaced into attacks on children.

(6) Sadistic men:
These men tend to be isolated socially. They develop egosyntonic, pleasurable, sadistic fantasies which may be understood in terms of a very disturbed background with a rejecting mother. As discussed by MacCulloch *et al*[54] the fantasies give way to assaults which escalate into sadistic attacks with mutilation and rape. These sadistic men are characterized by their hostility to women, their guilt over normal sexual behaviour, a need to possess and to dominate the victim, and pre-occupation with their mother's sexuality. These men are also the ones most likely to repeat the rape – become serial rapists.

(7) Mental illness:
Rape may occur (rarely) as a result of mental illness. It may, for example, be the result of delusional states (see above), organic states or, possibly, states of high excitement as in mania.

(8) Mental retardation:
Some rapists are mentally retarded people experiencing a high level of sexual frustration, coupled with a great sense of anger arising from particular difficulties, e.g. failure to be able to make a success of their lives, a failure to come to terms with their own mental handicap. They seem to feel a deep sense of anger with their inability to get a girlfriend, have a job and make a success. This anger becomes a driving force in the rape.

Rape and murder
Rape may be associated with murder in two main ways:

(1) The rapist may kill his victim either to silence her (if she is screaming) or to avoid detection.

(2) The murder may be part of a compulsive, sadistic act associated with mutilation of the victim.

Assessment of the offender
In order to assess the rapist it is essential that:

(1) A full history is obtained from the patient including the growth of his fantasies, previous sexual behaviour and any assaults. The offender will tend to deny or trivialize his behaviour, as do all sex offenders[55]. There will be a tendency to rationalize it and place responsibility on to the victim.
(2) An objective account of the offence is obtained. This is best obtained by insisting on seeing the written statements, which will be presented to court, from witnesses and from the victim.
(3) An objective account is obtained of the offender's past offences from the police with particular attention to the details of the offences (what actually happened in the previous 'assault').
(4) An objective account of the patient's previous behaviour and management is obtained – from relatives, if possible. Any social reports prepared on the offender by probation officers should be consulted. The probation officer may have been able to see relatives and obtain information not available easily to the psychiatrist.

Prognosis
A follow-up[56] of men charged with rape showed that 90% were not convicted of a second rape (though it is known that the offences of many sexual offenders remain undetected). However, 15% were re-convicted of a sexual assault and 17% of a violent offence within a 22-year follow-up. The factors relating to re-offending are – as with most other offences – a reflection of:

(1) The number of previous offences.
(2) The age of the offender (offending tends to fall off with age though less than it does with ordinary offenders). Some sexual offenders go on offending well past middle age, especially paedophiles and there was a gap of many years between offences in some instances.

Also of importance though less so than the first two factors are:

(3) Predisposing factors, such as despondency, difficulties at work, difficulties at home.
(4) Presence of temptation, e.g. paedophiles working with children.
(5) The presence of a related mental illness, e.g. a relapsing psychosis.
(6) The persistence of abnormal fantasies.

Management of the rapist
Clearly this must reflect the underlying cause. In the mentally ill,

admission to hospital under hospital order would be an appropriate recommendation. In some cases, the court may feel that a restriction order will also be appropriate – particularly to ensure adequate aftercare. Subnormal patients may also be referred to hospital, but this may, in the case of rape, often be a special hospital.

Those who meet the criteria of psychopathic disorder could also be recommended for a hospital order. Such orders tend to be made in those cases where the offender convinces the doctor that he is aware of psychological difficulty for which he desires psychiatric help. Nevertheless, the majority of rapists will receive a prison sentence.

The treatment approaches which have been used with rapists are essentially psychological ones. They revolve around improving the subject's self-control through self-awareness as well as improving social functioning using individual and group approaches. Antilibidinal treatment (see Chapter 12) may be used where the patient is aware of his sexual drive being a major factor in the motivation. It seems most useful when psychological treatments have been unsuccessful. It may also be useful at times of stress when the offender's fantasies may temporarily increase. Regular attention, understanding, and consideration in the care of such patients will be the basis for the rapport and understanding between the patient and doctor. The patient must feel able to report to the doctor any inclinations or impulses he has to re-offend. Similarly, the doctor must keep a very sensitive eye on the patient and not fail to check, by asking directly, the state of the fantasy life of the patient. This requires tactful but persistent questioning.

There is enormous difficulty in assessing when a patient is safe to be released to the community. The assessment will be made from:

(1) What the patient says of himself.
(2) What other people observe in his behaviour, e.g. his interest in disturbing pornography.
(3) The results of psychological testing where his arousal can be measured under laboratory conditions when exposed to appropriate erotic material (see Chapter 12).
(4) The continuance of factors which were relevant to the rape, e.g. aggressive behaviour, psychosis, presence of rape fantasies.

When a rapist has become an inpatient and there is anxiety about his dangerousness then he will tend to be detained in the hospital for a long time. Sometimes these periods far exceed the time he might have been detained had he received a simple prison sentence.

The victims of rape
In recent years it has become clear that the victims of rape suffer severe trauma – not only in the experience of the rape itself but also by the police investigation and social and family consequences. The victim, from the

time of making the complaint, must be handled calmly and sensitively with due respect for her privacy and feelings. Women police officers and women doctors who have received training in this field should be involved in the initial questioning and investigation. Afterwards, the victim may benefit from specialist counselling e.g. at a rape crisis centre to help her over the trauma of the offence. Victims may respond immediately with anxiety and depression as well as feelings of shock, disbelief, guilt or self-blame with intrusive thoughts. Some may have a reaction of such severity as to require psychiatric attention[57]. For the majority, there will be a period of resolution over months. Long-term studies, however,[58] show that up to 20% will be more susceptible to symptoms of anxiety and depression (which may be delayed for some years) and disturbed sexual and interpersonal relationships. It is not known how much these symptoms are due to associated factors, such as bad or cruel parenting. Factors which are associated with poor resolution include prior psychological or medical problems, lower socioeconomic status, repeated assaults, and alcohol or drug abuse.

Indecent assault

This offence covers behaviour which may be merely touching to behaviour of rape-like attacks falling just short of rape. The majority of such offences are likely to be minor, the offenders male, and the victims aged less than 16 years. There will be, as with rape and homosexual offences, a wide range of 'causes'.

Indecent exposure

Definition
Although classified as a sexual offence, indecent exposure was defined originally by the Vagrancy Act 1824: 'A person openly, lewdly and obscenely exposes his person with the intent to insult any female should be deemed a rogue and a vagabond'. Subsequent amendments and rulings classify that it is an offence to expose in public or private places, and 'person' means 'penis'[59].

Incidence
Only a small fraction of cases come to court and this number is falling as the behaviour is not now regarded as seriously as it was. It is the commonest sexual offence committed by adults with 3000 convictions per year. Less than 1% are dealt with under the Mental Health Act 1983[59]. Some 80% of first offenders are not re-arrested within five years.

Classification
(1) Exhibitionists (see Chapter 12): people who derive sexual pleasure or satisfaction of neurotic urges from indecently exposing.
(2) Indecent exposure as a symptom (rare) of mental disorder, e.g. psychosis, dementia, subnormality.
(3) Indecent exposure as part of homosexual soliciting.

Incest

Definition
Though regarded as an offence against God, incest did not become a crime in England until 1908. Bluglass[60] has outlined the legal and clinical aspects. It is an offence for a man to have sexual intercourse with a woman whom he knows to be his grand-daughter, daughter, sister (or half-sister) or mother. It is an offence for a woman over 16 to permit a man she knows to be her grand-father, father, brother, (or half-brother) or son to have sexual intercourse with her by consent.

Incidence
Incest and child sexual abuse have very recently become a focus of attention and it is now realized that the extent of such abuse is much greater than previously thought. In one New Zealand study, 4% of women stated they had experienced intrafamilial abuse[61]. In a later study,[62] the figure was 12.5%. In 1991 there were only 389 offences of incest in England and Wales recorded which must be a gross under-representation of all incest. In part, this may reflect the difficulty in diagnosis of incest, especially with a very young child. A diagnosis of sexual abuse based solely on 'signs' of sexual assault (bruising, laceration etc) has been questioned. Confirmatory evidence should be sought (an account from the child, evidence of a disordered family, etc). Most convictions (75%) are for father (or step-father)–daughter incest.

Types of incest

(a) FATHER–DAUGHTER INCEST

Types of father
(1) Aggressive psychopath: This father will tend to be in his forties and abuse alcohol. He is likely to have a history of criminal offences, to be violent and irritable. He probably has a poor work record with a great deal of unemployment. He will claim to have a high sex drive. His offences will involve several daughters at the same time and concurrently with a normal sexual relationship with his wife and mistress. It is likely that he will have come from a broken home himself.

(2) Inadequate psychopath: This sort of father will also have had an unsatisfactory childhood and a poor work record associated with nebulous complaints such as backache or neurotic disorders. The wife tends to become the breadwinner and the husband takes on house-wifely duties. He trades on his daughter's sympathy as the poor, hard-done-by father. He gradually seduces the daughter.
(3) 'Normal' father: Here incest arises due to close association between father and daughter in association with the illness or absence of the mother.

Predisposing factors
Factors which may lead or encourage father–daughter incest include:

(1) The daughter acting as a surrogate mother, following the loss of mother.
(2) Children having learning difficulties which put them more at-risk (more easily intimidated and misled).
(3) Social isolation of the family, especially with a family history of incest.
(4) Marital disharmony.
(5) Alcoholism.
(6) Gross overcrowding.
(7) Presence of wife who gives tacit encouragement or acceptance to the incest as opposed to those wives who are truly deceived.

Effect of the incest on the daughter
This is very variable and will reflect:

(1) The personality of the daughter.
(2) The nature of the incest – an aggressive assault would have a different effect from the sexualization of an affectionate relationship – and the quality of the general parenting in the family. The moral standards of the family and the group to which they belong have a big influence on the reactions of the daughter to the incest. In some groups the incest may be accepted without demur.

In a New Zealand study[62] just over half of the women who had experienced intrafamilial abuse reported long-term effects on their emotions or nerves. The following reactions may develop:

(1) Psychotic reaction (very rare).
(2) Neurotic reactions (depression, anxiety), bulimia and a subsequent tendency to self-injury.
(3) A personality disorder with conduct disorder (however, this may reflect gross generalized disturbance between the parents and the parents and the child, rather than the actual incest itself).
(4) Aversion to adult sexual behaviour.

(5) Amoral promiscuity or sexualized behaviour.
(6) No long-term effect.

(b) BROTHER–SISTER INCEST
This is rarely reported. Where it occurs it may be associated with reduced parental supervision, particularly absence of the father.

(c) MOTHER–SON INCEST
This is very rarely reported. It was thought to be almost always associated with severe mental illness (psychosis) on the part of the mother but there have been reports recently of incest committed by non-psychotic women as well as reports of sexual abuse of children by women[63].

Genetics of incest
Reports of incestuous conceptions suggest a very high increase of abnormalities or neonatal death due to the increased chances of recessive gene pairing.

The mental state of the offender in incest
Clearly any psychiatric disorder, in theory, could be associated with incest, but in practice the majority of male offenders will suffer, if anything, from personality difficulties – psychiatric illnesses are very rare. The principal problem lies in assisting the child, and in the family dynamics. Specialist clinics are spreading to deal with this problem.

Other sexual offences against children

Offences against children (apart from incest) include:

(1) Unlawful sexual intercourse with a girl less than 13 years. In such a case it is no defence for the girl to consent or the male to believe her over 16 years. The majority of the victims are aged 12 years.
(2) Unlawful sexual intercourse with a girl under 16 years but over 13 years. In such a case it is a defence if there has been a marriage ceremony and the man reasonably believed the girl to be his wife. It is also a defence if the man (if under 24 years of age) has no previous similar convictions, and reasonably believed the girl to be over 16 years.
(3) Indecency with children. This offence involves inviting or inciting a child to perform masturbatory activity upon an adult. It only becomes an assault if there is actual or threatened force.
     It is also an offence to take an indecent photograph or film of a child or to publish, show or possess such a film.
(4) Defilement of girls – e.g. encouraging children into prostitution.

(5) Any other offence (e.g. buggery, assault) where a child is the victim.

The principle 'causes' behind sex offences with children:

(1) Adolescent boys or mentally handicapped males making clumsy immature sexual approaches.
(2) Males with paedophilic sexual impulses (see Chapter 12).
(3) Aggressive amoral psychopaths indiscriminately using the children as sex objects.
(4) Susceptible men undermined by stress, mental illness or organic brain disorder, giving way to impulses normally alien to them.
(5) Stepfathers assaulting their stepchildren as a reflection of their personality, attitudes or disturbed family dynamics.
(6) Women sometimes with paedophilic impulses (not commonly reported) – sometimes reflecting their own very disturbed past of abuse, and sometimes under the influence of a man.
(7) The causes of incest (see above).

Incidence
Official police statistics grossly under-represent the actual levels. Surveys are difficult to do and face the problem of defining abuse. More recent surveys show more abuse. The Mori Poll (1984) found in the UK that 12% of women and 8% of men had had an unwanted sexual approach in childhood (only 0.7% sexual intercourse) but for most it only happened once. Some 1% felt damaged. On the other hand, a later study of 1500 New Zealand women[61] found 60% had had some form of unwanted sexual (genital) approach in childhood including 10% who had experienced a clear sexual assault, and 5–8% rape.

Effects of sexual abuse on children
It is unclear whether the disturbances are due to the abuse *per se*; due to associated factors such as chaotic family; separations from family; or due to parental and social reactions to knowledge of the abuse (anxiety in parents, persecution at school). It is unclear what proportion of victims suffer which symptoms and what proportion are unharmed. The severity of the psychological distress will reflect in part the dissonance between the behaviour, and the moral and social standards surrounding the child. It is said that the following disturbances may occur:

(1) Whilst the abuse persists secretly: The children may react with emotional disturbance. There may be depression with nightmares and suicidal ideas. There may be a neurotic reaction with anxiety, phobias, tensions and stomach aches. There may be behavioural disturbance (running away, outbursts of anger, fireraising, soiling, bed-wetting). On the other hand, they may behave promiscuously with other children or with adults without obvious distress.

(2) After the abuse has been discovered by others: The child may react with anxiety or guilt and there may be features of a post-traumatic stress disorder with dreams, anxieties, intrusive thoughts and avoidance behaviour.

(3) Long-term effects: These include[64]:

    (a) Long term emotional disturbance: Depression has been described in adults abused as children and may occur with anxiety in some 20%. An affective change may underlie the development of a self-damaging lifestyle with self-mutilation, eating disorders and somatization disorder. Clinically, symptoms of post-traumatic stress disorder are common, as are feelings of guilt.

    (b) Long-term disturbed sexual function: There seems to be two main disturbances – a withdrawal from sexual contact or the development of increased sexual activity going on to promiscuity.

    (c) Disturbed interpersonal behaviour: There may be loss of trust in others, a fear of close relationships, and hostility to adults, including parents. On the other hand, there may be a series of unsatisfactory relationships including very early marriage – perhaps in a vain search for a relationship which will lead to a resolution of early pain. There may be, because of this, an increased vulnerability to relationships which lead to further abuse. There may be an attraction to men resembling the original offender perhaps in the same attempt to resolve the problem.

    (d) Disturbed social behaviour: There may be a drift into antisocial behaviour and, more specifically, into prostitution. There is some suspicion that some victims of abuse (both male and female) are more likely to be perpetrators of abuse in their turn.

Prevention of offending against children

Protection of children

Arrangements have to be made to try and protect children from those who have been convicted of offences. Current practice is based on the Home Office and the Department of Health and Social Security circular (LAC(78)22): 'Release of prisoners convicted of offences against children in the home', the Department booklet (1981) *Review Leave Arrangements for Special Hospital Patients* and the development of good practice in Departments of Social Work. When releasing such a prisoner, the prison welfare officer (with the prisoner's knowledge) alerts the directors of Social Services both in the area to which the offender is going and the area in which the children were victimized. The prison medical officer may alert the prisoner's general practitioner about the offender's mental state and treatment needs. The relevant chiefs of probation are also informed, in case the offender wishes to make use of probation help. The directors in both areas should then check that no children are at risk. Care proceedings may be invoked where risk exists.

Similar precautionary steps are taken by the hospital social work and medical departments when an offender is released from a special hospital. It is regarded as good practice to do the same from a regional secure unit or ordinary psychiatric hospital. Offenders should be discouraged from living in situations which put themselves or children at risk. It is good practice to obtain the patient's permission for these disclosures but they may be made without permission. Employers advertising for paid or voluntary staff to work in close proximity to children are guided by the Department of Health and Social Security circular (LAC (86) 10): 'Protection of children. Disclosure of criminal background of those with access to children'. Applicants can be required to declare all their past offences and sign an agreement for police and Department of Health records to be searched. Applicants for such posts receive no benefit from the Rehabilitation of Offenders Act (1974) which allows certain convictions to be treated as spent.

Education of children
Children should be taught through the school and through the home the points to look out for. They should be taught to refuse invitations from strangers, to learn to say 'no' and to develop an open relationship with their parents so that they can speak of these matters. The parents, in turn, should provide suitable supervision of the children.

Prognosis of sexual offending

It is known that far more sex offences are committed than are known about. Careful questioning of 561 deviants suggested that the rate of offending might be 20–150 times the arrest rate[65]. Further, the majority claimed several deviations and might move from one to another through life.

Soothill and Gibbens[66] found that amongst serious sex offenders (offences against children under 13 years) followed up over 22 years (and with allowances made for the number free and at risk) the arrest risk for any criminal offence was around 50%. Half of those were a sex or violence offence, most of which were serious. The chances of reconviction for any offence reflected the number of previous convictions. Some 10% of first offenders re-offended, 22% of those with three or more offences and 47% of those with two previous convictions – a surprising and unexplained finding. The most important finding was that sexual offending might recur at any time during the 22 year follow-up – reflecting a persisting predisposition and the effect of chance circumstances. Ordinary recidivists with a long record who are convicted of a 'one off' opportunistic, minor, out-of-character sexual offence are not usually convicted of a further sexual offence.

References

(1) Cordess, C. (1990) Criminal poisoning and the psychopathology of the poisoner. *Journal of Forensic Psychiatry* **1**, 213–26.

(2) Holden, A. (1974) *The St. Albans Poisoner: The Life and Crimes of Graham Young.* Hodder and Stoughton, London.

(3) Walmsley, R. (1986) *Personal Violence. Home Office Research Study 89.* HMSO, London.

(4) Home Office (1991) Notifiable Offences, England and Wales, 1991. *Home Office Statistical Bulletin 2/92.*

(5) Hough, M. & Mayhew, P. (1983) *The British Crime Survey. Home Office Research Study 76.* HMSO, London.

(6) Brizer, D.A. & Crowner, M. (1989) Predicting careers of criminal violence: descriptive data and predispositional factors. In Brizer, A. and Crown, M. (eds) *Current Approaches to the Prediction of Violence.* American Psychiatric Press, Washington.

(7) d'Orban, P.J. & O'Connor, A. (1989) Women who kill parents. *British Journal of Psychiatry* **154**, 27–33.

(8) Bornstein, P.H., Hamilton, S.B. & McFall, M.E. (1981) Modification of adult aggression: a critical review of theory, research, and practise. *Progress in Behaviour Modification* **12**, 299–50.

(9) Glynn Owens, R. & Bogshaw, M. (1985) First steps in the functional analysis of aggression. In Karas, E. (ed.) *Current Issues in Clinical Psychology,* Vol. 2. Plenum Press, New York and London.

(10) Lorenz, K. (1966) *On Aggression.* Harcourt, New York.

(11) Dollard, J., Doob, L.W., Miller, N.E., Mowrer, O.H. & Sears, R.R. (1939) *Frustration and Aggression.* Yale University Press, New Haven, Connecticut.

(12) Bandura, A. (1977) *Social Learning Theory.* Prentice Hall, Englewood Cliffs, NJ.

(13) Hodge, J.E. (1992) Addiction to violence: a new model of psychopathy. *Criminal Behaviour and Mental Health* **2**, 212–23.

(14) Widon, C.S. (1989) The cycle of violence. *Science* **244**, 160–6.

(15) Toch, H (1969). *Violent Men.* Aldine, Chicago, Illinois.

(16) Megargee, E.I (1966) Undercontrolled and overcontrolled personality types in extreme antisocial aggression. *Psychological Monographs,* **80**, Whole no. 611.

(17) Blackburn, R. (1986) Patterns of personality deviation among violent offenders: replications and extension of an empirical taxonomy. *British Journal of Criminology* **26**, 254–69.

(18) Wolfgang, M.E. & Ferracuti, F. (1967) *The Subculture of Violence.* Barnes and Noble, New York.

(19) Bluglass, R. (1979) The psychiatric assessment of homicide. *British Journal of Hospital Medicine* **22**, 366–77.

(20) Gayford, J.J. (1979) Battered wives. *British Journal of Hospital Medicine* November, 496–503.

(21) Shepherd, J., Irish, M. & Scully, C. (1988) Alcohol Intoxication and severity of injury in victims of assault. *British Medical Journal* **296**, 1299.

(22) Virkkunen, M. (1992) Brain serotonin and violent behaviour. *Journal of Forensic Psychiatry* **3**, 171–4.

(23) Berger, P.A. & Gulevitch, C.D. (1981). Violence and mental illness. In Hamburg, D.A. and Trudeau, M.B. (eds) *Biobehavioural Aspects of Aggression*. Alan R. Liss Inc, New York.

(24) Taylor, P. (1982) Schizophrenia and violence. In Gunn, J. and Farrington, D.P. (eds) *Abnormal Offenders, Delinquency and the Criminal Justice System*. John Wiley, Chichester.

(25) Rappeport, J.R. & Lassen, G. (1965) Dangerousness–arrest rate comparisons of discharged patients and the general population. *American Journal of Psychiatry* **121**, 776–83.

(26) Zitrin, A., Hardesty, A.S. & Burdock, E.L. (1976) Socially disruptive behaviour of ex-mental patients. *American Journal of Psychiatry* **133**, 142–6.

(27) Sosowsky, L. (1980) Explaining the increased arrest rates among mental patients: a cautionary note. *American Journal of Psychiatry* **137**, 1115–6.

(28) Guze, S.B. (1976) *Criminality and Psychiatric Disorders*. Oxford University Press, New York.

(29) Cloninger, C. & Guze, S.B. (1970) Female criminals: their personal, familial and social backgrounds. *Archives of General Psychiatry* **23**, 554–8.

(30) Taylor, P.J. & Gunn, J. (1984) Violence and psychosis I – risk of violence amongst psychotic men. *British Medical Journal* **288**, 1945–9.

(31) Taylor, P.J. & Gunn, J. (1984) Violence and psychosis II – effect of psychiatric diagnosis on conviction and sentencing of offenders. *British Medical Journal* **289**, 9–12.

(32) Humphreys, M.S., Johnstone, E.C., MacMillan, J.F. & Taylor, P.J. (1992) Dangerous behaviour preceding first admissions for schizophrenia. *British Journal of Psychiatry* **161**, 501–5.

(33) Hafner, H. & Boker, W. (1973) Mentally disordered violent offenders. *Social Psychiatry* **8**, 220–9.

(34) Teplin, L.A. (1985) The criminality of the mentally ill: a dangerous misconception. *American Journal of Psychiatry* **142:5**, 593–9.

(35) Lindquist, P. & Allebeck, P. (1990) Schizophrenia and crime. *British Journal of Psychiatry* **157**, 345–50.

(36) Coid, B., Lewis, S.W. & Reveley, A.M. (1993) A twin study of psychosis and criminality. *British Journal of Psychiatry* **162**, 87–92.

(37) Taylor, P.J. (1985) Motives for offending among violent and psychotic men. *British Journal of Psychiatry* **147**, 491–8.

(38) Coid, J. (1983) The epidemiology of abnormal homicide and murder followed by suicide. *Psychological Medicine* **13**, 855–60.

(39) Fenwick, P. (1990) Automatism, medicine and the law. *Psychological Medicine, Monograph Supplement* **17**.

(40) Prenky, R.A., Burgess, A.W. *et al.* (1989) The presumptive role of fantasy in serial sexual homicide. *American Journal of Psychiatry* **146**, 887–91.

(41) Black, D. & Caplan, T. (1988) Father kills Mother. *British Journal of Psychiatry* **153**, 624–30.

(42) Fraser, K.A. (1988) Bereavement in those who have killed. *Medicine, Science and the Law* **28**, 127–30.

(43) Shapland, J., Willmore, J., Duff, P. (1985) Victims in the criminal justice system. *Cambridge Studies in Criminology LIII*, Gower, Aldershot.

(44) Smith, L.J.F. (1989) Domestic violence: an overview of the literature. *Home Office Research Study 107*. HMSO, London.

(45) Oliver, J.E. (1988) Successive generations of child maltreatment. *British Journal of Psychiatry* **153**, 543–53.

(46) Scott, P.D. (1977) Non-accidental injury in children: memorandum of evidence to the Parliamentary Select Committee on violence in the family. *British Journal of Psychiatry* **131**, 366–80.

(47) West, D.J., Roy, C. & Nichols, F.L. (1978) Understanding sexual attacks. Heinemann, London.

(48) Fisher, W.a. & Borak, A. (1991) Pornography, erotica and behaviour: more questions than answers. *International Journal of Law and Psychiatry* **14**, 65–83.

(49) Chiswick, D. (1983) Sex crimes. *British Journal of Psychiatry* **143**, 236–42.

(50) Mezey, G. & King, M. (1989) The effect of sexual assault on men: a survey of 22 victims. *Psychological Medicine* **19**, 205–9.

(51) Grubin, D. & Gunn, J. (1990) *The Imprisoned Rapist and Rape*. Department of Forensic Psychiatry, Institute of Psychiatry, London.

(52) Grubin, D. (1992) The classification of rapists. *Prison Service Journal* **85**, 45–55.

(53) MacDonald, J.M. (1971) *Rape: Offenders and their Victims*. Charles Thomas, Springfield, Illinois.

(54) MacCulloch, M.J., Snowden, P.R., Wood, P.J.W. & Mills, H.E. (1983) Sadistic fantasy, sadistic behaviour and offending. *British Journal of Psychiatry* **143**, 20–29.

(55) Kennedy, H.G. & Grubin, D.H. (1992) Patterns of denial in sex offenders. *Psychological Medicine* **22**, 191–6.

(56) Soothill, K.L., Jack, A. & Gibbens, T.C.N. (1976) Rape: a 22-year cohort study. *Medicine, Science and the Law* **16**, 62–69.

(57) Mezey, G.C. & Taylor, P.S. (1988) Psychological reaction of women who have been raped. *British Journal of Psychiatry* **152**, 330–9.

(58) Mullen, P.E. (1990) The long term influence of sexual assault on the mental health of victims. *Journal of Forensic Psychiatry* **1**, 13–31.

(59) Gayford, J.J. (1981) Indecent exposure: a review of the literature. *Medicine, Science and the Law* **21**, 233–42.

(60) Bluglass, R. (1979) Incest. *British Journal of Hospital Medicine* August, 152–7.

(61) Mullen, P.E., Romans-Clarkson, S.E., Walton, V.A. & Herbison, G.P. (1988) The impact of sexual and physical abuse on women's, mental health. *Lancet* i, 841–5.

(62) Bushnell J.A., Wells, J.E. & Oakley-Browne, M.A. (1992) Long-term effects of intrafamilial sexual abuse in childhood. *Acta Psychiatrica Scandinavica* **85**, 136–42.

(63) Wilkins, R. (1990) Women who sexually abuse children. *British Medical Journal* **300**, 1153–4.

(64) Sheldrick, C. (1991) Adult sequelae of child sexual abuse. *British Journal of Child Psychiatry* **158**. (suppl. 10) 55–62.

(65) Abel, G.G., Booker, J.V., Mittkeman, M., Cunningham-Rarhner, J. & Romleau, J.L. (1987) Self-reported sex crimes of non-incarcerated paedophiliacs. *Journal of Interpersonal Violence* **2**, 3–25.

(66) Soothill, K.L. & Gibbens, T.C.N. (1978) Recidivism of sexual offenders: a re-appraisal. *British Journal of Criminology* **18**, 267–76.

Chapter 8

Mental Illness and Forensic Psychiatry: The Functional Psychoses and Neuroses

Introduction

The legal term 'mental illness' as used in the Mental Health Act 1983 is undefined. It is used to cover the psychoses (organic and functional), neurotic disorders and various organic disorders. This chapter will deal with the functional psychoses and neuroses. The following chapter will deal with the organic brain syndromes.

For the first part of this century it was generally asserted that the mentally ill were less likely than normal to commit crimes, but in recent years evidence has appeared (see Chapter 7) suggesting that this is no longer so and that, in fact, the opposite may be the case. Whether or not someone with mental illness commits a criminal act depends not only on that person's characteristics (nature of the illness, previous personality, age, sex, and social pressures) but also whether the ill person is free in the community rather than detained in a hospital, and whether or not he is receiving effective treatment and supervision.

When a mentally ill person commits a criminal act he may be 'excused' by those around him – especially if he is already in psychiatric hands, and the case then not reported to the police. If the police become involved, they in turn may choose not to prosecute but simply ensure that the person receives appropriate health care. The decision whether or not to prosecute will depend in part on the readiness of the psychiatric services to take over the case. Where there is no help to be obtained from the services then the police may feel obliged to prosecute where otherwise they might wish not to. The more serious the case, the more likely that prosecution will proceed. Clearly, all these variables have to be borne in mind when interpreting statistics.

Functional psychoses and crime

Classification

The traditional division of psychotic and neurotic has not been used in ICD 10. Disorders are grouped into themes, e.g. mood disorders. The revised third edition of the *Diagnostics and Statistical Manual of Mental Disorders* does retain the division. ICD 10 recognizes:

(1) Schizophrenia (sub-divided into various forms), schizotypal and delusional disorders (F 20–F 29) that include those delusional states that are not organic nor yet clearly schizophrenia.
(2) Mood (affective) disorders (F 30–F 39).

The DSM IIIR classifies them under traditional headings:

(1) Schizophrenia – subdivided into various forms (295).
(2) Mood disorders (296).
(3) Delusional (paranoid) disorders (297).
(4) Psychotic disorders, not elsewhere classified which includes various reactive psychoses, schizophreniform and schizoaffective psychosis (298).

Schizophrenia

Definition

Both the ICD 10 and the DSM IIIR refer to delusions (bizarre, grandiose, persecutory), disordered thinking (e.g. interrupted and illogical flow of thought; incomprehensible speech), disturbed perceptions (e.g. hallucinations, feelings of passivity, ideas of reference), disturbed mood, disturbance of movements (e.g. catatonia, excitement, stupor), and deterioration in personality and functioning. The ICD 10 requires that the major symptoms be present for one month.

Schizophrenia and crime

There is little evidence about the overall incidence of crime among schizophrenics. How great the incidence may seem to be would depend not only on detection rates and arrest rates but on the treatment facilities, e.g. the extent to which the ill are institutionalized. Studies have concentrated on violent behaviour as this is easier to identify. The evidence reviewed in Chapter 7 suggests that serious crime is clearly more common than in the normal population especially violence.

The relationship of offending to the illness

There is no evidence to show that schizophrenics have any special pattern of offending. Teplin[1] found overall that the pattern of offending behaviour in seriously mentally disturbed offenders was the same as for the general population. Unfortunately, the study does not give the diagnoses of the disturbed offenders. The extent to which schizophrenics are reacting directly to their hallucinations or delusions, or to the stresses which occur as a result of their illness, has been discussed in Chapter 7. Virkkunen[2,3], studying a group of Finnish schizophrenics guilty of serious violence and a group guilty of arson, found that only one-third offended directly as a result of their hallucinations or delusions. The remaining two-thirds offended because of problems arising from the stresses produced within the family and was thought to account for the fact that near relatives or associates were frequently the victims of schizophrenic violence. It is interesting to note that schizophrenia was the commonest (74%) diagnosis amongst 58 Broadmoor patients who had killed their mothers. Green[4] argues that this incidence of schizophrenia is typical for this rare offence of matricide. He was, of course, examining a very biased sample.

Taylor[5] reviewing schizophrenia and violence came to the following tentative conclusions that:

(1) Schizophrenia disposes the patients to violence though the overall numbers are small.
(2) Paranoid schizophrenia and catatonic excitement are the subgroups most likely to be associated with violence.
(3) The violence leading to arrest is more common as a late accompaniment of the illness (after months or years) even though the patient may have been in treatment in the past. On the other hand, Humphreys *et al*[6] found that 20% of new schizophrenics exhibited life-threatening behaviour to others, though this frequently did not lead to arrest (see Chapter 7). It may be that hospitals and relatives are simply more tolerant of violence when the illness starts.
(4) The violence is more common in those patients who have recurrent exacerbations rather than those who are continuously ill.
(5) At the time of the offence the offender had generally lost all insight. The offence is often preceded by attempts to confirm or check delusional ideas or by steps taken by the patient to protect himself from the 'aggressor'. In a small number the violence may be the direct result of command hallucinations[7].
(6) Bizarre violence to another correlates more with psychopathy or personality than schizophrenia. Bizarre violence to self (e.g. enucleation of the eye), however, is strongly associated with schizophrenia.
(7) Violence may not always be directly related to current psychopathology, other factors such as the personality structure (and the damage caused to it by the illness) and the social setting may be equally important – partly echoing Virkkunen's observations.

Medicolegal aspects of schizophrenia

Schizophrenia is clearly a condition where a psychiatric disposal is required. It is not necessary that there be a direct link between the psychotic experiences and the offence; it is quite sufficient for the subject to be ill. Generally, in practice, if the crime is not linked to positive psychotic features it will be linked to the deterioration in the patient's personality caused by the illness. Although it is, of course, possible to come across subjects whose offence is part of a life-long pattern of criminality and who have, incidentally, developed schizophrenia, it is proper to offer psychiatric treatment if the subject currently requires it. This does not always happen, especially where hospital facilities are unsatisfactory. If, on the other hand, the subject offends as part of his criminal career whilst in full remission, then he is held responsible for his actions. The schizophrenia may be so severe as to render a subject unfit to plead. The illness is regarded as a basis for diminished responsibility in cases of homicide and may even bring the subject within the McNaughten Rules.

Paranoid (delusional) disorders

Definition

The paranoid or delusional disorders are characterized by persistent persecutory delusions (including delusional jealousy) with an absence of other evidence of schizophrenia, such as thought disorder, hallucinations, or inappropriate emotional responses. There must be an absence of organic causes. The paranoid states are subdivided into acute and chronic states, *folie à deux* and atypical paranoid states.

Paranoid states and the incidence of crime

The incidence of crime in this group of disorders is unknown. Criminal acts may follow from the delusional beliefs. A well-recognized association is that of homicide associated with delusional jealousy.

Delusional jealousy: Othello syndrome

In this illness, delusions of infidelity of the spouse are the central dominating symptom. This disorder is one of a group of disorders characterized by irrational and/or disproportionate jealousy. The group, reviewed by Mullen and Maack, and Tarrier *et al.*[8,9] is known sometimes as morbid or pathological jealousy.

Clinical picture of delusional jealousy
Delusions of infidelity develop after a few years of marriage. The development of the delusions is associated with irritability, despondency, aggression and severe preoccupation. It occurs in males more often than females. With the development of the delusion the subject searches obsessively for confirmatory evidence, e.g. searching the spouse's belongings, clothes, or bedsheets. The subject makes persistent attempts to extract a 'confession' by questioning, wheedling, or intimidation. Tension builds up resulting in violence or even homicide. The innocent accused spouse may attempt to assuage the subject by 'confessing' but the interrogation then becomes even more persistent.

Differential diagnosis
Similar delusional states may arise in

(1) Schizophrenia.
(2) Depression.
(3) Alcoholism or drug abuse (e.g. amphetamine and cocaine in their various forms).
(4) Organic states, including other addictions and cerebral disorders.

The delusional state of jealousy has to be distinguished from:

(1) Unreasonable and excessive jealousy from neurotic causes (as seen in some personality-disordered subjects) in which the subject has a very strong anxiety that the spouse is being unfaithful. It is sometimes difficult to distinguish this from a delusional state for there may be similar preoccupations and persistent interrogation.
(2) Excessive jealousy by a subject as a reaction to provocative behaviour by his spouse.

Medicolegal aspects
Where the cause of the jealousy rests in the delusional state, the underlying mental illness can form the basis of a recommendation for psychiatric treatment or the basis for a defence of diminished responsibility in cases of homicide. Where the jealousy is not delusional but has a neurotic cause then the medicolegal aspects are much less clear. There may be an associated personality disorder which falls into the 'psychopathic disorder' group. There may be other disturbances which may be classifiable as mental illness. Excessive jealousy to a provocative spouse would not, without underlying illness, be grounds for a medical defence.

In a delusional jealousy very careful consideration has to be given to the security aspect of psychiatric care. The persistence of the disorder and its potential dangerousness is well known. The patient must be carefully assessed for co-operativeness, and the risk of absconding and committing a violent offence. When the subject is known to be uncooperative, to have made violent attacks on the spouse, and to have absconded, he should be treated initially in some degree of security. Treatment may be difficult. Medication (antipsychotic or antidepressant) and cognitive therapy[9] may offer the best chance of improvement.

Mood disorders (affective psychoses)

Definition

The serious mood disorders are characterized by a severe disturbance of mood (depression and anxiety or elation and excitement) possibly accompanied by any of the following: delusions, perplexity, disturbed attitude to self, disorders of perception and behaviour – all in keeping with the subject's prevailing mood. Predominantly depressed, or manic, or mixed (circular) forms are recognized.

Incidence of mood disorders and crime

The mood disorders appear less frequently than expected among violent offenders as a whole[10]. Amongst the 4% of offenders remanded for psychiatric reports[11], 25% of the males and 46% of the females had a depressive state.

Relation of offending to mood disorders

Depressive and manic states can lead directly to offending. Although any offence may be committed because of an affective disorder, several well-known associations are recognized:

(1) *Depression and homicide:* Severe depression can lead the subject to the view that everything is hopeless, that there is no further purpose in living and that death is the only solution. In some cases the homicide will be followed by suicide. The rate of suicide after homicide has varied in different studies[12]. West[13] found that a high proportion of the suicides were associated with a mental abnormality of which depression was a prominent condition.

(2) *Depression and infanticide:* In such a case the killing of the child may arise directly from delusions or hallucinations. On the other hand, the violent act may arise from the irritability associated with the disturbed affective state.

(3) *Depression and theft:* In severe depression there are several possible associations with theft:
  (a) theft may represent a regressive, comforting act,
  (b) theft may be an attempt to draw attention to the plight of the subject,

    (c) the theft may not be a true theft but an absent-minded act in the distracted state of depression.

(4) *Depression and sexual offences:* Sexual offending in some men seems to be associated with depression as though the offending has a comforting effect on the man. Alternatively, the depression may have a disinhibiting effect undermining the subject's normal self-control.

(5) *Depression and arson:* In this association the arson may be an attempt to destroy something due to feelings of hopelessness and despair, or the arson may, through its destructive effects, reduce the subject's feeling of tension and dysphoria.

(6) *Depression, alcoholism and offending:* Prolonged alcohol abuse may induce feelings of depression or depression may lead to alcohol abuse. The disinhibiting combination of alcohol and depression may then lead to offending.

(7) *Depression and the explosive personality:* Personality-disordered people often seem less able to cope with depressive feelings. The tension engendered by the discomfort of the depression may be followed by outbursts of violence or destructive behaviour.

(8) *Depression and the adolescent offender:* In this association the depression may be masked. Acting out histrionic behaviour may be seen, as may conduct disorder such as persistent stealing. There is usually a history of normal behaviour and personality in the past.

(9) *Depression relieved by the offence:* A number of writers have drawn attention to the phenomena of depression and tension appearing to be relieved by a violent act. A history of depression is obtained up to the act but afterwards the subject appears free of it. Clinically, this is seen mostly in personality disordered subjects.

(10) *Manic states and offending:* In mania, the patient may be subject to elation with hallucinations or grandiose delusions which may lead to offending. This can take any form, from a violent attack on someone who dares to frustrate the subject, to the taking of objects in a disinhibited, grandiose way.

Medicolegal aspects of major mood disorder

The major mood disorders are grounds for a psychiatric defence and should lead to a psychiatric recommendation. In severe cases – particularly in mania – the disorder may be so serious as to make the subject unfit to plead. In homicide cases, a plea of diminished responsibility would normally be appropriate and where delusions or hallucinatory experiences have been present the subject may fall within the McNaughten Rules. Which hospital takes the patient depends on whether the patient is violent, uncooperative and determined to repeat the behaviour.

Other non-organic psychoses

Definition

This category includes a small group of psychoses (mood or delusional disorders), generally of an acute and transient nature and often appearing clinically to be largely, or wholly, attributable to a recent life experience (a reactive psychosis).

Medicolegal aspects

The relation of the illness to the offending is the same as with other psychotic illness. Despite the reactive nature of these illnesses they are such as to form the basis of a psychiatric defence.

The neuroses and crime

Definition

The ICD 10 brings together neurotic, stress-related and somatoform disorders in one large group (F 40–49) though depression of a neurotic type is classified with the mood disorders (F 32). The ICD 10 recognizes:

(1) Phobic anxiety disorders (F 40) including agoraphobia, social phobias, specific phobias.
(2) Other anxiety disorders (e.g. panic, mixed states) (F 41) including panic disorders, generalized anxiety, mixed anxiety and depression.
(3) Obsessive–compulsive disorder (F 42).
(4) Reactions to severe stress and adjustment disorders (F 43) including acute stress reaction, post-traumatic stress disorder, adjustment disorder.
(5) Dissociative (conversion) disorders (F 44) including dissociative amnesia, dissociative fugue, dissociative stupor, trance and possession states, dissociative disorders of movement and sensation. This group also includes 'Ganser syndrome' (see below) and 'multiple personality disorder'. The ICD 10 reports that controversy exists about the extent to which multiple personality is iatrogenic or culture-specific. The diagnosis is rarely made in England[14] though it is used in the USA even as a psychiatric defence. In England it is likely to be perceived as a dissociative reaction, possibly iatrogenic, to deal with dysphoria arising in a person with substantial personality difficulties[15].
(6) Somatoform disorders (F 45) including somatization syndrome, hypochondriacal syndrome, and other somatoform syndromes.

(7) Other neurotic disorders (F 48) including neurasthenia, depersonalization-derealization syndrome and various specific neurotic disorders such as Koro and Dhats syndromes.

The DSM IIIR refers to anxiety states which are subdivided into panic disorders (300.01) and generalized anxiety (300.02). Other 'neurotic' conditions include acute reactions to stress (308) and adjustment disorder (309) which includes post-traumatic stress disorder (309.80).

Incidence of crime in neuroses

The incidence is unknown. In a study of shoplifters[16] some 10% were found to be neurotic but there was no control study. Gunn *et al*.[17] gave a primary diagnosis of neurosis to 5% of a prison population but it is difficult to know how this would compare with the general population.

The relation of neuroses to crime

Clinically, the most common neurotic conditions seen amongst offenders are anxiety states and neurotic depressions. Phobic and compulsive states seem the least common.

Neuroses and homicide
A reactive neurotic state (depression and/or anxiety) may be so severe that the concomitant tension leads to a homicidal outburst even where the previous personality was good:

> A young man of excellent personality was cast into a state of depression and tension as a result of his wife's persistent histrionic, provocative behaviour which included dramatic threats of suicide, hypochondriasis and extraordinary demanding and unreasonable behaviour. He sought medical help but nevertheless suddenly snapped and killed her. He made a successful plea of diminished responsibility on the grounds of his illness and was placed on probation.

The neurotic condition may have considerable impact when combined with personality disorders, e.g. a neurotic depressive reaction in a person of explosive or antisocial personality. It may disinhibit the subject in a tense situation so that a homicidal outburst occurs, either to destroy the source of the frustration or to displace the tension onto an innocent person:

> A young man treated for neurotic and personality difficulties as a child and adolescent formed several unstable heterosexual relationships. A recurrence of tension and depression followed several difficulties. His tension was heightened by a rejection from his current girlfriend whom he then raped and killed. His plea of diminished responsibility was unsuccessful.

Neuroses and theft
Stealing may certainly be associated with neurotic depressive states (as has been shown in shoplifting) – perhaps to draw attention to the subject's plight or as a comforting activity. Such motivation is also seen in stealing by unhappy and disturbed children. The tension associated with the neurotic state may lead to stealing as a psychologically destructive act. Anger is displaced onto the shop or society or indirectly onto the relatives by the embarrassment caused by the act. The subject may reveal a history of depression though in some the associated behaviour disorder may be so gross as to divert attention from the underlying mental state:

> A subnormal girl became depressed when aged 14 years following a death at home which coincided with an unsuccessful change of school. She began not only to steal but to show severe antisocial behaviour in general as well as self-mutilation. The depression was overlooked and she was treated as a naughty, defiant child and received escalating punishments culminating in prison. Eventually, her condition was diagnosed and she responded rapidly to anti-depressant therapy.

Neuroses and sexual offences
In some men intermittent indecent exposure, intermittent paedophilia and intermittent sexual assaults may be associated with neurotic states of tension, depression or anxiety. Such men may have a propensity for such behaviour but normally they are able to control or suppress it. The neurotic state appears to have a disinhibiting influence. The sexual offence may be a way of reducing tension by displacing aggression or it may be a regressive comforting act or even a way of seeking punishment.

Neuroses and arson
An association between neurotic states and arson is well recognized – particularly with states of tension. The fire may be a way of getting rid of tension, relieving depressive feelings or symbolically destroying the source of pain, e.g. the depressed man who set fire to his marital bed.

Neuroses and alcohol-related offences
Alcohol may induce a melancholic state. Alternatively, neurotic conditions (e.g. depression or anxiety) may precipitate, in the susceptible, a bout of alcohol abuse. This combination may lead to offending, the alcohol serving to disinhibit the subject.

Neuroses and imprisonment
Being imprisoned, either on remand or after conviction, may produce neurotic symptoms in the offender, e.g. anxiety or depression. It is therefore very important to separate the symptoms which occur after arrest, with any disorder which preceded it and was relevant to the

offence. There is one particular syndrome, *Ganser Syndrome*, which has been described as a reaction to imprisonment – classified in ICD 10 as a form of dissociative disorder (F 44.8).

Ganser in 1897[18] described three prisoners who had become mentally disturbed with:

(1) An inability to answer correctly the simplest questions even though their reply indicated some understanding of the question (Q. 'How many legs has a horse?' A. 'Three'; Q. 'An elephant?' A. 'Five').
(2) Clouding of consciousness, (i.e. disorientated in place and time, distracted, perplexed, slow to respond and vacant as if lost in dreams).
(3) Hysterical conversion syndromes, (e.g. widespread loss of pain over the entire body or areas hypersensitive to pain).
(4) Hallucinations, (visual and/or auditory).
(5) A temporary abrupt end to the disturbance with a loss of all symptoms and a return of total clarity to be followed by a deep depression and a recurrence of symptoms.

Ganser was certain that the condition was not malingering but a genuine illness which he believed was hysterical in nature. He notes that his three cases had been preceded by an illness (typhus and two cases of head injury). The exact nature of the condition has been debated ever since. It is a rare condition in its full blown syndrome and occurs in people other than prisoners though individual features may occur with any mental disorder[19]. It has been said to be a true transient psychosis or even malingering but probably the most commonly accepted English view is that it is a hysterical reaction resulting from a state of depression[20]. It is to be distinguished from malingering, pseudodementia, schizophrenia, and drug-induced states.

Medicolegal aspects of neurotic illness

Where there is a clear-cut neurotic illness underlying the offending which is uncomplicated by any antisocial personality disorder, the courts will generally wish to accept a recommendation for psychiatric treatment. Such consideration may even extend to the most serious of crimes, as in the young depressed man charged with the murder of his wife. Where the neurotic condition complicates a psychopathic disorder then the court's anxiety for the safety of the public or the court's lack of sympathy may lead, in serious cases, to a prison sentence. In cases where the public is not at-risk (e.g. the depressed shoplifter) and where hospital is not required, then outpatient treatment as a condition of probation is commonly used.

Assessing offenders for mental disturbance

The screening process

As it would be impossible for psychiatrists to check the mental state of every offender, a filtering process is used which is both formal and informal. This filtering process begins from the time of the offence. The arresting police may recognize a mental abnormality or the offender (or relative) may give a history of it. Similarly, the solicitor or probation officer may discover the abnormality. The behaviour of the offender in court may arouse suspicion or his offence may strike the court as bizarre and requiring psychiatric explanation. Certain offences in particular seem to prompt a referral for a psychiatric report, e.g. arson and sexual offences. If the offender is remanded in custody, prison officers may observe bizarre behaviour within the prison which leads them to ask for a medical opinion. Each prisoner, on admission to prison, is examined briefly at reception by a doctor and it may be there that mental disturbance is detected. The prison doctor may discover mental abnormality if he is asked to provide a court report. This network appears to catch the majority of seriously mentally disturbed offenders. Once a patient has been so recognized, the next state is to involve a psychiatrist from the catchment area hospital or, in appropriate cases, a psychiatrist from a regional secure unit, or special hospital. Discussion would then occur between the psychiatrists as to the best way of managing the case.

Common problems in the screening process

How efficient is the system and what are the snags involved? Some attempt has been made to measure the court's efficiency in these matters. Gibbons et al.[11] studied the practices in Wessex and London and found overall that less than 4–5% of offenders were remanded for reports, half of which received a psychiatric recommendation. London referred more cases for reports than Wessex, but doctors in Wessex recommended more patients to have psychiatric treatment than did those in London. What is not known is how many offenders had a mental disorder not noticed by the courts. Donovan and O'Brien[21], forensic psychiatrists, sat in court listening to a series of cases, noting the ones they would have referred for a report, and comparing their findings with those actually referred. Although they would have referred more cases than the court did, it is still not clear whether they would have identified more cases requiring treatment.

Over-referral of cases
In the past (perhaps less now) most remanded offenders referred for a

report in custody did not have a treatable psychiatric disorder[22,23]. Common reasons for this include:

(1) The assumption that persistent antisocial behaviour must indicate a treatable psychiatric disorder, e.g. a man who persistently committed property offences and abused drugs was referred on the basis that 'he must need help'. In fact no disorder other than persistent intractable antisocial attitudes was detectable. Although he suffered from a psychopathic disorder (antisocial personality) he was unlikely to benefit from hospital treatment.
(2) The belief that the severity or nature of the offence (e.g. some bizarre, sadistic offences, such as multiple murders) must indicate mental illness.
(3) Deliberate malingering by the offender. This may occur especially among neurotic, histrionic or personality disordered offenders though it is a rare phenomenon.

> A delinquent youth suffered brain injury from a road traffic accident after which he developed epilepsy. When later arrested, yet again for shoplifting, he claimed to have been confused by a fit. Independent evidence was inconsistent with this. It seemed likely, on this occasion, that he was trying to deceive.

(4) Mistaking irrational behaviour due to intoxication or drugs to be a symptom of mental illness.

Missed cases
Cases of mental illness may be missed for the following reasons:

(1) The mentally ill person is misdiagnosed as 'psychopathic' due to persistent bad behaviour which actually arises from the illness. This seems to be a common presentation to regional secure units of young people who have had schizophrenia diagnosed some years before, the illness fails to be brought totally under control or breaks down when the person returns to the community. The deterioration in social state and personality caused by the illness is associated with deteriorating behaviour, uncooperativeness in hospital and unpleasant behaviour in the home. More obvious positive symptoms may recede with time and the clinical picture is clouded by misbehaviour. Study of the medical notes reveals how a change in diagnosis occurs over the years from schizophrenia to personality disorder. However, a very careful history and present state examination clarifies this situation.
(2) The patient may deliberately hide his symptoms: This occasionally happens, particularly with patients who have had previous experience of hospital care. They have learned which symptoms interest psychiatrists and are anxious to avoid (through lack of insight) further hospitalization. They will therefore deceive the doctor.

> A man developed a paranoid psychosis in which he believed he was being persecuted by a former housemaster of an approved school. He returned to the approved school and made an attempt to kill the man by hurling a brick at him through a window. He hid the true motivation from those who saw him and passed it off as an attempt of burglary. The true motivation only became apparent during his subsequent prison sentence when his illness increased in severity and the man was no longer able to contain his symptoms.

(3) Sometimes the positive features of a mental illness only gradually emerge after the offence: The offence may appear at the time to be a little strange but becomes fully understandable when the offender's illness becomes apparent, the offence having occurred in the prodromal stage of the illness when there was a disturbance of psychological functioning but before clear delusions and hallucinations developed.

> A man killed his brother for no clear reason. There had been some tension between them and he was found guilty of murder. Shortly after sentence a full blown delusional symptom of persecution evolved which involved his brother and his family. This seemed a better explanation of the crime.

(4) Doctor's error: Clearly some cases must be missed by inexperienced practitioners failing to detect difficult cases, or experienced practitioners making a mistake. Both occur and to a degree are inevitable, though training and experience should keep this error down to a minimum.

Deciding disposal

The bulk of offenders are dealt with by their catchment area hospital. However, it has to be borne in mind that the number who are sentenced to a hospital order (less than 1000 per annum in England and Wales) is relatively tiny.

Similarly, of those with minor mental illness, such as the depressed man caught shoplifting, the bulk will be dealt with by the catchment area hospital at an outpatient level, either on a voluntary basis or as a condition of probation. Patients taken into treatment will predominantly suffer from mental illness, only a minority will suffer from mental subnormality and psychopathic disorder. The level of security that the patient requires will be decided by the psychiatrists after discussion with each other and will reflect local practice. The factors which are always considered in deciding security levels include:

(1) Dangerousness: An estimation of dangerousness is a very controversial subject (see Chapter 14). However, where increased dangerousness is a factor – especially dangerousness to the public – then increased security will be required. In general, where a patient is

likely to abscond and be an immediate grave danger to others, then he most certainly should be considered for a special hospital. If once admitted to an ordinary hospital ward he would no longer represent a danger to others then the catchment area hospital may be expected to look after him.

(2) Co-operativeness: Clearly a co-operative patient can be easily managed in a local hospital. If the lack of co-operation is only in connection with medication this may be overcome through the powers given to the doctor by the Mental Health Act 1983. If the uncooperativeness takes the form of repetitive absconding, antisocial behaviour within the ward, etc. then some degree of security may become necessary. Repetitive absconding or dangerous behaviour within the ward may be the basis for referral to a regional secure unit or special hospital.

(3) Local reputation: The patient's reputation may be so bad because of previous bad behaviour that the nurses lose the will or ability to manage the case and referral to another unit or regional secure unit may be appropriate.

(4) Local facilities: A number of hospitals have developed 'intensive care' wards with high staffing and a variable degree of security. Other hospitals have very well-developed acute admission wards which claim to manage those patients who would have been sent to an intensive care ward. On the other hand, some hospitals lack both intensive care wards and well-staffed acute admission wards. The latter hospitals tend to refer more to the regional secure unit than the others. The number of secure beds available to the hospital has been shown to relate to the willingness of the hospital to take on forensic cases[24].

(5) Attitude of the consultant and nursing staff: Staff attitudes towards forensic patients do differ. This is reflected in their willingness to take on such cases, whether from the courts[22,23] or from special hospital[24,25].

Treatment and management

Inpatient care

Patients who come before the courts vary considerably in their ease of management. Management is said to be easy when a patient has insight into the fact that he is ill, and accepts treatment which works rapidly without side-effects. A difficult case would be a psychotic patient with heightened negative emotions who refuses to co-operate, tries to abscond and fights staff and other patients.

Violent behaviour in a psychotic patient will arise due to the effects of delusions and hallucinations or anger and frustration. The latter reflects the patient's heightened irritability caused by the illness. Violence can be kept to a minimum by a sensitive, tactful, non-confronting approach. Reasoning may be helpful when explaining limits and house rules but it is useless and aggravating to argue about delusions or psychotic experiences. Medication should be given as soon as possible to bring the psychosis under control. When possible this should be done by trying to persuade the patient to accept it, perhaps in terms of reducing his tension or protecting him from the persecutory experiences. Later, as insight is gained, so a proper explanation of the illness can be given.

A clear inverse correlation has been found between the likelihood of violence and serum levels of medication[26]. In practice some patients will require much higher doses than is normally recommended. Because of the dangers (particularly cardiac arrhythmias and neurological side-effects), this must be discussed with relatives (and the patient, if possible). In very disturbed cases, doses equivalent to chlorpromazine 100–200 mg orally every hour may be required. Droperidol is a very useful drug in this situation and probably safer than chlorpromazine. There are some reports (supported by clinical experience) that severe agitation in delusional psychosis or mania may be more easily settled by combining the anti-psychotic medication with a short course of lorazepam[27] (combined with ECT in mania). An awareness of side-effects and sensitivity to the patient's account of unwanted effects are particularly important when dealing in these high doses.

If there is an outburst of violence requiring physical control, it may be necessary to isolate the patient in a secure room until he has calmed down. These episodes must be carefully documented and there must be agreed procedures for the use of seclusion, as well as for observation and exercise (see also Chapter 16 on the ethics of physical control). Nursing staff will be helped to look after persistently difficult patients by devising individually tailored nursing management programmes under the guidance of a psychologist or similarly trained person. Similar programmes using behaviour therapy principles may improve behaviour (aggression, hygiene etc.) in even the most ill patient, including those whose condition is unresponsive to medication.

At the point of maximum improvement full insight may still not be gained. For the most severe cases, there may be no improvement and long-stay care will be inevitable. Nevertheless, in the majority of cases a degree of improvement may be expected such that the patient can progress to the community – though this may take months to achieve. Where the patient has behaved dangerously because of his illness and is likely to do so again, then gauging the time for discharge can be difficult. It is perfectly possible to safely release patients who have not gained full insight, but whose illness has come under sufficient control that they no longer currently feel threatened, and their emotional state has changed from irritability and hostility to one of co-operativeness, warmth and friendliness. A degree of legal control may be useful[28] for successful after-care to ensure that treatment and supervision continues. This is obtained by the use of restriction orders, treatment as a condition of probation, or trial leave.

After-care

Good after-care cannot depend on the co-operation of the patient alone. Positive action from members of the treatment team is essential. In the case of restriction order patients detailed instructions for good practice are issued by the Home Office in an endeavour to avoid the tragedy of a further breakdown in the community and all that that may entail. The people involved in after-care include the responsible medical officer, the social worker, often a community nurse, a general practitioner, the family or landlady, the employer and the inpatient staff of the unit or hospital who looked after the patient.

It is essential that those who will be regularly in contact with the patient are instructed on the background of the case before the patient moves into the community. They should have come to know the patient and be made aware of the principal signs and symptoms which may herald a breakdown. A clear and easy system of communication must be available from the community to the responsible medical officer and/or unit. The responsible medical officer, community nurse and nursing staff must provide 24-hour cover with whom the community-based workers (social worker, probation officer, general practitioner) and family and patient can liaise. It must also be possible for the unit to re-admit the patient rapidly, if necessary.

Those in charge of the case must have arrangements to cover the worst situation (e.g. the responsible medical officer on holiday, the social worker has just left, the new social worker has not taken over, the sister in charge of the unit is ill...). This is the setting for disaster and all workers must therefore be sure that their deputies or successors are conversant with the cases and have the power to take action. Intervention must be swift and positive recognizing the increased chance (up to five times) of re-offending or suicide in this group[29]. *One of the commonest complaints of relatives is that they are unable to make the professionals react quickly enough to a rapidly deteriorating condition.*

Case histories

Four case histories of mental illness are given in order to illustrate the way cases are managed. Cases presenting difficulty have been chosen as these best illustrate all the points.

Case 1 – Schizophrenia and dangerous behaviour

The patient, a young man from an intact and supportive family, developed paranoid schizophrenia when aged 17 years. His delusions and hallucinations caused him to believe that workmates were insulting and laughing at him. Initially, he hid his delusions but his illness came to light two to three years later and a series of psychiatric hospital admissions followed. Each admission produced a reduction or disappearance of his symptoms but once an outpatient he would stop his medication sooner or later and his condition would relapse. During one such relapse he drove his car at a group of youths thinking they were insulting him. The patient was charged with attempted murder. The police quickly realized that he was seriously mentally ill (confirmed by the police surgeon).

Choice one: At this point the police, technically, had several possible courses of action. These included:

(1) Continuing to detain the man and bringing him before the magistrates' court the next day, and then allowing the court to decide on how to proceed. This is by far the commonest pattern in the case of serious offences like this.
(2) Taking him to a psychiatric hospital under section 136 of the Mental Health Act 1983 for detention and observation. This disposal is used commonly when the offence is very minor or where there has been a simple disturbance. Whether this section is used depends very much on local practice and custom – being more frequent in metropolitan areas.
(3) Having the patient assessed in the police station by two doctors and a social worker in order to have him admitted to hospital under an observation or treatment order. This is rarely used in a case as serious as this but might be in cases of lesser dangerousness. The prosecution could then proceed by summonsing the patient to court at a later date.
(4) Let the patient return home on police bail – clearly not appropriate here.

In this case the first option was adopted and the patient was brought to court the following day. The court was informed of the charge and the defence solicitors had the opportunity to tell the court about the defendant.

Choice Two: The magistrates' court at this point (or at any subsequent appearance in court) has several choices. These will be facilitated if there is a court-based diversion scheme in operation. The court can:

(1) Allow remand on bail to hospital or local regional secure unit if a hospital was willing to take the patient.
(2) Make an order under section 35 of the Mental Health Act 1983 for assessment in a hospital, if a medical officer makes this recommendation to the court and a bed is available in the hospital.

(3) Remand the patient in custody, in which case the prison medical service would pick up the case.

In this particular case, the patient was remanded in custody for three weeks but on his next court appearance, having been assessed by the local psychiatrist, he was remanded on bail to his hospital as he was willing to go voluntarily. However, in hospital, despite treatment, the patient remained paranoid and incorporated the staff in his delusions of persecution resulting in two fierce attacks on staff. The hospital felt it unsafe to continue looking after him.

Choice three: The hospital had the following choices:

(1) To declare at the next court appearance their unwillingness to continue the bail arrangement and thus have the patient remanded in custody.
(2) To make arrangements for the patient to be treated in a different unit, e.g. a regional secure unit and recommend this to the court as a change of bail conditions.

In fact, the first course was adopted due to the lack of beds in the regional secure unit. In custody, the patient was placed in the prison hospital. Here, medication was offered and accepted leading to an improvement in his mental state. Had the patient remained very disturbed and uncooperative with treatment, the prison medical service could have pursued several courses – to:

(1) Begin treatment against the patient's will (under the powers given by common law) if the patient represented an immediate danger to himself or others.
(2) Recommend to the crown court (a possibility not available to a magistrates' court) a transfer to hospital for treatment under section 36, if arrangements could be made in a suitable hospital, e.g. the regional secure unit.
(3) Have two doctors recommend to the Home Office that the patient be transferred to a named hospital under section 48 if arrangements could be made.

In the event, the patient continued to improve in the prison hospital. Because of the improvement the question of fitness to plead was not a problem. In due course the court requested a psychiatric report from the prison medical service. By this time the regional secure unit had a bed available for the patient. At this point a number of recommendations could have been made to the court by the doctors in order to continue treatment if the patient was found guilty. The choices were:

(1) A simple treatment order under section 37 in hospital.
(2) A treatment order with a restriction order (sections 37 and 41)

(proposed in order to make treatment a condition of discharge and thus prevent further relapse in the community).

(3) Treatment as a condition of probation with the patient returning to the community. The court would need to be assured that such arrangements would be safe for the general public.

(4) Treatment on a voluntary outpatient or inpatient basis if the patient was willing to co-operate. The court could then give a sentence such as a conditional discharge. However, in a case as serious as this the court would probably expect a period in a psychiatric hospital on section 37 to ensure that the patient had properly recovered.

In this case, a hospital order with a restriction order (unlimited in time) was made. The patient went from court to the prison hospital as a place of safety and was then transferred to the regional secure unit within 28 days.

In the regional secure unit the patient's improvement continued. He quickly lost what remained of his feelings of persecution. His mood, which, at the time of the offence, had been tense, hostile, irritable and explosive, became relaxed, warm and friendly. He was then allowed unaccompanied parole within the hospital grounds (movement within the hospital or its grounds does not require Home Office permission). Permission for escorted day leave outside the hospital grounds was obtained from the Home Office, once the Home Office had been convinced of the improvements. Finally, permission for conditional discharge was obtained and the patient returned to his family. The negotiations for these moves can be very prolonged due to the cautious approach adopted by the Home Office (see Chapter 15).

In this case the patient's consent to treatment was never a problem. At three months he was able and willing to give consent otherwise a second opinion from The Mental Health Act Commission would have had to be obtained. At six months the patient made his first application for a Mental Health Review Tribunal.

In preparation for the patient's conditional discharge, his parents, as the prospective carers, were informed of the need for continued medication and the signs of early breakdown. In his case the regional secure unit continued his after-care because it was felt to be a safer way of managing his case. The social worker from the unit became the supervising social worker which had the advantage that he was already cognisant with the case. A unit doctor saw the patient on a regular basis and a community nurse from the unit visited the patient's home weekly or fortnightly. The parents could contact the community nurse, social worker or unit at any time. The patient continued in this way for some months but he relapsed after his medication was reduced at his request. The early signs of breakdown (suspiciousness, withdrawal, irritability) were first noted by the parents who reported it to the community nurse. She saw him immediately and he was voluntarily admitted that day, the patient having insight at this early stage, although the insight was lost as the illness developed. An informal re-admission of the patient is perfectly possible even though on a conditional discharge.

Had the patient refused to be admitted then two choices would have been open to the responsible medical officer. He could:

(1) Re-admit the patient using section 2 or 3 of the Mental Health Act.
(2) Ask the Home Office to formally recall the patient.

The former method is the least restrictive of the two and leaves the management of the patient in the responsible medical officer's hands. The latter method takes the management of the patient out of the responsible medical officer's hands and returns it to the Home Office. The responsible medical officer would then have had to make application again for all the stages of rehabilitation as he did following the original admission.

Back in the unit the patient's condition came under control though high doses of medication were necessary (above British National Formulary levels). It seems to be the experience of regional secure units that there are a number of patients who require these high doses to control their psychosis.

Case 2 – Schizophrenia – Not Guilty by Reason of Insanity

A man of 56 stabbed his father to death in the middle of the night then called the neighbours to witness the fact. It was immediately apparent that the defendant had the delusion that his father and relatives were trying to kill him. After arrest he followed the same course as Case 1 ending up remanded in custody and being looked after by the prison medical service. The local psychiatrist felt that the facilities at his disposal were not secure enough to look after the patient. He feared that the patient might abscond and attack his relatives or incorporate the staff or other patients in his delusions and attack them.

Remand to hospital for assessment (section 35) or treatment (section 36) was possible before conviction but not afterwards in the case of those charged with murder. It would, if necessary, have been possible to have applied for a transfer direction under section 48. In this case a period of assessment was not needed. The patient had a paranoid psychosis which had begun some ten years before. The illness had suddenly flared up three weeks before the offence. Early in the remand the patient agreed to accept medication whilst in the prison hospital. His delusional state remitted promptly but he then developed a depression in reaction to his offence and his predicament, again treated by the prison doctor. Most of the remand period up to his trial (some six months) was occupied by his treatment in prison and the preparation of psychiatric reports. In view of the worries of caring for him in his local hospital he was accepted in the regional secure unit.

In making the psychiatric assessment for the court the following possibilities had to be considered:

(1) Was the patient fit to plead and stand trial?
(2) Did he fit the McNaughten Rules?
(3) Did he have diminished responsibility?
(4) Did he still require psychiatric treatment and, if so, where?

In this case he was clearly fit to plead and the only problem was whether or not he met the McNaughten Rules (Chapter 3). The psychiatrist believed that he met the condition of the third rule (relating the offence to the delusion) and this plea was successful. Had it not been, a plea of diminished responsibility could have been offered which certainly would have been accepted. The Secretary of State at the Home Office was informed of the findings of the court. The patient was transferred to the regional secure unit to be looked after as though on a hospital order with a restriction, unlimited in time. His management in hospital from then on followed that of Case 1. Because of the special verdict he was allowed to apply for a Mental Health Review Tribunal within the first six months. Eventually permission was obtained for transfer to the rehabilitation unit of a local psychiatric hospital preceding conditional discharge to a group home.

Case 3 – Schizophrenia – Unfit to Plead

A man of 23 years had a history of antisocial behaviour and drug abuse from his late teens. He developed a paranoid psychosis (schizophrenia precipitated by drug abuse) at the age of 20 years. He had several hospital admissions precipitated by bizarre or aggressive behaviour. His admissions to the local hospital were marked by his uncooperative behaviour whilst psychotic, his tendency to abscond and the regularity with which he abandoned treatment once he had become an outpatient. This was followed by his condition relapsing and a recurrence of the cycle.

The offence of wounding occurred during a period in the community whilst off medication. A policeman approached the defendant to ask an innocent question. The defendant responded with a vicious knife attack. His arrest and appearance in magistrates' court followed the procedure for Case 1 and he was remanded in custody. In the prison he was immediately found to be grossly thought disordered, paranoid, hostile and irritable. His thought disorder was such that he could not instruct his solicitor. It was felt that the patient would be too difficult to look after in the open condition of the local hospital. Meanwhile the patient refused all medical help from the prison doctors.

The prison doctors had to consider the following possibilities:

(1) Submit reports that the patient was not fit to plead.
(2) Apply for the transfer of the patient for treatment under sections 48 and 49, Mental Health Act 1983.
(3) Apply to the crown court (to which the patient was eventually committed) for a remand to hospital for treatment under section 36, Mental Health Act 1983.

Course (2) or (3) would have been the most appropriate but due to a lack of beds in the regional secure unit at the time and the belief that the case was not serious enough for a special hospital, the first course was adopted. The patient was in due course found not fit to plead and was transferred (after a further wait) to the regional secure unit. Here his psychotic condition rapidly responded to treatment (which could be given without his consent in the first three months) so that within two months he was fit to go to trial. The choices available to the responsible medical officer were:

(1) To inform the Home Office of the improvement but recommend that the patient stay in hospital until the court case.
(2) Recommend to the Home Office the patient's transfer back to prison (to continue medication there, the patient now consenting to treatment).

The first recommendation was offered and accepted by the Home Office.

When the court was able to give a date for the trial, the Home Office issued a warrant for the hospital to return the patient to prison to await trial. In the meantime, an agreement had been reached directly between the psychiatrists at the regional secure unit and the catchment area hospital to recommend to the court, in the case of the man being found guilty, that he should continue treatment in the local psychiatric hospital on a hospital order (section 37) and because of his lack of co-operation in the past, when in the community, coupled with his previous dangerous behaviour, a restriction order was also recommended. Under the Criminal Procedure (Insanity and Unfitness to Plead) Act 1991, an 'insanity' plea might have been successful. The court would certainly have made the same order.

Case 4 – Depression – Treatment on a voluntary basis

A man of 36 years of previous excellent personality had had a very good career in the services despite a serious injury shortly after he joined. He was, however, retired on medical grounds due to a disabling physical illness. Just before this he had been involved in extremely dangerous action under fire when many people were killed. In this action he had a position of key responsibility for the lives of others. Following his medical discharge to civilian life he developed a depressive illness and post-traumatic stress disorder with anxiety, sadness, tearfulness and recurrent dreams about his experiences under fire. His depression continued undiagnosed for some three years but came to notice after his arrest for shoplifting. The police granted bail to his home. The magistrates' court continued bail as he had somewhere to live and his offence was not one which required him to be remanded in custody. The solicitor referred the defendant to a local psychiatrist for an assessment because the offence was so out of character. At the psychiatric interview it became clear that the defendant was seriously depressed. Treatment by medication and psychotherapy was immediately started as an outpatient.

The psychiatrist had to consider the following:

(1) Fitness to plead: Clearly this was not a factor in this case.
(2) Presence of mental illness: Clearly he had a depression but not of psychotic proportions.
(3) The relationship of the illness to the offence: The patient asserted that he had been distracted due to the depression and had no intent to steal (therefore no crime had been committed). The psychiatrist felt the man's mental state at the time of the offence was compatible with such a view.

Certainly the illness was a major factor in the behaviour of the defendant and therefore the court could be expected to find it a major mitigating factor, even if they rejected the plea of lack of intent. The psychiatrist offered treatment on a voluntary outpatient basis. The treatment (if the man had been found guilty) could have been given as a condition of probation. After-care would then have been a combination of psychiatric treatment in conjunction with probation support. Had the man dropped out of treatment the psychiatrist would have had the responsibility of informing the probation officer who would have had the choice of taking the man back to court for breach of probation.

In fact, in this case, when the prosecution received the psychiatric report they chose not to proceed and the prosecution was dropped. The prosecution was following the Code for Crown Prosecutors which gives guidance on the discretion which can be applied to appropriate cases associated with mental disorder. Broadly this guidance advises against prosecution where there is clear evidence of mental illness which might worsen under the strain of prosecution and outweigh the interests of justice.

Conclusion

Although the above cases cannot cover all the eventualities they serve to illustrate how the law offers numerous opportunities to bring mentally ill offenders into treatment. Where there is failure to do so, this is generally due to lack of facilities, not due to lack of legal opportunities.

References

(1) Teplin, L.A. (1985) The criminality of the mentally ill: a dangerous misconception. *American Journal of Psychiatry* **142:5**, 593–9.
(2) Virkkunen, M. (1974) Observation on violence in schizophrenia. *Acta Psychiatrica Scandinavica* **50**, 145–51.

(3) Virkkunen, M. (1974) On arson committed by schizophrenics. *Acta Psychiatrica Scandinavica* **50**, 152–60.

(4) Green, C.M. (1981) Matricide by sons. *Medicine, Science and the Law* **21**, 207–14.

(5) Taylor, P.J. (1982) Schizophrenia and violence. In Gunn, J. and Farrington, D.P. (eds) *Abnormal Offenders, Delinquency and the Criminal Justice System*. John Wiley and Sons, Chichester.

(6) Humphreys, M.S., Johnston, E.C., MacMillan, J.F. & Taylor, P.J. (1992) Dangerous behaviour preceding first admissions for schizophrenia. *British Journal of Psychiatry* **161**, 501–5.

(7) Rogers, R., Gillis, J.R., Turner, R.E. and Frise-Smith, T. (1990) The clinical presentation of command hallucinations in a forensic population. *American Journal of Psychiatry* **147**, 1304–7.

(8) Mullen, P.E. & Maack, L.H. (1985) Jealousy, pathological jealousy and aggression. In Farringdon, D.P. and Gunn, J. (eds) *Aggression and Dangerousness*. John Wiley and Sons, Chichester.

(9) Tarrier, N., Beckett, R., Harwood, S. & Bishay, N. (1990) Morbid jealousy: a review and cognitive-behavioural formulation. *British Journal of Psychiatry* **157**, 319–26.

(10) Hafner, H. & Boker, W. (1973) Mentally disordered violent offenders. *Social Psychiatry* **8**, 220–9.

(11) Gibbens, T.C.N., Soothill, K.L. & Pope, P.J. (1977) Medical remands in the criminal court. *Maudsley Monograph No. 25*. Oxford University Press, Oxford.

(12) Coid, J. (1983) The epidemiology of abnormal homicide and murder followed by suicide. *Psychological Medicine* **13**, 855–60.

(13) West, D.J. (1965) *Murder followed by suicide*. Heinemann, London.

(14) Mersky, H. (1992) The manufacture of personalities. *British Journal of Psychiatry* **160**, 327–40.

(15) Fahy, T.A., Abas, M. & Brown, J.C. (1989) Multiple personality. *British Journal of Psychiatry* **154**, 99–101.

(16) Gibbens, T.C.N. & Prince, J. (1962). The Institute for the Study and Treatment of Delinquency, London.

(17) Gunn, J., Maden, A. & Swinton, M. (1991) Treatment needs of prisoners with psychiatric disorder. *British Medical Journal* **303**, 338–41.

(18) Ganser, S.J.M. (1897) A peculiar hysterical state. Reproduced in translation in *British Journal of Criminology* (1963), **5** 120–6.

(19) Whitlock, F.A. (1967) The Ganser syndrome. *British Journal of Psychiatry* **113**, 19–29.

(20) Trethowan, W.H. (1979) Some rarer psychiatric disorders. In Gaind, R.N. and Hudson, B.L. (eds). *Current Themes in Psychiatry*. MacMillan Press Ltd, London and Basingstoke.

(21) Donovan, W.M. & O'Brien, K.P. (1981) Psychiatric court reports – too many or too few? *Medicine, Science and the Law* **12**, 153–8.

(22) Bowden, P. (1978) Men remanded into custody for medical reports: the selection for treatment. *British Journal of Psychiatry* **133**, 320–31.

(23) Bowden, P. (1978) Men remanded into custody for medical reports: the outcome of the treatment recommendation. *British Journal of Psychiatry* **133**, 332–8.

(24) Bowden, P. (1975) Liberty and psychiatry. *British Medical Journal* **2**, 94–6.

(25) Dell, S. (1982) Transfer of special hospital patients into National Health

Service hospitals. In Gunn, J. & Farrington, D.P. (eds), *Abnormal Offenders, Delinquency and the Criminal Justice System.* John W Riley and Sons Ltd, Chichester.

(26) Yesavage, J.A. (1982) Inpatient violence and the schizophrenic patient: an inverse correlation between danger-related events and neuroleptic levels. *Biological Psychiatry* **17**, 1331–7.

(27) Editorial (1991) Management of behavioural emergencies. *Drug and Therapeutic Bulletin* **29**, 62–4.

(28) Acres, D.I. (1975) The after care of special hospital patients. In *Report of the Committee on Mentally Abnormal Offenders.* Cmnd. 624. HMSO, London.

(29) Robertson, G. (1987) Mentally abnormal offenders manner of death. *British Medical Journal* **295**, 632–4.

Chapter 9

Mental Illness and Forensic Psychiatry: Organic Brain Syndromes

Introduction

Brain damage or dysfunction may be caused by a multitude of factors, including difficulties during birth, infections, trauma, tumour, cerebrovascular disorders, neurological disease, endocrine and metabolic disorders, vitamin deficiencies and toxic disorders. These various conditions, depending on their extent and site of action, may cause a number of organic brain syndromes including:

(1) Dementia (DSM IIIR and ICD 10 F 00–03).
(2) Delirium (confusional state) (DSM IIIR and ICD 10 F 05).
(3) Epilepsy and its associated psychiatric conditions.
(4) Organic personality syndrome (DSM IIIR and ICD 10 F 07).
(5) Organic psychoses –
    (a) Organic delusional syndrome (DSM IIIR, ICD 10 F 06.2)
    (b) Organic hallucinosis (DSM IIIR, ICD 10 F 06.0)
    (c) Organic mood disorder (DSM IIIR, ICD 10 F 06.3)
(6) Substance-induced organic disorders.
(7) Amnesic syndrome (DSM III and ICD 10 F 04)

This chapter will deal with some aspects of organic disorder in order to illustrate the working of forensic psychiatry in this field.

Dementia and forensic psychiatry

The ICD 10 gives the essential features of dementia as decline in memory and thinking. There is impaired thinking and reasoning, and impaired flow of ideas and reasoning – but with evidence of clear consciousness. The DSM IIIR includes the following features:

(1) Memory impairment for long- and short-term memory.
(2) One of the following:
    (a) impaired abstract thinking,
    (b) impaired judgement,

(c) other disturbances of higher cortical function, e.g. aphasia,
(d) personality change.
(3) That (1) and (2) combine to interfere with work or social activities.

To differentiate it from delirium or intoxication the state of consciousness should not be clouded. There must be evidence of a specific organic factor which is aetiologically related to the disturbance, or an organic factor can be presumed. The effect of the dementia may be to increase the subject's irritability, aggressiveness and suspiciousness (which may lead to violence), or it may lead to disinhibition (leading to offences such as unwanted sexual behaviour) or forgetfulness (leading to behaviour such as absent-minded shoplifting).

Dementia and the law

Dementia, of which there are a number of varieties (primary, pre-senile, post-alcoholic, etc.) clearly falls under the definition of mental illness as defined in the Mental Health Act 1983. Dementia, therefore, can be used as a basis of a recommendation for treatment under the appropriate section of the Mental Health Act. The court is interested in the extent of the dementia and how it affects the offender's judgement and behaviour. The severity would be of relevance to the degree of mitigation or responsibility:

A married man of age 63 has shown increasing signs of dementia over two years with a loss of intellectual abilities, impaired memory, deterioration of personality with increasing irascibility and paranoid ideas. He was a man of previously good personality. He had enjoyed a good relationship with his wife, children and his work had gone well. His declining mental state, particularly his irascibility, led to considerable stress as he began to react with violence when irritated or frustrated by his wife. One particular morning an argument developed and in an explosive reaction he fatally beat his wife on the head with a heavy object. He was subsequently arrested and charged with murder.

Psychometric assessment on remand confirmed a dementia which was evident clinically and from the history obtained from the family. The first question to be considered was his fitness to plead. In his case he was not so demented as to fulfil these criteria. The second question was the extent of his responsibility at the time of the offence. He did not fall within the McNaughten Rules as he knew what he was doing and that it was wrong. He was not acting under any delusion at the time so that aspect of the McNaughten Rules did not have to be considered. He did, however, have a mental abnormality (dementia) which was considered by the psychiatrist to diminish substantially his responsibility – a view accepted by the prosecution. The defendant therefore pleaded not guilty to murder but guilty to manslaughter on the grounds of his diminished responsibility and this was accepted by the court. The psychiatrist recommended detention in hospital under section 37 on the grounds of his mental illness. The judge, however, in view of the offence coupled with a previous history of irascible behaviour made a restriction order under section

41 unlimited in time. The defendant's behaviour did not rule out his management in an ordinary hospital and the court took up the offer of a bed in the
catchment area hospital.

Had the offence been a less serious one, e.g. theft or assault, the case might
have gone differently. In the first place, at the time of his arrest, the police
might have sought a place in a psychiatric hospital if they had recognized
that the subject was mentally disturbed. They might have requested a
psychiatrist to consider admission under a civil section whilst the subject
was still in the police station or they might have used section 136 if it had
been appropriate. If the offender had appeared in a court then a court
diversion scheme might have led to his diversion to hospital. The bail
period before trial might therefore have been spent in hospital. In minor
cases, the charges might have been dropped. On the other hand, had the
offender only committed a very minor offence he might simply have been
allowed bail.

If the case had proceeded and had been a minor one, e.g. shoplifting,
then outpatient care might have been appropriate (voluntarily or as a
condition of probation) provided that the subject could manage to look
after himself sufficiently well or there were others who could assist him.

The dementia may be associated with other mental disturbances, such
as depression or paranoia, and these in themselves may lead to antisocial
behaviour. The important point is to always consider the possibility of
dementia in any older offender particularly where there has been a
previous history of a good personality.

Delirium and forensic psychiatry

This is a state, due to many organic causes, of clouded consciousness
coupled with confusion, disorientation, possibly with delusions, vivid
hallucinations or illusions. It is this state of mind, not the underlying
cause, which forms the basis of a medical defence. But offending in a state
of organic delirium must be very rare. The appropriate disposal would
depend on the clinical need. What defence was adopted would depend on
the situation. It might be appropriate to plead not guilty because of lack of
intent, or to ask for a hospital order (or some other form of treatment) on
the grounds of mental illness, or to plead, insanity under the McNaughten
Rules.

Epilepsy, its associated psychiatric conditions and forensic psychiatry

Epilepsy is classified in the ICD 10 and DSM IIIR as a disease of the
nervous system and *is not a mental disorder* but it becomes important

because of its effects on the mental state of the subject. Epilepsy is divided[1,2] into:

(1) Generalized epilepsy: A generalized discharge of all cells leading to a sudden unconsciousness with no aura. Two types are recognized:
   (a) grand-mal attack (primary and secondary),
   (b) petit-mal attack (petit-mal absence, akinetic seizures, generalized myoclonic jerks).
   The grand-mal attack is associated with a tonic phase followed by a clonic phase and a period of unconsciousness lasting several minutes. In the petit-mal attack there is only momentary lapses of consciousness, the patient immediately resuming normal activity. An 'absence' is evident to the observer only by transient blankness of facial expression and perhaps a slight twitching of limbs or eye-lids; an akinetic seizure by a sudden fall; and a myoclonic jerk by a flung-out limb.
(2) Focal (partial) epilepsy: Such seizures begin in part of the brain and may spread to involve the whole brain. Whilst they involve only part of the brain then there may be a conscious sensation (aura). The nature of the sensation gives a clue to where the discharge is coming from. Focal epilepsy is divided into:
   (a) simple partial (focal) seizures without impairment of consciousness,
   (b) complex partial (focal) seizures with complex movements and impairment of consciousness (generally arising in the temporal lobe).
   In either partial form the seizure may spread to involve the whole brain causing a grand-mal fit (secondary generalized epilepsy).

Epilepsy and behaviour

Epilepsy becomes important forensically for its effects on consciousness (which may be associated with offending) and its possible aetiological association with behavioural disturbance (including offending) between fits.

Disturbance of consciousness associated with a fit
The following alterations of consciousness have been described by Fenton[1] and Lishman[2]:

(1) *The aura:* In this state part of the brain is discharging abnormally and the subject is aware of various experiences depending on the part of the brain discharging. Typically, auras include involuntary movements of limbs, discreet sensations, emotions, various hallucinations and intrusive thoughts. The aura may or may not progress to a fully

developed seizure. The subject may have no recall of the aura afterwards.

(2) *Total unconsciousness:* This may be extremely brief as in petit-mal or last several minutes as in a grand-mal fit. A state of stupor has been described in petit-mal due to rapidly repeated fits.

(3) *Epileptic automatism:* Complex and semi-purposive activity may accompany an abnormal disturbance of brain electrical activity – commonly from the temporal lobe (a variety of complex partial seizure). The activity occurs in a state of clouded consciousness, though the individual retains control of posture and muscle tone. The automatism lasts usually a few seconds or minutes, mostly less than five minutes, though rarely it can be prolonged (psychomotor status). The subject appears to the observer to be dazed or the behaviour is inappropriate to the situation in some way. The episode may culminate in a grand-mal fit. The subject usually has an impaired memory of the automatism. Theoretically, an 'offence' could be committed in this state if, for example, the subject had a knife in his hand at the start of the automatism and he continued cutting movements.

(4) *Fugues:* This is disturbed behaviour resembling a complex epileptic automatism but lasting much longer (hours or days) in which journeys may be accomplished, purchases may be made, etc. Nevertheless the behaviour usually appears abnormal in some way. The subject has no memory of the event. Differentiating epileptic fugues from psychogenic fugues may be very difficult, and indeed there may be overlap. A history of fits, an abnormal EEG, and a previous history of fugues will assist in diagnosis.

(5) *Twilight states:* Lishman[2] recommends that this term be reserved for episodes of prolonged abnormal subjective experiences lasting up to several hours with impaired consciousness – dream-like, absent-minded behaviour, and slowness of reaction. The degree of reaction to the environment is very variable. The subject experiences strong feelings of panic, terror, anger or ecstasy. He may sit quietly through the attack or show sudden outbursts of aggressive or destructive behaviour. He may be very irritable and react with an outburst of rage to any interference which could result in an 'offence'. The experience is accompanied by disturbed brain electrical activity often with a temporal lobe focus. The state may terminate with a grand-mal fit.

(6) *Post-ictal states:* After the fit (ictus) proper there may be a failure to regain full consciousness. The subject appears confused and clumsy. The subject is in an irritable state and aggressive behaviour (which could lead to an offence) can occur, in which case it is usually a reaction to unwanted interference by others.

Sometimes a post-ictal twilight state may occur lasting hours or days with retardation, hallucinations and affective disturbance, or a-post-ictal paranoid psychosis may occur.

Disturbance of behaviour between fits

There is a complex relation between epilepsy and disturbed behaviour between fits[3]. This may be due to:

(1) Changes in the brain which caused the epilepsy or changes in the brain following severe epilepsy or the medication.
(2) Psychological effects of suffering the disease of epilepsy.
(3) Any associated mental impairment.
(4) Any associated mental illness.

As a result of the above factors the subject may experience:

(1) Changes in emotional state or personality.
(2) Mental illness-like states.
(3) A degree of mental retardation.
(4) Disturbed sexual behaviour.

Changes in emotional state, behaviour and personality:

(1) Prodromata of fits: Some subjects (most commonly with temporal lobe epilepsy) are aware of an altered emotional state in the hours or days before a grand-mal attack. This state is usually disagreeable with heightened irritability, tension and sullenness. This emotional state may be associated with difficult behaviour. It is possible that an assault might occur in such a state.
(2) Behaviour disorder in epileptic children: It has been shown that children with epilepsy are more likely than normal to show antisocial behaviour[4]. Such behaviour is not directly linked with seizures but is likely to be due to the complex interaction of multiple factors, such as brain dysfunction, adverse family influences, type of fit (temporal lobe epilepsy has a greater effect), the psychological reaction of the child to his illness, the effects of medication, and the effects of hospitalization or placement in institutions.
(3) Personality disorder in epileptics: There was a traditional idea that epileptics were constitutionally handicapped with personalities characterized by egocentricity, resentment and aggression. Such traits described in the past amongst institutionalized patients are now understood to be a product of brain injury, medication, institutionalization, etc. Nowadays, only a very small proportion of epileptics have such marked personality difficulties, and these, when seen, often appear to be understandable in terms of neurological damage, treatment and life experience. Of this group a number have marked aggressive traits:

> A young man developed grand-mal epilepsy as an infant (which was extremely difficult to control) and it was necessary to place him in a residential school for epileptics. He showed, from an early age, traits of aggression and resentment which escalated with time resulting in his

suspension from school and his placement in special institutions. These placements were also unsuccessful because of his aggression and he was returned to his home in his teens. At home his behaviour varied between an immature desire to please with bursts of resentful, hostile, violent behaviour. After one such outburst he was admitted to a psychiatric hospital in the hope of modifying his personality. There were long periods of what seemed conforming behaviour but it later became clear that he was hiding weapons and indulging in sly, destructive activity. He bore grudges and acted on them when the opportunity presented. The culmination of this was two near homicidal attacks on other patients committed in revenge for minor slights. He was transferred to a special hospital on a treatment order (section 3, Mental Health Act 1983) classified as suffering from psychopathic disorder (the disorder having arisen in conjunction with epilepsy). Because he was already in hospital he was not charged with the assaults.

Mental illness-like states

There are many clinical pictures and classifications but these are still unsatisfactory. All, theoretically, could be associated with offending. The following have been described[2]:

(1) Hallucinations and/or grossly disordered emotional states occurring in association with the seizure, either during the aura or in one of the other disturbances of consciousness.
(2) Paranoid hallucinatory states following grand-mal seizures lasting two to three weeks and accompanied by clouding of consciousness.
(3) Transient schizophrenia-like episodes which are self-limiting and occur between fits. They present a very variable picture, some patients remain fully alert whilst others have a clouded consciousness. Some are followed by amnesia and others by normal recall. Some are related to abnormal EEGs and others to normalization of the EEG (which becomes abnormal when the psychosis stops). Some are related to medication.
(4) Chronic schizophrenia-like psychoses identical to paranoid schizophrenia. This has been described in association with a history of epilepsy (usually temporal lobe epilepsy) longer than 14 years.
(5) Depressive states and neurotic states. These seem to be commoner in those with temporal lobe epilepsy. They are often short-lived and self-limiting. However, it must not be forgotten that there is a raised suicide rate amongst epileptics.

Mental retardation and epilepsy

Epilepsy is much commoner amongst subjects with retardation. This reflects the underlying brain disorder which has caused both conditions. Severe fits may, of course, lead to brain damage which may worsen the mental retardation. Some 50% of severely mentally retarded subjects have had an epileptic fit.

Sexual dysfunction and epilepsy

It is said that low libido and impotence are common complaints but these are thought to be due to poor social skills resulting from the sheltered life of an epileptic, frequent fits and the effects of heavy medication.

Fetishism and transvestism have been shown to be associated with temporal lobe epilepsy in certain rare cases. Case reports have claimed that operative removal of a temporal lobe focus has cured a fetishism[5]. Whether there was any true direct link with the temporal lobe lesion or whether the sexual disorder was due to distorted human relationships because of the subject suffering from epilepsy, is uncertain.

Epilepsy, the law and the Mental Health Act 1983

Although epilepsy itself is not regarded as a mental disorder, clearly it can, as described above, be intimately associated with mental disorder. The mental disorder forms the basis of any defence or mitigation, and for any recommendations for treatment under the Mental Health Act.

However, the courts have insisted in the past that severe disturbance of consciousness associated with epilepsy should be regarded as a disease of the mind[6].

Sullivan committed an act of serious violence in a confusional state following a seizure. A plea of non-insane automatism was submitted. It was ruled (supported by the Court of Appeal and later by the House of Lords) that this was insane automatism which would result in the verdict of not guilty by reason of insanity. At that time (1984) the Court would have had no option but to detain Sullivan under sections 37 and 41 Mental Health Act 1983 as though he were insane under the Criminal Justice (Insanity) Act 1964. As a result of the publicity and pressure, a change in the law was occasioned resulting in the present Criminal Procedure (Insanity and Unfitness to Plead) Act 1991 which gives the Judge discretion in disposal after a finding of insanity (see Chapter 3).

However the courts may be changing their view. In a recent case[6], a plea of sane automatism for an offence committed during a fit was successful on the basis that the epilepsy in that case (and hence the associated abnormal mental state) was brought on by an external cause (stress). The finding of sane automatism led to an acquittal. However, under the new Criminal Procedure (Insanity and Unfitness to Plead) Act 1991 a plea of insane automatism could be safely made in the expectation of being sent for treatment to an appropriate establishment under supervision.

Epilepsy and crime

In the nineteenth century it was believed that epilepsy or a tendency to epilepsy was a feature of many criminals. Crimes committed in blind fury were particularly thought to represent an epileptic process. Modern studies refute this view. A number of studies of epileptics attending outpatient clinics have failed to demonstrate excessive criminality in the patients. However, a more complete study by Gudmundsson[7] of all the epileptics in Iceland showed a small excess of criminality amongst the male epileptics. Gunn[8] has shown that the incidence of epilepsy in English prisons is higher than in the general population: 7–8 prisoners per thousand had epilepsy compared to 4–5 people per thousand of the general population. In a study[9] of 158 epileptic prisoners there was no convincing evidence of offending in a state of automatism though nine offended just before or just after a fit. In a study of 32 epileptics in special hospital[9], two were probably in a post-confusional state at the time of the offence. In short, whilst epilepsy may well be a factor leading to antisocial behaviour in some cases, the association is not common among epileptics and it is rare to offend at the time of the fit. The association of offending and epilepsy is summarized by Gunn[8]:

(1) The offence may occur in a disturbed state induced directly by a fit. This appears to be rare.
(2) The offences and the fit may be coincidental.
(3) The brain damage which caused the epilepsy may have led to personality problems resulting in antisocial behaviour.
(4) The subject may have developed strong antisocial attitudes as a result of the difficulties he has experienced in life as a result of his illness.
(5) An early deprived childhood environment may have both engendered antisocial attitudes and exposed the subject to epileptogenic features.
(6) Antisocial subjects may expose themselves to dangerous situations and sustain more head injuries than normal which may cause epilepsy.

Electroencephalographic changes, epilepsy and crimes of violence

Violence is probably unusual in direct association with a fit[10]. Usually any violence associated with the fit occurs in the post-confusional state and involves attacks on people who may be interfering. Violence can also occur (very rarely) in an epileptic automatism[11]. It has also been described associated with amygdaloid discharges (responding to amygdaloid ablation). Most violence committed by epileptics, however, seems to occur between fits. There is argument whether there is a raised incidence and surveys give varying results. In a study[10] of 31 subjects with temporal lobe epilepsy referred to an epileptic clinic, 14 were found to have a history of aggression. The violence was generally mild and did not correlate with electroencephalographic (EEG) or computerized axial tomography (CAT) scan findings. The behaviour *did* correlate with maleness, behavioural disturbance since childhood (often leading to residential schooling), adult personality problems, and dull intelligence. Violence may occur, of course, where there is an associated psychosis.

It has been asserted that EEG changes are commoner amongst violent offenders. Evidence for this is based on a classical study which found that the incidence of EEG abnormalities was greater if the murder was impulsive or lacked motive[12,13]. Williams[14] claimed that impulsive violent men had an increased incidence of temporal lobe abnormalities. Nevertheless, caution has been expressed about these findings as they are not supported by all studies. Gunn and Bonn[15], for example, did not find that temporal lobe epilepsy was associated with violence. Lishman's study of head injury subjects[16] found that frontal lobe lesions were the commonest lesion to be associated with aggression. Driver *et al.*[17] failed to find any significant difference between the EEGs of murderers and the EEGs of non-violent subjects when the examiner of the EEGs had no knowledge of the subjects.

Assessing the offending epileptic

Hindler[11] has summarized guidance to making the difficult judgement of whether the claim by a subject, that his offence occurred in a disturbed state due to an epileptic phenomenon is likely to be true. Before such a claim is supported there should be:

(1) A past history of definite epileptic attacks, not just vague *déjà-vu* phenomena.
(2) A history of the abnormal behaviour appearing suddenly, being of short duration (minutes) and never entirely appropriate for the circumstances.
(3) Amnesia (partial or total) for the event though not for more than a few minutes before the attack.
(4) Detection by observers of a clouding of consciousness with inappropriate movements, lack of awareness of surroundings, aimless wandering and a dazed expression. There will often be little attempt to conceal the crime.
(5) No motive for the crime.
(6) EEG studies are compatible.

If these criteria are met, then there are grounds for:

(1) A defence of sane or insane automatism.
(2) A plea of not guilty through lack of intent.
(3) Mitigation on the grounds of an acute temporary mental illness (organic confusional state) with a recommendation for treatment as an inpatient or outpatient as appropriate.

The majority of Mental Health Act orders on epileptic subjects, however, will be based on the associated disorders (such as personality disorder) where the disorder is sufficiently severe to bring it within the Mental Health Act definitions.

Organic personality syndrome

The DSM IIIR defines organic personality syndrome (F 310.10) as a change in personality due to an organic factor with at least one of the following:

(1) Affective instability.
(2) Recurrent outbursts of disproportionate aggression or rage.
(3) Marked impairment of social judgement.
(4) Marked apathy and indifference.
(5) Suspiciousness or paranoid ideation.

It should be differentiated from delirium, dementia, organic affective states or organic psychosis. The ICD 10 has similar criteria (F 07.0) but adds 'inability to persevere with goal-directed behaviour, alteration in rate and flow of language and altered sexual behaviour'.

Organic personality syndrome and behaviour

The reasons for this condition coming to the attention of the forensic psychiatrist arise from the loss of normal controls, increased egocentricity and loss of normal social sensitivity. People of previously good personality will present with an out-of-character offence. The history will show the development of an organic cerebral state. Frontal lobe damage is most likely to be associated with such a picture, and particularly right frontal lobe damage. The behaviour of the subjects reflects their previous personality, their emotional reaction to their loss of ability as well as the loss of brain function.

Organic personality syndrome and the law

The organic personality syndrome will be accepted by the court as a mental illness. The illness may then be used in mitigation and perhaps as the basis of a treatment order. Problems arise in knowing how to deal with the person of somewhat antisocial personality who sustains brain damage which exacerbates his antisocial attitudes and behaviour. The subject may be very difficult to manage in ordinary psychiatric hospitals due to the long-standing antisocial attitudes, increased impulsiveness and lack of concern. The case may be complicated by the anger and depression the subject feels about the illness. There is a temptation to describe such a patient as having a psychopathic disorder which is not amenable to treatment in order to pass his care over to the penal system. Whilst this may be appropriate in milder cases it really reflects a lack of specialized psychiatric units with the ability to take on the problem.

> A normal schoolboy from a good family sustained a serious head injury with considerable brain damage. He was in intensive care for a prolonged period and unconscious for many weeks. He eventually regained consciousness but had a hemiparesis which only partially resolved. His intellectual functioning was severely damaged. The worst problem, however, was the change in his personality. From being pleasant, normal and conforming he became a resentful, aggressive, demanding youth with no regard for other people's feelings. When frustrated he would react rapidly and aggressively. When things went his way he was cheerfully oblivious to anyone else's feelings. He soon began to commit impulsive antisocial acts to the extent that it became impossible to leave him unattended.
>
> He was admitted to conventional psychiatric hospital where his resentment of discipline led to considerable discord with the staff. His difficult behaviour was controlled either with heavy medication or the use of secure wards. Eventually he was placed in a special unit where he showed some response to behavioural techniques used in a very controlled regime. However, once back in the community his behaviour gradually deteriorated again and he was arrested for impulsively making a determined attempt to assault a married woman.
>
> By this stage he had exhausted the facilities of conventional psychiatric hospitals who might have managed a less severely disturbed subject. The extent of his assault and his destructive behaviour had by this stage reached such a magnitude that a place was offered by a special hospital. The court accepted a recommendation for a hospital order on the basis of his suffering from the mental illness of organic brain syndrome.

A claim has been made that an organic basis underlies the behaviour of certain aggressive people which has been called the *episodic dyscontrol syndrome*[18]. The underlying concept is that there is a neurological deficit of the controlling mechanisms which results in over-reactive explosive behaviour. It is asserted that supportive psychotherapy plus treatment with certain anti epileptic drugs, e.g. phenytoin, with or without phenothiazines, can be very helpful. The concept has not received widespread acceptance in England. Its proponents argue that the syndrome occurs principally in males from seriously disturbed backgrounds. There is a life-long history of violent outbursts on minimal provocation, with minor neurological dysfunction (soft signs), a high incidence of abnormal EEGs, particularly with temporal lobe abnormalities, an 'aura' (hyperacusis, visual illusions, numbness, nausea), headaches or drowsiness after the attack, and remorse for the attack. The condition is exacerbated by alcohol and diazepam. Opponents of the concept[1] argue that the episodic dyscontrol syndrome is merely a convenient label for impulsive aggressive antisocial personalities, the EEG changes are very unspecific and the behaviour is understandable in terms of the subject's damaging early life experiences.

A similar claim has been made for *attention deficit disorder with hyperactivity*. This condition is recognized in children as hyperkinetic disorder of childhood (ICD 10 F 90) or attention deficit hyperactivity disorder (DSM IIIR – 314.01). It has been asserted that the condition is due to minimal brain damage and can persist into adult life and present with impulsive character disorders, irritability, lability, explosiveness and violence. Evidence suggests that a third of cases will develop an antisocial disorder as a child and that the majority of these will become criminal adults[19]. As in children, a therapeutic effect can be obtained with stimulant medication[20].

Organic psychoses

Definition

The DMS IIIR recognizes an 'organic delusional syndrome' with delusions as a prominent feature secondary to an organic cause, an 'organic hallucinosis' with persistent or recurring hallucinations occurs due to a specific organic factor and an 'organic mood disorder'. The ICD 10 recognizes the same groups – F 06. The clinical picture is that of a severe psychotic condition arising from an organic cause. The behaviour of the subject simply reflects the psychosis and its content, e.g. a paranoid state may lead to suspicious, hostile behaviour.

Organic psychoses and the law

The psychoses can clearly be accepted as a mental illness within the meaning of the Mental Health Act 1983 and thus can form the basis of a treatment order and can be considered as a factor in mitigation, etc. Where the illness occurs after a head injury, or other trauma, there may also be grounds for compensation.

> A young man of previously good personality suffered a severe head injury at work. He was in hospital for some months and made a slow recovery. Although he was able to return to his home he appeared unable to concentrate on his work as well as he had before and his general behaviour became bizarre. He was sent for a psychiatric assessment one year after his injury. At that point it became clear that he had developed a severe paranoid psychosis believing that his lodgers and neighbours were spying on him. His attitude towards his lodgers had become increasingly suspicious and unpleasant to the point that they left. Over the subsequent months his condition deteriorated so that compulsory admission to psychiatric hospital became necessary.
> It was argued successfully in the High Court that his psychotic condition was

a result of the head injury and substantial compensation was paid. Of course, had the subject committed any offence as a result of his psychotic state then the psychotic state would have acted as mitigation on the grounds of mental illness in the normal way.

Substance-induced organic disorders

Definition

There are disorders induced by any substance, of which the most common is alcohol. Various drugs (sedatives, stimulants, hallucinogens, etc.) may be used legally or illegally and may induce disorders of mental function including:

(1) Intoxication: due to an excess of the drug with altered mood, altered motor abilities and altered psychological functioning.
(2) Idiosyncratic intoxication: Where an apparent intoxication is induced by very small amounts due to an idiosyncratic reaction on the part of the subject. A variety of effects, including delirium and autonomic changes, may be observed.
(3) Withdrawal effects: A variety of effects may be induced by suddenly stopping a drug to which the subject has become addicted. These effects will include delirium, autonomic changes, depression, anxiety, tremors.
(4) Mental illness: This may be associated with drug use in several ways:
　(a) as a direct effect of the drug, e.g. amphetamines and their derivatives, cocaine, lysergic acid, or a medication such as steroids,
　(b) as an effect of a sudden withdrawal of a drug, e.g. paranoid psychosis after alcohol withdrawal,
　(c) due to the chronic effects of drug use, e.g. alcoholic dementia.

Substance-induced disorders and the law

Intoxication
The Mental Health Act 1983 specifically excludes simple alcohol or drug abuse from the conditions which make a person subject to Mental Health Act orders. Generally speaking, if a person takes an illegal drug (including alcohol) he is held responsible for any actions he commits whilst intoxicated by the drug. The fact that it has disinhibited him or caused him to be amnesic for the occasion will be no excuse. Exceptions to this include (1) to (4). 'Involuntary intoxication' covers (1) to (3) and can lead to an acquittal[21]. Exceptions are:

(1) Deception: Where a man is being tricked into taking a substance without his knowledge (a difficult thing to prove).

(2) Idiosyncratic response: A person's reaction is quite idiosyncratic and could not be anticipated, e.g. gross intoxication following a very small amount of the substance. It has been claimed that some individuals show 'pathological intoxication' (ICD 10 F1x.07) ('Mania a Poitu') on very small doses of alcohol – particularly if there is some pre-existing brain damage. Following a small amount of alcohol there is a brief, severe aggressive outburst in a state of disorientation and even psychosis followed by sleep and amnesia. This claim has both supporters and detractors[2]. The situation is unresolved but the defence has been tried in court where the clinical picture justified it.

(3) Untoward reaction: A person had an untoward reaction to a medication prescribed by a doctor. A person befuddled with medication walked out of a shop with goods he had not paid for. A plea of not guilty because of lack of intent (due to 'involuntary intoxication') was offered. It was argued that the drug, taken in good faith, had led to the state of confusion in which the act occurred.

> A man attacked his cohabitee when suffering from a temporary paranoid psychosis ascribed to the steroid medication he was then receiving. He was found not guilty[21] due to 'involuntary intoxication' (which, presumably, would affect his ability to form intent.

Edwards[22] points out that there must be a clear relationship between the medication and the act. The unwanted reaction should be authoritatively documented, the act should not be a manifestation of the illness the patient suffers from, no other substances which could have caused the reaction should have been taken, taking the medication and the reaction should be appropriately related in time, and the reaction should disappear when the medication is stopped.

(4) Incapable of intent: Here, the degree of intoxication is such that the subject becomes incapable of forming intent. Courts have been very sceptical of such a defence for fear that a successful plea would encourage similar pleas from any criminal who offended when in drink. It has now been ruled[23] that for crimes of basic intent (e.g. manslaughter, assault and unlawful wounding) the accused will not be acquitted if, having knowingly and willingly taken drink or drugs, he deprived himself of the ability to exercise self-control or became unconscious of what he was doing. In crimes of specific intent (e.g. murder or theft) there would still be a defence available of 'no intent'. In the case of murder, the charge might then be reduced to manslaughter.

> Lipman took lysergic whilst in bed with a girl friend. Lysergic acid induced a temporary state in which he believed he was fighting off snakes which were attacking him. He 'awoke' to find that he had killed his girlfriend. Although charged with murder Lipman was found guilty of manslaughter, a finding confirmed by the Court of Appeal in Lipman (1969) 53 Cr. App. R. 60.

It is quite common for offenders who were heavily intoxicated at the time to claim that they had no memory for the offence and that it 'was all due to the drink'. A study of the relevant statements nearly always confirms that the subject's behaviour was perfectly understandable in terms of the situation, even though intoxicated. In such a case, it is no defence to plead the effects of the intoxication. Nevertheless, after conviction, courts will often take a sympathetic view of people anxious to rid themselves of dependence on alcohol or drugs, and make probation orders with conditions of treatment for the dependency provided it seems appropriate in that particular case and the offence is not too serious.

Psychiatrists may be asked in a particular case what effect alcohol, taken perhaps on top of medication, may have had on the mental state or degree of intoxication. The blood level of alcohol varies with sex, type of drink (fizzy drinks absorb more rapidly), food in the stomach, body build, and rate of gastric emptying (affected by some drugs). There is euphoria at 30 mg/100 ml, impaired driving at 50, dysarthria at 160, with loss of consciousness possible over this figure and death over 400 mg/100 ml. The risk of a road accident is more than double at 80 mg/100 ml and is more than tenfold at 160. Alcohol is metabolized at about 15 mg/100 ml/ hour but this varies considerably. Heavy drinkers metabolize more quickly unless there is liver damage, which slows the rate. Nevertheless, the Court of Appeal has allowed a back calculation to be made from a known blood level and given as evidence. The psychiatrist might be asked to comment on the factors which might have influenced this.

Withdrawal disorders

A court may accept, in mitigation, a disorder of mind induced by substance withdrawal, certainly where this disorder could not reasonably have been anticipated by the subject.

> A married man who drank heavily on shore returned to his ship having promised his wife he would stop drinking. This he did, only to develop an acute, paranoid illness with auditory hallucinations and delusions. He believed his life was in danger from his shipmates and he therefore set fire to the ship to 'escape them'. He was subsequently charged with arson on the high seas. The court accepted that he had been ill at the time and made an order for treatment as a condition of probation (he had, with medication, recovered from his illness by the time of his trial). He was therefore able to receive continued medication and supervision as an outpatient.

Mental illness associated with substance abuse

Where an offence has been committed while the subject is suffering from a substance-induced mental illness then the courts seem to be ready to consider accepting this in mitigation and to be willing to make a treatment order if recommended to do so by the doctors – if it seems a fair and sensible disposal. On the other hand, psychiatrists are sometimes unwilling to accept as a patient someone who has had only a temporary disorder from substance abuse, especially where the patient is of anti-social inclination. The difficulty with this view is that in some people various drugs seem to precipitate a mental illness which does not rapidly clear up but which begins to take on all the features of a chronic psychosis (e.g. schizophrenia) for which hospital and after-care is needed.

Organic amnesia

Amnesia may have psychological causes (see Chapter 3) or be organic. Organic amnesia may be divided[2,24] into

(1) 'Amnesic' syndrome with focal pathological lesions: Pathological examination shows brain damage, particularly to the mamillary bodies, posterior hypothalamus, and the grey matter around the third and fourth ventricles, and the aqueduct. Occasionally, there are bilateral hippocampal lesions. The causes of this focal damage includes tumours, thiamine deficiency (as in Wernickes encephalopathy and Korsakoffs psychosis) and infarcts. There is an inability to lay down new memory from the time of the event (anterograde amnesia) and loss of old memory (retrograde amnesia) without confusion or loss of attention.
(2) Amnesia caused by diffuse brain damage as in dementia (e.g. Alzheimer's disease), toxic confusional state, head injury, or hypoglycaemia.

Amnesia and the law

The inability to recall an offence is no defence in itself (see Chapter 3). In the above case the patient could be said to suffer from the mental illness of an organic brain syndrome causing confusion or very severe memory loss. The question of fitness to plead might be raised. The patient might be unable, because of his illness, to comprehend the trial and its relevance to him. Certainly, the illness would be sufficiently severe for it to mitigate sentence and it would constitute grounds, in a case of homicide, for diminished responsibility if not for a plea of insanity or automatism.

Sleep disorders and the law

Offending can occur during sleep, in which case a defence of automatism is appropriate though it is unclear whether this will be recognized as sane or insane automatism (see Chapter 3). Three forms are recognized:

(1) Sleepwalking: This occurs during stage IV slow-wave sleep – not REM sleep where the body is normally paralysed[2]. There may be partial arousal in which complex actions are possible including violent attacks.

To make the diagnosis of sleepwalking there should be previous episodes of it confirmed by observers. The behaviour is usually banal and stereotyped. There is normally no memory for the episode (though some writers believe that partial recall is possible). Some may respond to simple commands during the episode. The episodes usually last several minutes to half an hour (occasionally longer) and then the subject returns to bed. Episodes may be precipitated by tension or family discord. Certain drugs may precipitate an episode (hypnotics, various psychoactive drugs and possibly alcohol). A disturbed personality is not uncommon and some have suggested that sleepwalking may be akin to hysterical dissociation[25].

Management and treatment is by: (1) advising the subject to sleep with doors and windows locked and (2) prescribing drugs which suppress stages III–IV sleep (such as diazepam).

(2) Night terrors: These also occur in stage III–IV sleep. The subject wakes with intense fear and anxiety with autonomic arousal. The subject may run around screaming and may injure others.
(3) Awaking from deep sleep: A state similar to a night terror may be precipitated by being awakened suddenly from a deep sleep particularly in a threatening situation. The subject may then react violently.

References

(1) Fenton, G.W. (1984) Epilepsy, mental abnormality and criminal behaviour. In Craft, M. and Craft, A. (eds) *Mentally Abnormal Offenders*. Ballière Tindall, Eastbourne.
(2) Lishman, W.A. (1987) *Organic Psychiatry: The Psychological Consequences of Cerebral Disorder* (2nd edn). Blackwell Scientific Publications, Oxford.
(3) Gunn, J. (1977) *Epileptics in Prison*. Academic Press, London.
(4) Rutter, M., Graham, P.J. & Yule, W. (1970) *A Neuropsychiatric Study in Childhood*. Heinemann, London.
(5) Falconer, M.A. (1973) Reversibility by temporal lobe behavioural resection of the behavioural abnormalities of temporal lobe epilepsy. *New England Journal of Medicine* **289**, 450–5.
(6) Brahams, D. (1990) Epilepsy is no longer a disease of the mind. *Lancet* **336**, 869.
(7) Gudmundsson, G. (1966) Epilepsy in Iceland: A clinical and epidemiological investigation. *Acta Neurologica Scandinavica*, Supplement **25**, 7–124.
(8) Gunn, J.C. (1969) The prevalence of epilepsy among prisoners. *Proceedings of the Royal Society of Medicine* **62**, 60–3.
(9) Gunn, J.C. & Fenton, G.W. (1971) Epilepsy, automatism and crime. *Lancet* i, 1173–6.
(10) Hertzberg, J.L. & Fenwick, P.B.C. (1988) The aetiology of aggression in temporal lobe epilepsy. *British Journal of Psychiatry* **153**, 50–5.
(11) Hindler, C.G. (1989) Epilepsy and violence. *British Journal of Psychiatry* **155**, 246–9.

(12) Stafford-Clark, D. & Taylor, F.H. (1949) Clinical and electroencephalographic studies of prisoners charged with murder. *Journal of Neurology, Neurosurgery and Psychiatry* **12**, 325–30

(13) Hill, D. & Pond, D.A. (1952) Reflections of one hundred capital cases submitted to electroencephalography. *Journal of Mental Science* **98**, 23–43.

(14) Williams, D. (1969) Neural factors related to habitual aggression. *Brain* **92**, 503–20.

(15) Gunn, J.C. & Bonn, J. (1971) Criminality and violence in epileptic prisoners. *British Journal of Psychiatry* **118**, 337–43.

(16) Lishman, W.A. (1968) Brain damage in relation to psychiatric disability after head injury. *British Journal of Psychiatry* **114**, 373–410.

(17) Driver, M.V., West, L.R. & Faulk, M. (1974) Clinical and EEG studies of prisoners charged with murder. *British Journal of Psychiatry* **125**, 583–7.

(18) Bach-Y-Rita, G., Lion, J.R., Climent, C.E. & Ervin, F.R. (1971) Episodic dyscontrol: a study of 130 violent patients. *American Journal of Psychiatry* **127**, 1473–8.

(19) Mannuzza, S., Klein, R.G., Bonagura, N., Malloy, P., Giampino, T. & Addalli, K.A. (1991) Hyperactive children almost grown up. *Archives of General Psychiatry* **48**, 77–83.

(20) Wender, P.H. Reimherr, F.W. & Wood, D.R. (1981) Attention deficit disorder ('minimal brain dysfunction') in adults. *Archives of General Psychiatry* **38**, 449–56.

(21) d'Orban, P.T. (1989) Steroid-induced psychosis. *Lancet* **ii**, 694.

(22) Edwards, J.G. (1992) Antidepressants and murder. *Psychiatric Bulletin* **16**, 537–9.

(23) Legal Correspondent (1976) Intoxication and crime. *British Medical Journal* **1**, 1286–7.

(24) Stone, J.H. (1992) Memory disorder in offenders and victims. *Criminal Behaviour and Mental Health* **2**, 342–56.

(25) Crisp, A.H., Matthews, B.M., Oakey, M. & Crutchfield, M. (1990) Sleepwalking, night terrors and consciousness. *British Medical Journal* **300**, 360–2.

Chapter 10

Psychopathic Disorder and Forensic Psychiatry

Introduction

Walker[1], quoting Pinel shows how for many years there has been a tradition for psychiatrists to regard people with grossly disordered personalities, characterized by aggression and irresponsibility, as being subjects for psychiatric treatment. What has changed over time has been the understanding and diagnostic titles. These have included[2] *manie sans delire*, moral insanity, moral imbecility, psychopathy, degenerate constitution, congenital delinquency, constitutional inferiority, moral deficiency, and sociopathy, as well as other terms.

The term 'psychopathy' originated in the late nineteenth century in Germany[1,3] and was used originally (and still is on the Continent) to embrace all disorders of personality. It was in the USA that the term first became restricted to those showing antisocial behaviour and it was with this meaning that it was imported into England. It became incorporated into statute in the Mental Health Act 1959 as 'psychopathic disorder'. This generic term replaced the older terms 'moral insanity' and 'moral defect' which had been incorporated into the Mental Deficiency Acts. Despite the controversy about its value, the term continues in the Mental Health Act 1983 (see Chapter 3). The Butler Report[3] points out that the legal term psychopathic disorder' carries no implication that psychopathic disorder is a single entity – rather it is a generic term adopted for the purpose of legal categorization and capable of covering a number of specific diagnoses. On the other hand, reliable specific diagnoses in this area are still to be developed!

The legal term is used to cover a number of personality disorders in the ICD 10 and DSM IIIR plus a number of other categories[4]. Although the ICD 10 dissocial personality disorder (F 60.2) and DSM IIIR antisocial personality (301.7) are the equivalent of the clinician's use of the term 'psychopathic personality', the legal term psychopathic disorder has also been used to cover some people with ICD 10 paranoid personality (F 60.0), emotionally unstable personality disorder (including impulsive and borderline types F 60.30 F 60.31) and DSM III borderline personality disorder (301.83) and schizoid personality disorder (ICD 10, F 60.1). In fact, remembering the Mental Health Act, it includes any personality disorder which results in 'seriously irresponsible or abnormally aggressive behaviour'. Furthermore, some men with sexual deviations in conjunction with a disordered personality have been classified legally as psychopathic disorder although, in psychiatric terms, they fall into DSM IIIR and ICD 10 groups such as sexual sadism/sadomasochism, paedophilia and exhibitionism.

The confusion about the meaning and interpretation of the term 'psychopathic disorder' is demonstrated in attempts to assess the incidence of the disorder. What are the investigators looking for, what are the cut-off points in a particular trait, are there any crucial features which must be present? A comparison of studies of the incidence of mental disorder in prison[5,6] found a considerable difference between surveys of the incidence of psychopathic disorder varying from 5.5% to 78%. Gunn *et al.*[7] in his study of Grendon Prison inmates, all with a diagnosis of psychopathic disorder, were unable to demonstrate 'syndromes' of psychopathy, i.e. personality traits did not form recognizable clusters. They found the official (British and American) descriptions too vague to be useful which led to a lack of inter-rater reliability. They felt forced to eschew the terms 'personality disorder' and 'psychopathy' and study specific neurotic traits. Similar conclusions were reached by Walton and Presly[8,9] in their study of personality disorders.

Some, wanting to preserve the concept of personality disorder but recognizing the unsatisfactory nature of having many subtypes, suggest having a few broad clusters only. Tyrer[10] proposes three clusters, (1) the erratic, (2) the flamboyant or dramatic (including the antisocial, borderline, sadistic, histrionic and narcissistic) and (3) the anxious or fearful cluster.

Blackburn[11] argues that many descriptions of personality fail because they confuse social behaviour (theft, violence) with personality and temperamental traits. This leads to confusion about treatment. He offers a model of personality deviation based on the traits of dominance-submission and hostility-friendliness. Normality would be a proper balance between them. Disorder would be a rigid inflexible dependence on only one part. The antisocial personality depends rigidly on a mixture of dominance and hostility. The theory leads logically to a cognitive therapy approach in which the patients' distorted expectation of others can be challenged.

Because of the problem of definition, the Butler Committee recommended the abandonment of the term. Nevertheless, the term was retained in the Mental Health Act 1983 despite these difficulties – although with two very important practical changes. First, it is now clear under the present Act that the diagnosis of psychopathic disorder is not in itself sufficient to lead to a hospital order, it is also necessary to show that medical treatment is likely to alleviate or prevent deterioration in the subject's condition before an order can be made; second, it is now possible to use a civil order for treatment in case of psychopathic disorder (provided the treatment conditions are met) at any age, and not, as existed under the previous Act, just for those under the age of 21 years.

Clinical features of psychopathic disorder

As the legal term psychopathic disorder is used generically there can be no single clinical description. One can list the main conditions encompassed by the term. In practice, the conditions blend into each other and any one person may have features from several.

(1) Antisocial Personality DSM IIIR (301.70) or dissocial personality disorder ICD 10 (F 60.2)

The DSM IIIR diagnosis is made after 18 years. It includes an onset, before the age of 15, of three of the following: truancy, initiating fights, using weapons, forcing someone into sexual activity, physical cruelty to animals or people, destroying other people's property, deliberate fire raising, lying, stealing, or robbery. This childhood behaviour is then followed from the age of 15 by at least four of the following: inability to sustain consistent work behaviour, failure to accept social norms with respect to lawful behaviour, inability to maintain a monogamous relationship for more than a year, irritability and aggressiveness, failure to honour financial obligations, impulsivity, disregard for the truth, recklessness for own or other's safety, and lack of remorse. Finally, the antisocial behaviour must not be due to severe mental retardation, schizophrenia or other mental illness. The ICD 10 describes only adult traits (callousness, disregard for others, incapacity to maintain relationships, low tolerance of frustration, lack of guilt, tendency to blame others). It observes that childhood behavioural disorder is frequently though not invariably present.

There have been several attempts to produce classifications of antisocial personality but none has received universal acceptance. Henderson[12] spoke of aggressive (violent aggressive personalities), inadequate (liars, swindlers, impulsive wanderers, hysterics and neurotics) and creative (considerable talent combined with egocentric and antisocial attitudes) psychopaths. The classification has had some popularity but it is recognized that subjects change from one group to another or have features of all groups.

Antisocial personalities have been divided into *primary* and *secondary* *(neurotic) psychopaths*. The syndrome of a primary psychopath has been described by Cleckley[13]. At first sight the subject appears normal, charming, intelligent and articulate with low anxiety. The history, however, reveals extremely egocentric, impulsive and bizarre behaviour, which, in the long run, is against the subject's interest. Legal confrontation may be avoided indefinitely because of the subject's intelligence and charm, and prominent positions in society may be attained until the true picture emerges. Although the subject will learn to give a history of early psychological trauma as this interests psychiatrists, in fact, investigation fails to support this. The behaviour is not understandable in ordinary psychological terms. Cleckley postulates that such psychopaths have an inherent disorder of brain function by which emotions (e.g. guilt) and words are dissociated. Cleckley considered, therefore, that primary psychopathy is quite untreatable. The concept of a primary psychopath has been widely accepted in some research and psychological faculties but has not, in England, received much support from clinicians. Secondary psychopaths resemble the description of antisocial personality in DSM IIIR with prominent anxiety. Their personality is understood largely in terms of psychological traumas experienced in early life (parental and childhood deprivation, bad models, bad environment, etc.) as discussed in Chapter 5.

(2) Emotionally unstable personality disorder ICD 10 (F 60.3)

There is no exact equivalent in the DSM IIIR. This personality is characterized by a marked tendency to act impulsively together with affective instability. Outbursts of anger, often associated with violence, are easily aroused. Two variants are described – the impulsive and the borderline type (see below).

(3) Borderline personality DSM IIIR (302.83), (ICD 10 F 60.31 Borderline type of emotionally unstable personality disorder)

The DSM IIIR gives the fuller description. This is a relatively new concept which has not so far been widely accepted in the UK. The diagnosis is based on the long-term presence of at least five of the following which cause significant impairment in social or occupational functioning:

(1) Unstable and intense interpersonal relationships alternating from over-idealization to devaluation.
(2) Impulsivity in at least two areas of self-damaging activities, e.g. gambling, sexual behaviour, substance abuse, shoplifting, overeating, reckless driving.
(3) Affective instability with marked shifts of mood over hours or days.
(4) Inappropriate, intense anger or lack of control of anger.
(5) Recurrent suicidal threats, gestures, or self-mutilation.

(6) Identity disturbance with uncertainty and doubts about self-image, gender identity, long-term goals and loyalties.

(7) Chronic feelings of emptiness or boredom.

(8) Frantic efforts to avoid real or imagined abandonment.

These patients include some of the most difficult to manage. They have a tendency, almost pathognomonic, to involve staff in their intense emotional relationships causing splitting amongst staff as a result of their idealization or devaluation: 'You are the only one who understands me, if only the others were like you'. There are dangers for staff who become over involved in such a situation[14]. Professional behaviour must be maintained. Staff programmes (with supervision) to guide in managing the patient can be a great help.

(4) Schizoid personality disorder ICD 10 (F 60.1)

The personality is characterized by emotional coldness or detachment with a limited capacity to express warmth. There is indifference to others and an excessive preoccupation with fantasy and introspection. There is a marked insensitivity to social norms.

(5) Sexual Sadism DSM IIIR (302.84), ICD 10 (F 65.5)

(6) Paedophilia DSM IIIR (302.20), ICD 10 (F 65.4)

In both these latter groups, discussed in Chapter 12, psychiatrists have made recommendations for treatment under the category of 'psychopathic disorder' where the sexual deviation has been seen as part of a personality disorder. (Sexual deviation on its own is not grounds for compulsory detention under the Mental Health Act 1983.) Psychiatrists seem more likely to make recommendations for treatment in this group when the subject himself convincingly requests psychiatric help to rid himself of unwanted sexual behaviour. In the past it was also possible that treatment recommendations had been made because it had been felt that a treatment order combined with a restriction order would give better protection to the public than a simple prison sentence. However, the difficulty of treating sexual deviations, the difficulty of gauging the right time for release from hospital (with the subsequent political repercussions if the patient re-offends) and the relatively high re-offending rate seems to be having an effect on psychiatry's attitude to psychopathic disorder in general, so that there has been a steady fall in the use of this category.

Intercurrent mental illness and psychopathic disorder

It is common experience in prisons and secure hospitals to observe relatively brief periods of mental illness in subjects with psychopathic disorder[4]. They seem to occur in all the severe disorders of personality, usually at times of stress, but other times for no clear reason. The illness is usually either a marked affective disturbance or a schizophreniform psychosis. Coid[15] studied 72 female patients with borderline personality disorder in special hospital. He described a cyclical pattern of affective disturbance (often seemingly endogenous in origin) with anxiety, anger, depression and tension as the principal features. After a build up of these symptoms (over hours or days) a compulsion to act out criminal (e.g. fire raising) or self-destructive behaviour. Acting-out would be followed by a temporary relief of symptoms. The cycle would then be repeated.

The management of these disturbed periods is difficult. This is partly due to the tensions and stress placed on the staff by the patient and partly by the difficulty of bringing the conditions under control (a combination of neuroleptics, carbamazapine and monoamine oxidase inhibitors within a structured setting may be required). In the *psychotic periods* there is usually a paranoid state with delusional and hallucinatory experiences. The subject may react to the psychotic experiences (commonly paranoid ideas and auditory hallucinations) with a similar tension, hostility and destructiveness as may occur in an affective disturbance and with similar difficulties in management, though recovery with antipsychotic medication tends to be good. A number of such subjects become more stable if they take antipsychotic medication regularly at which times relatively small doses may be sufficient.

Self-mutilation and psychopathic disorder

Recurrent self-mutilation is a well-known feature in patients with a diagnosis of psychopathic disorder, though clinical experience suggests that it is most common in the secondary (neurotic) psychopath and those with borderline personality. The principal form is multiple cuts to the skin, commonly on the forearm, but occasionally elsewhere. It is allied to burning oneself (often with a cigarette end) and repeated mild overdoses. Coid[15] postulates that such patients suffer from a chronic cyclical mood disorder which causes these periods of tension and dysphoria.

Incidence of self-mutilation

The incidence is unknown. It is particularly common in closed institutions where there is high emotion. There is often a histrionic, imitative quality to the behaviour in that it seems to be learned from others and may occur in epidemics. Although it occurs in both sexes, from a clinical point of view, it seems to be commoner in women.

Aetiology and clinical features

It is frequently stated that such self-mutilation is attention-seeking behaviour. This is incorrect. Rather, it should be properly described as tension-reducing behaviour. A common pattern is for the subject to experience a period of considerable tension seemingly precipitated by rejection, frustration or perceived damage to self-esteem, or perhaps due to a cyclical mood disorder for which a rationalization is sought. The subject then retires to a private place (a toilet, a quiet part of the building) and makes several cuts. The subject may tell the staff or the staff become aware of the behaviour because of the severity of the bleeding. Sometimes the cuts may be hidden from view and are discovered by accident later. The cuts vary in thickness from mere scratches to skin-thickness cuts. No pain is felt when the cuts are made. The patient will describe how feelings of tension and anger are relieved by seeing the skin part or seeing the accompanying bleeding. This relief is only temporary, however, and further mutilation may well occur. Indeed, this same tension, anger or resentment plays a part in the reaction of some patients to the attempts of doctors and nurses to treat the condition. They may, in severe cases, destroy the bandaging or pull the stitches out and repeat the cutting or attack their helpers.

Typically the syndrome is associated with feelings of emptiness or despair, mood swings, disorders of eating (anorexia or bulimia), drug or alcohol abuse, confusion of sexual identity and menstrual complaints.

Treatment

Managing the patient at this stage is particularly trying as the staff become a focus for primitive feelings of anger and hostility which well-up in the patient. The aim of all treatment and management techniques should be to reduce the tension by attention to the areas of frustration and to help the subject to get his feelings under control. There are many approaches to the problem which is a measure of the difficulty in dealing with it. There is frequently no clear, right answer. Approaches which have been tried (after attending to the wounds) include:

(1) Isolating the patient in a firm 'We won't tolerate that behaviour here' approach. The difficulty with this is that it is very easy to provoke a spiral of defiant, destructive behaviour.
(2) Give intensive individual attention 'Let's talk this through and learn to express our feelings verbally'. This approach may come to grief if the patient refuses to do so and reacts violently to the staff.
(3) Giving medication. Various drugs (see below) may be helpful in reducing tension. They are usually combined with (4).
(4) Adopting a structured behavioural based nursing management

approach, perceiving self-mutilation as maladaptive behaviour: 'We will discourage this inappropriate behaviour but encourage more appropriate responses by scientifically applied reinforcers and aversive stimuli'. Skilfully done, with warmth and concern, this approach can be effective in some cases but great care must be taken that it is not used as a cover for a punitive repressive approach. At best, it provides a structured, calm, warm, consistent milieu in which tension may rapidly fall. The nursing programme of management must be orchestrated by someone with adequate training and who is not directly involved with the patient, e.g. a psychologist or a behaviour therapy-trained nurse therapist.

Differential diagnosis

Self-mutilation of this type has to be distinguished from:

(1) True attempts at suicide.
(2) The bizarre mutilations which may occur in a psychotic state under the influence of delusions or hallucinations, e.g. poking out an eye or genital mutilation.
(3) Self-immolation for idealistic or psychotic reasons.
(4) Overdoses or suicidal gestures aimed at manipulating others, usually a spouse, boyfriend or the institution.
(5) Deliberate self-harm to intimidate others, e.g. prisoners who will go on hunger strike in order to force the authority to give way.
(6) Overdoses which are aimed at drawing attention to one's plight.

Medicolegal aspects of psychopathic disorder

Psychopathic disorder (without a superimposed mental illness) is not a cause of being unfit to plead, being unfit to stand trial or grounds for an insanity defence. It may be used in mitigation either to get a reduced sentence, to support a hospital disposal or to form the grounds for a plea of diminished responsibility in cases of homicide. In the latter case, whilst a successful plea might in the past have led to a hospital order, nowadays, it is more likely to be followed by a prison sentence which may in fact be a life sentence[16]. This reflects, in part, the psychiatrists' disillusionment in their ability to treat this disorder.

An assessment of the case requires a most careful collecting of data going back as far as possible (school reports, child guidance clinic reports, social and probation reports, medical and psychiatric reports), as well as a careful study of statements and previous offending. Information from relatives is very helpful. The clinical problem will often be to clarify the extent to which there was a superimposed mental dysfunction at the time of the offence caused by an illness (e.g. depression), self-induced intoxication (drugs, alcohol) or stress with an excessive emotional reaction. Only illness is likely to be accepted as a mitigating factor.

The following cases illustrate the relationship of the law to the psychopathic offender.

Case histories:

Case A

A man of 40 years from a broken and severely discordant home, had a history of childhood temper tantrum, fighting, lying and repeated violations of rules at home and school. After leaving school, he failed to sustain himself in work. There was repeated offending, violence, impulsivity and a total lack of truthfulness. Psychiatrists noted his antisocial personality and their expectations of dangerous behaviour. When aged 37 years he successfully presented himself as a considerate, charming, man to a widow and married her. Once they had set up home he reverted to his usual behaviour, drinking heavily and treating her, as he had others, violently and without any consideration. Inevitably, she left him. He reacted with rage and depression, drinking too much, making numerous attempts to contact her and speaking of suicide and despair. He finally met up with her having brought a knife. He confronted her and then lethally stabbed her. He then waited for the police to arrive.

Psychiatric assessment for the court demonstrated that he fell within the Mental Health Act 1983 definition of psychopathic disorder. It was also argued that at the time of the offence he had the mental illness of reactive depression. This combination of mental illness and psychopathic disorder was, it was argued, sufficient mental abnormality to substantially diminish his responsibility within the meaning of the Homicide Act 1957. However, it was not felt that treatment in a psychiatric hospital was likely to be beneficial and recommendations for psychiatric treatment were not made. The judge passed a life sentence, the court having accepted his plea of diminished responsibility.

The case illustrates a number of things: First, a finding of diminished responsibility may not lead to a lighter sentence or to a referral for psychiatric care but depends on the facts of the case; second, 'psychopathic disorder' can be put up as a 'mental abnormality' within the Homicide Act though usually it would be unsuccessful without some other mental disorder (in this case depression) being present.

Case B

Miss B was the second of four children. She had a good mother but her father was violent and alcoholic. As a child she was impulsive and labile in mood, and suffered from severe temper. Her relationships with others were intense (strong, brief attachments) and unstable (falling out and quarrelling). She failed to settle at school and truanted, both at primary and secondary schools and was suspended twice. When aged 14, she began a disastrous sexual affair with an older man. She abused drugs from her teens. She was placed by the court in a residential community home at the age of 14 but remained uncooperative and defiantly absconded a great deal.

To support her drug habit she persistently broke into chemist shops after which she frequently took overdoses. Interspersed with this she also cut herself badly at times of tension and despondency. The self-mutilation and overdoses led to psychiatric hospital admissions where she was usually tense, despairing, suicidal and hostile. There were times when she appeared to be in a paranoid state with hostile suspiciousness and complaints of auditory hallucinations. At other times she might appear with an appealing child-like dependence and vulnerability. Nevertheless, in hospital, she was usually an uncooperative patient. Relationships with her nurses and doctors were usually discordant with violence and frequent absconding followed by a repeat of the cycle of chemist break-ins and overdoses. She had many of the characteristics of a borderline personality as well as an antisocial personality.

She clearly met the criteria of the Mental Health Act 1983 for psychopathic disorder, the disorder of mind in her case being the disordered personality with severe emotional lability, impulsiveness and failure to form mature judgements or relationships. She was seriously irresponsible and abnormally aggressive both to herself and others. Finally, the psychiatrist advised the court that detention in a special hospital with a restriction order was the only psychiatric way he could see to control the patient and prevent her death. The court took up this recommendation and a hospital order was made on the grounds of psychopathic disorder. In special hospital she eventually became calm and sensible to the extent that, against medical advice, she was discharged absolutely by a Mental Health Review Tribunal.

On returning to the community she again became tense and despondent. She fell out with her parents, she abused her social workers, and alienated those who would befriend her. She began to mutilate herself even more and a series of informal admissions to psychiatric hospital followed. These were again marked by discordant relationships, violence and impulsive, angry absconding. Interspersed with admissions were a series of court appearances for minor shoplifting. At one such appearance the psychiatrist recommended detention in a regional secure unit. The psychiatric grounds on that occasion, however, were given as mental illness, i.e. the depression which she seemed to be suffering from at the time. It was felt that whilst hospital admission for the depression could have a clear purpose (alleviation of the depression), admission to treat her personality was unlikely to be successful. In her case, at the time, admitting for treatment of the illness (likely to be short- rather than long-term) was also much more acceptable to the patient. In practice, the admission dealt with both her depressive symptoms and controlled, for a period, her psychopathic behaviour.

There then followed a series of admissions to the unit associated with self-mutilation or expressions of depression from which she would recover and return to the community. The ability of the secure unit to control the patient through physical security and extra attention using nurse management programmes in conjunction with medication (major tranquilizers and monoamine oxidase inhibitors) facilitated her care. Nevertheless her stays were tempestuous and exhausting. With time, however, her behaviour gradually settled to a shadow of its former self.

The case illustrates how doctors use different aspects of the mental disturbance to tackle the case depending on the dangerousness of the situation, the facilities available and the views of the patient. Thus, as in this case, the same mental disturbance (psychopathy with severe affective disturbance) could be dealt with in legal terms either as psychopathy or mental illness and admissions were sometimes best managed informally and sometimes by detention under the Mental Health Act.

Case C

Mr C developed an antisocial personality. He was the last of 10 children of a very poor family. At 4 years he was placed in care in need of care and protection. Various foster parents found him too difficult to manage due to his stealing, deceit and hostility. He was a regular truant and was before the courts innumerable times. He was labelled an 'incorrigible rogue' by 17 years. In his twentieth year he was in the army but was invalided out due to 'mental disability'. He was thought (for reasons which were never clear) to have schizophrenia. Subsequently, in the next few years whenever he was before the court this diagnosis was resurrected and there were a serious of hospital admissions. All doctors reached the conclusion after admission that he did not suffer from mental illness though he was a tense, anti-authoritarian man, excessively suspicious and mistrustful of others and quite uncooperative with hospital. When his tension was extremely high he did seem, on some occasions, to have brief psychotic periods in which he genuinely appeared to experience paranoid delusions. These psychotic periods very rapidly cleared up (in a few days), once admitted to a ward, leaving everyone unclear as to whether the 'breakdown' had been genuine or was simply malingering. As he got older he became manifestly less tense and more evidently plausible and manipulative but without illness. The point came where further hospital care was refused, for, by this stage, he was using the hospital merely as a free hotel.

The case is of interest because of the brief 'psychotic' episodes. When these occurred they almost always caused disagreement between the staff. Some felt the patient to be malingering, others that the symptoms were genuine. Nevertheless, this 'psychotic' reaction is widely seen in prisons and special hospitals and does seem, in fact, to be genuine.

This situation has to be distinguished from the true schizophrenic who, in late teens or early twenties, has a clear schizophrenic breakdown with a subsequent deterioration in personality. The positive schizophrenic symptoms may become less visible with time, social skills deteriorate due to the severity of the illness, the patient remains (whilst untreated) suspicious, truculent, hostile and uncooperative. Such cases of mental illness may get misdiagnosed as psychopathic disorder. A careful history reveals the difference. In the illness cases there is a clear onset with a subsequent change and deterioration of personality. In the psychopathic disorder, as above, the features of psychopathy are present from an early age and are continuous with the present state. The schizophrenic case requires hospital care and many, though difficult to treat, will respond to appropriate treatment if it is sustained for long enough (months not weeks) and given sufficiently vigorously. The other situation which must be recognized is the 'psychopath' who subsequently develops a full-blown schizophrenic illness as well. This will be recognized by the quality and persistence of the psychotic symptoms. Differentiating it from a brief psychotic breakdown can be difficult initially. However, once recognized, the illness may require hospital treatment.

Case D

D was the second of three children. He came from an intact family though his father was said to be somewhat strict and frightening. He grew into a somewhat nervous, isolated child. He got on badly with teachers, did poorly at work and became involved with delinquent boys. He had brushes with the police but there were no convictions. Because of his nervousness and poor school performance he was referred to the Child Guidance Clinic and educational psychologist but without improvement. After leaving school he had several jobs as a semi-skilled worker but was unable to settle. He remained reserved, quiet and anxious with no special friends and a gross inability to form adult friendships. He became aware in his teens of an urge to indecently expose himself and of sadistic paedophilic feelings. As he got older he began a series of increasingly violent sexual assaults on pre-pubertal children. These began with seductive approaches but escalated to include physical intimidation and culminate in a savage sexual attack. At psychiatric interview, during remand, he described the development of his sadistic paedophilic thoughts and his dislike of them and requested psychiatric assistance. Consultation took place with psychiatrists from special hospital. The court was advised that D suffered from psychopathic disorder. His sexual offending was perceived as a symptom of his disturbed personality. A recommendation was made (and accepted by the courts) that D should be sent to a special hospital on a hospital order with a restriction order unlimited in time because of his dangerousness.

There are of course many similar subjects with many similar backgrounds who receive a prison sentence. The extent to which this is so needs to be studied but chance seems to play a considerable part in what happens. In this case, had D gone to prison, then it is possible that he would have been referred for treatment in prison, or even, (rather rare) transferred from prison to a hospital. Where the subject makes it clear by word or deed that he is not motivated to change his behaviour, treatment is unlikely to be offered.

The treatment of adults with psychopathic disorder

In 1959 at the time of the introduction of the legal term 'psychopathic disorder' there was considerable optimism that these disorders could be treated. Disillusionment has now set in and there is, at present, considerable pessimism about the psychiatrist's ability to treat those who fall within the psychopathic disorder group. It can be shown that the conduct displayed by a subject will improve in the appropriate setting. Unfortunately, there is little evidence that this improvement is maintained (other than for a relatively short time) once the subject leaves the helpful setting, although it is known that the disturbed behaviour will die down with age. Consequently, many psychopaths were detained in hospital simply to prevent re-offending. It is now questioned whether open-ended hospital detention is the way to do this[17]. Indeed, since the Judicial Review ruling (*R* v. *Cannon's Park Mental Health Review Tribunal, ex parte A, Times Law Report* 24.8.93) that tribunals should discharge those detained suffering from psychopathic disorder who are no longer amenable to treatment, prolonged detention of this type may no longer be legal. The Appeal Court has yet to judge on the issue (see page 60). This section will describe various examples of the treatment approaches which have been tried.

Treatment in prison

Historically prisons in many countries have tried various approaches to reform or rehabilitate the recidivist criminal using religious teaching, education, inculcating a work ethic, punitive methods, etc. Psychiatric approaches are typified by the following strategies.

(a) Herstedvester Treatment Centre, Denmark
This centre, opened in the 1930s, was a forerunner of prisons attempting to treat psychopaths by psychotherapeutic means. It was run by a psychiatrist, Dr Sturrup, and based on therapeutic community principles. Originally it relied heavily on the effect of an indeterminate sentence to motivate prisoners to take part so that they could earn their release by improving. The prison claimed to produce long-term improvements in its clients[18]. However, a comparative study, described in the Butler Committee Report[3], showed that there was no difference in the final re-offending rate of prisoners from Herstedvester compared to similar prisoners from an ordinary prison – despite the apparent improvement during treatment.

(b) Grendon Underwood Prison, England
This 200-bedded prison, planned in the 1930s, was set up in 1964 in the belief that criminality could be due to a neurosis which could be treated.

In practice, the prison was used for the treatment, by group therapy, of those offenders with psychopathic disorders who were able to make use of groups and were already serving a prison sentence. Referral to Grendon Prison is made after conviction by the prison medical service with the final selection being made by Grendon staff and based on the prisoner's intelligence, articulateness, willingness to accept groups and evidence of some personal achievement. Gunn[7] showed that attitudes and behaviour improved at Grendon compared with that in other prisons but that the beneficial effect of Grendon's regime was counteracted by the environment to which the prisoner returns on release. It was found that chance factors in the community (occupation, marriage) after release were as important in the ultimate outcome as the experience of Grendon itself. Overall, after ten years in the community, the re-offending rate of ex-Grendon inmates was the same as that of an equivalent group from ordinary prison[19] although the better-motivated and more intelligent may have been helped more. As a result, the regime has been modified. Treatment is now being tried with a more heterogenous group of inmates with psychopathic disorder.

(c) C Wing, Parkhurst Prison, England

This wing caters for men with psychopathic disorder characterized by high levels of tension, emotional lability, violence and disturbed behaviour (self-mutilation, impulsive attacks, tension-reducing destruction). Such men are unable to cope with ordinary prison regime and are too disordered (too impulsive or aggressive) to make a success of Grendon Prison. The regime aims to do no more than help these very disordered psychopathic inmates through their sentence. This is accomplished by being more flexible and giving more attention (medication and counselling) than in ordinary prison. The overall clinical impression is that violent and disruptive incidents are substantially reduced during the man's stay in the wing. There is no study of the long-term effects of the wing. A study of a similar unit in Barlinnie Prison, Scotland showed a rapid reduction in violent behaviour in the unit and a suggestion of reduced re-offending afterwards[20].

Treatment in hospital

(a) Conventional hospital

A conventional hospital tends to admit those with psychopathic disorder during periods of crises, i.e. during periods of depression, high anxiety or psychosis and this may be useful to prevent harm being done by the patient to himself or those around him. However, most hospitals find that they are unable to tolerate such patients on a long-term basis because of persistent disruptive, anti-authoritarian behaviour which they are unable to modify. It may be a reflection of this that there has been a reduction in recent years in the number of hospital orders made by the courts on those with psychopathic disorder.

(b) Special hospital
There has been a fall in the rate of admission of patients with psychopathic disorder so now only some 30 patients with psychopathic disorder are admitted to special hospital annually. This represents fewer than one in every two thousand offenders convicted of violent or sexual crimes. Grounds et al.[21] has described the treatment in Broadmoor Hospital of one group with psychotherapeutic methods, education, sexual and social training within the setting of the total institution. He lists the problems of treating such patients and discusses the view that a hospital disposal may not be the most appropriate one. Mawson[22] has argued that a prison disposal would be best with transfer of the patient from prison to hospital for a period of treatment when indicated. Dell et al.[16] found that in the absence of clear 'illness' criteria, the time spent in special hospital by psychopaths tends simply to reflect the severity of the offence.

(c) Regional secure units
Psychopathic disorder as the principal diagnosis forms a small proportion of the diagnoses of patients admitted to a regional secure unit. The bulk of these patients are admitted from a special hospital as part of an attempt to rehabilitate them into the community. A few may come directly from the courts, and these will tend to be in the borderline personality group. The psychiatric approach is similar to that in the special hospital. The extra attention and control which can be provided seems to be effective in reducing disturbed behaviour at least in the institution, as already demonstrated by Craft[23] in the field of subnormality.

(d) Henderson Hospital
This unit in the grounds of the Belmont Hospital, Sutton, was developed to treat patients with psychopathic disorder within the NHS. It does best with articulate, intelligent, younger psychopaths who have not been very criminal or violent. There is no controlled trial to demonstrate its efficacy, though claims have been made that it has a beneficial effect[24]. The unit is most famous for the development, under Maxwell Jones, of its therapeutic community approach.

(e) Van der Hoeven Clinic, Utrecht, Holland
This is one of several famous Dutch clinics run by psychiatrists to treat offenders with psychopathic disorder. This particular clinic is a therapeutic community (within a physically secure unit) which employs group psychotherapy in combination with educational rehabilitation and resocialization programmes. It is supported by a good parole system, and the prisoners stay there for about two years. Although the clinic asserts

that it is successful in producing long-term as well as short-term change, there is a dearth of controlled studies to support this claim.

Management in probation hostels

It has been shown that probation hostels differ from one another in their ability to improve probationers' behaviour whilst in the hostel. A lesson learned from the study was that hostels with a caring but firm atmosphere were the most effective[25]. The least effective were the permissive or negligent and uncaring hostels. Unfortunately, the improvements seen in the behaviour of the probationers during their stay in the hostel were not sustained after leaving. Two or three years later the re-offending rate was the same whatever the original hostel.

Individual psychotherapeutic treatments in the community

The most famous work on this approach was the Cambridge-Somerville Study, USA.[26]. It was an attempt to see if individual counselling would prevent the development of antisocial personality amongst youths at risk. The experiment compared a treated and untreated group. Treated youths were meant to see the same counsellor on a voluntary basis every week. Unfortunately, the experiment was disrupted by World War II as the counsellors were enlisted. As far as could be worked out in broad terms, however, those who received counselling did not do better than those who did not.

Other individual clinical approaches

Psychotherapy with borderline and narcissistic personality disorder has been reviewed by Higgitt and Fonagy[27]. The principal lesson is the need for a long-term commitment. Workers with each technique claim successes, but it is not clear which approach will work in any individual case without a trial.

Reality therapy
This is an attempt to teach social skills in a very practical way to delinquents dealing with here-and-now problems, rather than attempt to do any interpretative psychotherapy.

Supportive counselling
This is the backbone of probation and outpatient services. Firmness applied tactfully, coupled with acceptance and warmth is probably the most effective style, though there is no evidence that it can produce long-

term change. Clinically, it seems to be helpful to some subjects in assisting them in staying out of trouble – as long as they are receiving the counselling.

Psychoanalysis

Intensive psychotherapy has been used with some claims for success with borderline personality disorder. The treatment with psychoanalysis – which is very difficult – has to be very long-term and relies principally on interpreting transference reactions.

Family therapy

This intervention will expose family dynamics and appears to the workers involved to be a very powerful tool. Empirical studies of relative effectiveness are lacking.

Group therapy

A number of workers have found group work to be a useful approach and it is commonly used in institutions where personality disordered subjects are detained.

Cognitive therapies

Where anger and violence is a problem, psychological therapies based on the recognition of automatic thoughts combined with relaxation, general cognition and behavioural modification techniques, have achieved some success at modifying the violent behaviour – at least in the short term[28].

Treatment with medication

Medication may be helpful in management and treatment of those with a personality disorder characterized by tension and anxiety (e.g. secondary psychopaths or borderline personality)[29].

Anxiolytics

These may be useful in the short term for periods of anxiety or tension but paradoxical reactions have been reported with benzodiazepines leading to disinhibition and aggression[30].

Antidepressants

Persistent dysphoric mood and the atypical depression of the borderline state may respond to monoamine oxidase inhibitors[31] or to serotonin re-uptake inhibitors[32]. Lithium carbonate has appeared useful in some emotionally unstable aggressive patients[33] and aggressive mentally subnormal patients[23].

Major tranquillizers

Any of the major tranquillizers may be useful in reducing persistent tension; sometimes they seem to work in relatively low doses (e.g. flupenthixol 20 mg per month or less), but at times of high tension large doses may be required. Recent trials have shown the value of low-dose haloperidol[34] and thioxanthene[35] for long-term management.

Stimulants

It has long been known that amphetamines can produce a reduction in feelings of tension in some psychopaths[36,37] but the dangers of abuse and addiction outweigh any advantages. There have been some claims that pemoline is useful in the same way, reducing feelings of tension and dysphoria with a reduction in disturbed behaviour[38]. It has been postulated that the stimulants are useful where the sociopathic behaviour can be understood as an adult development of childhood hyperactivity with attention defect – so-called 'minimal brain dysfunction' in adults[38].

Anticonvulsants

In a double-blind-crossover trial, carbamazepine appeared[39] to reduce the incidence and seriousness of dyscontrol episodes (angry outbursts, violence, self-mutilation, suicide attempts) in 16 females with borderline personality – though the trial was only over six weeks. The authors point to the hypothesis that links the episodes of dyscontrol with a disorder of the limbic system and the similarity with the episodic dyscontrol syndrome.

There seems no way of recognizing beforehand which drug will be useful, if at all, in any particular case. Sometimes one does have the experience of finding a successful drug to help a patient over a long period of time which leads to improved behaviour and well-being. However, the gains with medication may be partial and only short-lived and other undesirable antisocial behaviour may continue. Nevertheless, drug treatment combined with psychological treatments (group therapies, individual therapy, behavioural-based nursing management programmes) form the cornerstone of the hospital management of the psychopath high in neurotic symptoms, tension and dysphoric mood[40,41]

References

(1) Walker, N. & McCabe, S. (1973) *Crime and Insanity in England*: Volume Two: *New Solutions and New Problems*. Edinburgh University Press, Edinburgh.
(2) Lewis, A. (1974) Psychopathic disorder: a most elusive category. *Psychological Medicine* **4**, 133–40.
(3) Home Office and Department of Health and Social Security (1975) *Report of*

the Committee on Mentally Abnormal Offenders (Butler Report). Cmnd. 6244. HMSO, London.

(4) Coid, J.W. (1992) DSM-III diagnosis in criminal psychopaths: a way forward. *Criminal Behaviour and Mental Health* **2**, 78–94.

(5) Faulk, M. (1976) A psychiatric study of men serving a sentence in Winchester Prison. *Medicine, Science and the Law* **16**, 244–51.

(6) Coid, J. (1984) How many psychiatric patients in prison? *British Journal of Psychiatry* **145**, 78–86.

(7) Gunn, J., Robertson, G., Dell, S. & Way, C. (1978) *Psychiatric Aspects of Imprisonment.* Academic Press, London.

(8) Walton, H.J. & Presley, A.S. (1973) Use of the category system in the diagnosis of abnormal personality. *British Journal of Psychiatry* **122**, 259–68.

(9) Presley, A.S. & Walton, H.J. (1973) Dimensions of abnormal personality. *British Journal of Psychiatry* **122**, 269–76.

(10) Tyrer, P. (1992) Flamboyant, erratic, dramatic, borderline, antisocial, sadistic, narcissistic, histrionic and impulsive personality disorders: who cares which? *Criminal Behaviour and Mental Health* **2**, 95–104.

(11) Blackburn, R. (1992) Criminal behaviour, personality disorder and mental illness: the origins of confusion. *Criminal Behaviour and Mental Health* **2**, 66–77.

(12) Henderson, D.K. (1939) *Psychopathic States.* Norton, New York.

(13) Cleckley, H. (1976) *The Mask of Sanity* (5th ed). The C V Mosby Co., St Louis.

(14) Gutheil, T.G. (1989) Borderline personality disorder. Boundary violations and patient–therapist sex: medicolegal pitfalls *American Journal of Psychiatry* **146**, 597–602.

(15) Coid, J.W. (1993) An affective syndrome in psychopaths with borderline personality disorder? *British Journal of Psychiatry* **162**, 641–50.

(16) Dell, S., Robertson, G. & Parker, E. (1987) Detention in Broadmoor: factors in length of stay. *British Journal of Psychiatry* **150**, 824–7.

(17) Robertson, G. (1992) Objections to the present system. *Criminal Behaviour and Mental Health* **2**, 114–23.

(18) Sturrup, G. (1968) *Treating the Untreatable, Chronic Criminals at Herstedvester.* John Hopkins, Baltimore.

(19) Robertson, G. & Gunn, J. (1987) A ten-year follow-up of men discharged from Grendon Prison. *British Journal of Psychiatry* **151**, 674–8.

(20) Cooke, D.J. (1989) Containing violent prisoners. *British Journal of Criminology* **29**, 129–43.

(21) Grounds, A.T., Quayle, M.T., France, J., Brett, T., Cox, M. & Hamilton, J.R. (1987) A unit for 'psychopathic disorder' patients in Broadmoor Hospital. *Medicine, Science and the Law* **27**, 21–31.

(22) Mawson, D. (1983) Psychopaths in special hospitals. *Bulletin of the Royal College of Psychiatrists* **7**, 178–81.

(23) Craft, M. (1984) Should one treat or gaol psychopaths. In Craft, M. and Craft, A. (eds) *Mentally Abnormal Offenders.* Ballière Tindall, Eastbourne.

(24) Whiteley, J.S. (1975) The psychopath and his treatment. *British Journal of Psychiatry* **121**, 159–59.

(25) Sinclair, I.A.C. (1971) *Hostels for Probationers.* HMSO, London.

(26) McCord, W. & McCord, J. (1959) *Origins of Crime.* Columbia University Press, New York.

(27) Higgitt, A. & Fonagy, P. (1992) Psychotherapy in borderline and narcissistic personality disorder. *British Journal of Psychiatry* **161**, 23–43.

(28) Levey, S. & Howells, K. (1990) Anger and its management. *Journal of Forensic Psychiatry* **1**, 305–27.

(29) Stein, G. (1992) Drug treatment of the personality disorders. *British Journal of Psychiatry* **161**, 167–84.

(30) Editorial (1975) Tranquillizers causing aggression. *British Medical Journal* **1**, 113–14.

(31) Cowdry, W.L. & Gardner, D.L. (1988) Pharmacotherapy of borderline personality disorder. *Archives of General Psychiatry* **45**, 111–19.

(32) Markovitz, P.J., Calabrese, J.R., Schulz, S.C. & Meltzer, H.Y. (1991) Fluoxitine in the treatment of borderline and schizotypal personality disorders. *American Journal of Psychiatry* **148**, 1064–7.

(33) Sheard, M.H., Marini, J.L., Bridgesci, C.I. & Wagner, E. (1976) The effect of lithium on impulsive aggressive behaviour in man. *American Journal of Psychiatry* **133**, 1409–13.

(34) Soloff, P.H., George, A., Nathan, R.S., Schulz, P.M., Ulrich, R.F. & Perel, J.M. (1986) Progress in the pharmacotherapy of borderline disorders. *Archives of General Psychiatry* **43**, 691–700.

(35) Goldberg, S.C., Schulz, S.C., Schulz, P.M., Resnick, R.J., Harner, R.M. & Friedel, R.O. (1986) Borderline and schizotypal personality disorders treated with low-dose thiothixene vs placebo. *Archives of General Psychiatry* **43**, 680–6.

(36) Hill, D. (1944) Amphetamine in psychopathic states. *British Journal of Addiction* **44**, 50–4.

(37) Richmond, J.S., Young, J.R. & Groves, J.E. (1978) Violent dyscontrol responsive to d-amphetamine. *American Journal of Psychiatry* **135**, 365–6.

(38) Wender, P.H., Reimherr, F.W. & Wood, D.R. (1981) Attention deficit disorder (minimal brain dysfunction) in adults. *Archives of General Psychiatry* **38**, 449–56.

(39) Gardner, D.L. & Cowdry, R.W. (1986) Positive effects of carbamazepine on behavioural dyscontrol in borderline personality disorder. *American Journal of Psychiatry* **143**, 519–22.

(40) Editorial (1986) Management of borderline personality disorder. *Lancet* **ii**, 846–7.

(41) Gunderson, J.G. (1986) Pharmacotherapy for patients with borderline personality disorder. *Archives of General Psychiatry* **43**, 698–700.

Chapter 11

Mental Retardation and Forensic Psychiatry

Introduction

The purpose of this chapter is to discuss:

(1) The clinical concept of mental retardation and its relation to the present legal concept of mental impairment (Mental Health Act 1983) and to the older legal term, mental subnormality (Mental Health Act 1959).
(2) The degree to which mental retardation contributes to offending.
(3) The pattern of particular crimes associated with mental retardation.
(4) Case histories to describe the ways in which the medical and legal systems interact.
(5) The facilities available for the mentally retarded offender.

Definition

The diagnosis of mental retardation in both the ICD 10 and the DSM IIIR requires an intelligence quotient (IQ) of less than 70 in regard to general intellectual functioning, accompanied by concurrent deficits or impairments in adaptive behaviour. The ICD 10 and the DSM IIIR both point out that where there are specific cognitive handicaps, e.g. in speech, the IQ assessment must be made on areas outside that handicap. The diagnosis is made by the level of functioning, without regard to its nature or causation. Any IQ tests should be validated for the particular culture of the subject. The DSM IIIR specifically requires that the onset be before the age of 18 years.

Mental retardation in both classificatory systems is divided into:

(1) Mild mental retardation (IQ 50–69)
(2) Moderate mental retardation (IQ 35–49)
(3) Severe mental retardation (IQ 20–34)
(4) Profound mental retardation (IQ under 20)

Where there is additional psychiatric disturbance or evidence of physical disease or injury, then an additional diagnosis must be made. Where there is a strong presumption of mental retardation due to the patient being untestable for various reasons (e.g. lack of co-operation) then the diagnosis of unspecified mental retardation may be used in both classifications. There are enormous variations in people's ability to cope in society, regardless of IQ. Some people with mild degrees of handicap may well be able to sustain themselves without assistance in society, people with greater degrees of handicap may only require minimal basic support. Retardation in itself does not automatically dictate whether help is required or what sort of help. The revolution which has occurred in this field at the present time is due to the realization that the mentally retarded can be more independent than had been previously accepted. It is now appreciated that the condition does not, in itself, demand the full panoply of medical supervision or nursing care.

Mental retardation and the Mental Health Act 1983

The question has to be asked: 'How the law should deal with offenders who are also mentally retarded'. Society has traditionally protected those with retardation from the full vigour of the law, allowing subnormality of intelligence to be submitted as a mitigating factor or, if severe enough, grounds for finding a person not guilty by reason of insanity. Whilst a number of mildly mentally retarded people are admitted to prison and do cope there it would be grotesque to imprison the more severely handicapped. On the other hand, there is a strongly held view that mental retardation should not, on its own, be grounds for committal to a psychiatric hospital unless there is a likelihood that some good will come of it. Too many people in the past have been sent to hospital, often on the basis of quite minor offences and held there for many years without any clear benefit. Similarly, there has been a tendency to classify people as subnormal on the basis of social inadequacy, lack of achievement and delinquency, even though they are not, strictly speaking, mentally retarded (i.e. do not have an IQ below 70). Parker[1] found over half the detained so-called severely subnormal and subnormal in a special hospital had IQs above the category they had been placed in. It might be argued that the mildly mentally handicapped, at least, should have the right of choice of a simple, quick penal measure rather than prolonged hospitalization. The Mental Health Act 1983 tried to resolve these conflicting forces. The new terms 'mental impairment' and 'severe mental impairment' were introduced with the intention to limit the effects of the Mental Health Act to the few mentally retarded people for whom detention in hospital is essential for treatment and for whom prison should be avoided[2]. Mental impairment means (in the Mental Health Act 1983) a state of arrested or incomplete development of mind (not amounting to severe mental impairment) which includes a *significant* impairment of intelligence and social functioning and is associated with abnormally aggressive or seriously irresponsible conduct. Severe mental impairment means (in the Mental Health Act 1983) a state of arrested or incomplete development of mind which includes a *severe* impairment of intelligence and social functioning and is associated with abnormally aggressive or irresponsible conduct. 'Significant' and 'severe' are undefined but the former seems to be, by usage, an IQ of 60–70 and the latter an IQ below 60. Falling into the definition of severe mental impairment is sufficient for a hospital order to be recommended. However, in the case of mental impairment, a hospital order cannot be recommended unless it is also the case that treatment is likely to alleviate or prevent deterioration in the subject's condition. It seems possible, therefore, that some mildly retarded subjects will be given penal sentences after offending on the grounds that a hospital has nothing to offer in the way of help, unless a guardianship or probation order is appropriate (see Chapter 3).

Of course, if an offender with mental retardation also suffers from a psychiatric illness (e.g. a psychosis) then that illness may form the basis of the psychiatric recommendation for compulsory detention.

Mental retardation and offending

The studies by West[3] show that a low IQ is one of the five major factors associated with the development of delinquent behaviour. Subjects with severe mental retardation are unlikely to be free in the community to get into trouble as they tend to be in the care of their families or institutions. Some very disturbed, severely impaired patients (often in hospital or residential communities) are violent or destructive. They may, through the sympathies of those around them, escape formal legal prosecution but steps may be taken to place them in appropriate specialist units, detained under the Mental Health Act. The most severe may be transferred to a special hospital. Subjects with mild retardation, on the other hand, may be much more mobile in the community and therefore in a position to offend.

A bigger problem arises from the group in the IQ range 70–85, the borderline subnormal group. Whilst most such subjects cope normally in the community, a number do not – due, perhaps, to a combination of personality problems exacerbated by dull intelligence. The end-result of their inadequacies and frustration may be antisocial activity. The borderline group does not fall within any of the Mental Health Act categories who may be detained and can only be dealt with under the Mental Health Act if they have a mental illness or a psychopathic disorder.

Estimating the extent to which those with lower intelligence contribute to the criminal statistics may be made in a number of ways. Studies of populations of children show a consistent statistical association between a low IQ and offending[4]. West found that 20% of those with an IQ below 90 become delinquent compared with only 9% of those with an IQ of 91–98 and 2% of those above 110. Delinquents on average have an IQ at least five points below the population norm. Studies of penal populations show a wide variation (1–45%) in estimates of the incidence of subnormality[5], though this may reflect the quality of the diagnosis, the prisons assessed, the year in which the assessment was done, and the quality of the services which might remove the mentally retarded from the penal system. Relying only on prison studies would produce debatable conclusions about the importance of retardation in criminality[6].

It has been argued that the mentally retarded may, in fact, not offend any more but simply be caught more easily. Although this may be a factor, self-report studies such as those by West[3] support the view that the mentally retarded do commit more offences. It has been thought that as there is a statistical association between low IQ and other criminogenic factors such as large families and low social status or associated physical problems, that there was no true effect of low IQ. Careful matching of samples, however, shows that a low IQ is a criminogenic factor in its own right[3]. It has been shown that a low IQ increases the chance of behavioural problems before the age of 3 years or before educational failure[7]. The combination of low IQ and behavioural problems will enhance the chances of a child then doing badly at school, with subsequent loss of esteem, emotional disturbance and antagonism to the school. Mental retardation may also be a criminogenic factor because the subject is less able, intellectually, to cope with stresses and therefore more easily frustrated and disappointed. It is possible that this leads to a greater inclination to react antisocially when things go wrong.

It is generally asserted that the mentally retarded, although capable of any offence, are more likely to commit sex or fire raising offences. This assertion derives largely from clinical practice and a study of the offences committed by mentally retarded offenders admitted to hospital[8] and should be treated with some caution, therefore.

Medicolegal assessment of the mentally retarded

The diagnosis may have been made before the offence was committed. However, any testing that has to be done requires great care and the services of a psychologist experienced in the field. It is very easy to obtain a false result due to the offender failing to give proper attention to the task. In a case of suspected mental retardation it is also important to consider the possibility of brain damage and chromosomal defects, as well as the possibility of a superimposed mental illness presenting in an unusual way[9].

In taking the history it has to be borne in mind that the subject is likely to be an unreliable historian with poor ability to recount past events accurately; objective accounts are, therefore, imperative. Considerable care must be taken not to intimidate or lead the subject in giving a false account. The Police and Criminal Evidence Act 1984 dictates that precautions to avoid these traps must be taken in police interviews, including having an independent person present at interview, e.g. a social worker or solicitor for the mentally retarded, and a psychiatrically experienced person present for the mentally ill.

The following questions must be asked:

(1) Is the offender fit to plead?

The answer cannot simply reflect the IQ score. It requires an examination of the offender's understanding (see Chapter 3). It is only likely to arise in cases of severe mental retardation. If the offence is a minor one it may be best dealt with under section 37 (3), Mental Health Act 1983 (making an order without a conviction).

(2) Is the mentally retarded patient also mentally impaired or severely mentally impaired within the Act?

If he is, then the question of whether a hospital or a guardianship order should be used will be raised; which is recommended will depend in part on the facilities available. The decision can only be made after discussion with the key workers in the field, the consultant in mental handicap and the social services department.

(3) Can the mental retardation be used as a mitigating factor?

The court will be anxious to assist and will usually be willing (the safety of the public allowing) to accept a psychiatric recommendation. In the case of an offender with mild mental retardation where mental impairment is not diagnosed then contact with a psychiatrist or other agency may be arranged as a condition of probation if it is felt that this will be helpful.

(4) In the more serious offences the question of insanity and, after homicide, diminished responsibility will have to be considered (see Chapter 3). The mental retardation would have to be severe before a plea of insanity would be successful. On the other hand, lesser degrees of mental retardation would be a condition which could form the grounds for a plea of diminished responsibility. The ultimate disposal will reflect the offence, the offender and the assessment of his dangerousness and treatability.

Case histories

The following histories illustrate the interaction between the law and the mentally retarded offender.

Case A Sexual aggression and mental retardation

Mr A was charged as his third offence (when aged 20 years) with the attempted rape of a 12-year-old girl. He had induced her to go into a field where he had demanded, with threats, that she undress. He then attempted to rape her. At this point he was discovered by passers-by and was duly arrested.

His first sexual offence had occurred 9 months before when he had indecently touched a woman in a supermarket. He received a conditional discharge for the offence. He committed a second offence three months later when he grabbed the breast of a woman in the street. At his appearance in court on that occasion it was decided, because of his repeated sexual offences and his demeanour in court (which suggested mental handicap), to seek a psychiatric opinion.

It was already known to the court, through a probation officer's report, that A came from a delinquent family. A's intellectual difficulties had been discovered at primary school and he had been sent to a school for the educationally subnormal until he was 16. He was found at the age of 11 years to have an IQ of 65. At school and at home he was a shy and socially awkward boy, much less bright than his siblings. He had been unable to obtain permanent work after leaving the school and had drifted into the habit of mixing with the fringes of a delinquent group and drinking heavily. At his psychiatric assessment after his second offence he was perceived as being a mildly mentally retarded young man lacking in confidence and social skills which, it was believed, accounted for his clumsy sexual behaviour. The alcohol abuse was also seen as a secondary effect of his poor social integration and was understood to be a disinhibiting factor at the time of his offences.

At the time of the second offence the possibilities open to the psychiatrist were as follows:

(1) To recommend treatment in hospital under section 37 on the grounds of mental impairment if the psychiatrist had also believed treatment would be likely to alleviate or prevent deterioration. His aggression, however, was not thought to be serious enough at that stage to require detention in hospital. A hospital order was not therefore recommended.

(2) To recommend treatment as an outpatient as a condition of probation. This was the option chosen. The psychiatrist believed that the counselling which he and the probation officer could provide, plus the increase in self-esteem which the patient might acquire from the interest taken in him, would be sufficient to assist the patient in preventing him re-offending.

(3) To recommend no psychiatric treatment. Technically under the Mental Health Act 1983 this would be possible – despite a diagnosis of mental retardation and impairment – and should be done if there is no confidence that psychiatric treatment would be useful. The court would then have to decide between the many options (custodial or non-custodial) remaining to it, depending on the severity of the offence.

The court accepted the recommendation of psychiatric treatment as a condition of probation and the patient began to attend. He proved regular in his attendance but remained shy and inarticulate. Four months later he was arrested for the attempted rape. On this occasion it became clear that he had been having fantasies of paedophilic rape for many years. He admitted to carrying a knife with him and of having fantasies of using it during a rape. It was clear therefore that some form of containment was required to protect others until his condition came under control.

The choices now open to the psychiatrist were as follows:

(1) To recommend a hospital order to a local subnormality hospital under section 37. The local psychiatrist believed that there was a grave danger that in an open hospital the offender would give way to his impulses again and attack someone on the hospital site. There was, therefore, no proposal for a local admission.

(2) Recommend a hospital order to a special hospital. The advantages include the safety of the procedure and the availability at special hospitals of psychologists with special experience in the treatment of sexual disorder as well as in the treatment of social malfunctioning. However, a difference of opinion arose between the local psychiatrist and the psychiatrist at the special hospital. The latter believed that the patient's behaviour could be understood as a reaction to the frustration arising from his social situation and intelligence. He believed that the patient would be best helped by admission to a mixed ward in an ordinary subnormality hospital. As a result of the disagreement between the doctors, the Department of Health and Social Security remained unconvinced that a special hospital bed was required and they refused to offer one.

> In the absence of a bed being made available either in a local or a special hospital the patient was given a prison sentence. The prison doctors felt it unreasonable to put the patient in the main prison and he was protected by being kept in the prison hospital. An educational programme and psychiatric counselling was arranged. At the same time an application for his transfer to a special hospital under section 47 (Mental Health Act 1983) was made emphasizing his escalating violence in the community, his mental retardation and his positive response to help given to him in prison. On this occasion the Department of Health and Social Security relented and a bed was made available to which he was transferred under section 47 of the Mental Health Act with a restriction order under section 49.
>
> In the special hospital general educational classes were continued and an intensive course of sexual education was begun. He was also given treatment by a behaviour therapist for his unwanted sexual impulses and he became involved in social skills training. When the date of his release from prison was reached, the doctors recommended his continued detention in hospital and the section 47/48 was converted into a nominal section 37 (without restrictions). In due course (some two years later) he reported the

hoped for improvement (loss of fantasies about small children and rape, replaced by fantasies of normal adult sexual intercourse). His general behaviour in hospital and his interaction with others indicated maturation in a social sense. He had also benefited from his formal ordinary education.

As he was now detained on a section 37 without a restriction order, arrangements for his transfer from the special hospital could be made without consulting the Home Office. He was transferred to the regional secure unit as a stepping stone to the community. It was assumed that intensive supervision in a regional secure unit would provide a check on his apparent improvement before his final return home, remembering the level of risk in such a case (see Chapter 7).

Comment

The case illustrates a number of points. The history demonstrates, what is often the case, that the misbehaviour is often associated with a number of factors of which low IQ is but one. In A's case, the other factors included low social class, large family (five children or more), a history of delinquency in the family and excessive use of alcohol. The factors underlying his sexual offending included his lack of social skills, his inability to get a girlfriend, coupled with the general frustrations of his life. He aspired to a normal existence but his failure to succeed produced tension and anger which was discharged when the attacked person became the focus of all his rage. These psychodynamic factors are, of course, seen in people with disordered personalities at all levels of intelligence. In most cases where the intelligence is normal the subject would not be protected from the legal process. A few might be picked out and diverted to a psychiatric field (though not always with a particularly good outcome) but the majority would not. This case shows how the law allows the mentally retarded to be protected from the full vigour of the penal sanction yet in the end the offender was detained for longer than his prison sentence.

Case B Theft and mental retardation

Miss B, aged 21, had an IQ of 67. She was referred to a regional secure unit because of persistent stealing, violence to others and self-mutilation. Attempts to modify her behaviour in conventional settings had been a failure. She had been supervised and treated at home, in subnormality hospital, in day centres and in hostels. In all these settings her misbehaviour had continued. She was admitted to the regional secure unit under section 3 of the Mental Health Act 1983 on the grounds of mental impairment.

Miss B had two successful older sisters of normal intelligence. Her father had been a steady worker on whom had fallen the task of bringing up his family after his wife developed a chronic severe illness when B was aged 2. His wife died when B was aged 17.

Miss B was slow to develop in walking and speech. She was found to be educationally subnormal at primary school and transferred to a school for the educationally subnormal when she was aged 8 years, staying there until she was aged 17 years. From an early age she showed behavioural difficulties including stealing and tempers. She was referred to a child guidance clinic but without improvement. Her behaviour in the community (particularly stealing from shops and at home) all became much worse after the death of her mother. She was then referred to a general psychiatrist and admitted to hospital. At the time of the admission it was thought that she was depressed following the death of her mother and was treated as such but without any improvement. In the psychiatric hospital she showed very egocentric behaviour with extremely poor tolerance of frustration. She was very manipulative and demanding in her dealings with others, totally dishonest and given to bullying and intimidation. She stole flagrantly and persistently. She ate voraciously and became grossly obese. She was tried again at home but her bad behaviour continued.

Day hospitals had no effect on her intolerable behaviour. She was then admitted to a local subnormality hospital but again the institution was unable to cope and she was therefore referred to the regional secure unit.

Her care in the regional secure unit depended on a programme of nurse management based on the principles of behaviour modification and designed and supervised by a psychologist. Gradually, her general behaviour improved, there was a reduction in her neurotic symptoms of tension and lability of mood and she formed some good relationships. She was introduced back into the community where she managed with a lot of support, though with a certain amount of misbehaviour. Eventually she was thought stable enough (but only just) to try again back in her own home.

Comment

The case again demonstrates how mental retardation may protect the subject from ordinary penal measures. Because of her handicap no one felt it proper to take her to court despite innumerable thefts and attacks on others. Had the police been called to one of the institutions about her behaviour it is extremely unlikely that they would have taken any action. They would have expected the psychiatric services to cope with the case unless her offending became extremely serious. Like patient A, her behaviour and its psychodynamics were not exclusive to those with retardation though her lower intelligence may have made her more vulnerable to the disturbing effects of her mother's illness and death. It has been suggested that her family may have overindulged her because of her handicaps though that sort of suggestion, often made at a late stage, is very difficult to substantiate. As in the previous case, the frustration of trying to lead an ordinary life, whilst being handicapped, may have contributed to her sense of outrage and injustice which played such a part in her stealing and bullying.

Case C Theft and borderline subnormality

Mr C was one of five children from an intact family. His father suffered from epilepsy and was a chronic respiratory invalid. His early development was unremarkable, except that he persistently wet the bed into adult life – despite all forms of therapy. He attended ordinary school but was considered backward and uncooperative. He left school at the age of 15 with no qualifications. He held his first job satisfactorily for some 4 years but then failed to settle into any more work.

He first came to psychiatric notice as a child because of his backwardness at school and bedwetting. He attended child guidance clinic intermittently for some 10 years. During that period his IQ was assessed at 80. As an adult, he was referred to a psychiatrist because of his bedwetting and depressive feelings. In his mid-twenties he was brought to psychiatric notice after being arrested for the theft of female underwear. He had a series of admissions after this because of repeated overdoses, wrist-cutting or complaints of feeling suicidal. In between admissions he was supported through outpatient clinics.

C was unable to sustain himself in work, or maintain friendships. His social and sexual skills were poor which in part accounted for his stealing female underwear for fetishistic reasons. He experienced periods of despondency and tension which were relieved by overdoses, self-mutilation or heavy drinking. His admissions and outpatient treatments were palliative only. His dullness of intelligence was not severe enough to bring him into the mentally impaired range. His appearances in court were dealt with by probation orders (with or without psychiatric supervision) community orders, or fines.

Case D Violence, depression and mental retardation

Miss D was charged with wounding with intent having attacked her mother with a garden ornament which caused serious head injuries. At the time D believed (falsely) that she, D, had a serious medical complaint and that, as she was going to die, it seemed better to take her mother with her.

She was the only child of a good family. Her early development, both physical and emotional were unremarkable. She attended ordinary school but was school-phobic and used to avoid school for long periods. She was intellectually slow and poor at her work. She left at 15 without qualifications. She was unemployed for some 18 months until she attempted, unsuccessfully, various unskilled jobs.

She married, at the age of 21, a man of 72 who died ten years later. At the age of 31 she married a second time to a man of 60 who died after two years of marriage. At this point Miss D became depressed and her behaviour became very disturbed. She became increasingly irritable and aggressive and began to complain of severe abdominal pain for which no physical cause could be found. She believed she had a terminal illness and this culminated in the attack on her mother.

Her description of the abdominal pain was bizarre: 'My stomach is ripping away', 'the lining of my stomach has passed through me'. She was distraught and agitated when seen on remand. The diagnosis of depression with nihilistic delusions in a mentally retarded girl (IQ 69) was made. She was admitted to psychiatric hospital on section 37 on the grounds of mental illness (depression). She was treated with ECT and antidepressants and made a remarkable recovery.

This case illustrates the interaction between the mental illness and mental retardation and demonstrated the bizarre symptomatology which can occur when the two occur together.

Treatment and management facilities for the mentally retarded offender

Community facilities

Social services
The social services have a responsibility to provide facilities for the mentally retarded in the community. In practice this will include:

(1) Support and guidance from the family.
(2) Provision of residential accommodation, either on a voluntary basis or on a guardianship order. The residential accommodation may include a variety of settings, including staffed homes or hostels, groups homes, sympathetic landladies and adult placement schemes. Social services may also provide day facilities and protected workshops.

Hospital services
The hospital services are increasingly moving to community-based services, the core of which is the community-based hospital unit. This is likely to be a small purpose-built unit in a residential area, staffed by NHS personnel and run on a multidisciplinary basis. Such a unit, if staffed appropriately with skilled supervision, can cope with very disturbed patients.

Local hospital services

Hospitals for the mentally impaired are in a state of flux. The old asylums are being abandoned and replaced by the (generally) much more satisfactory community arrangements, retaining only small units in the hospital for the very handicapped and dependent patient. There has, however, been some unease about the effect of these changes on the care of the mildly mentally retarded offender. The old locked villas which would have accepted such patients in the past are being closed, often with nothing in their place. It is true that the locally based hospital unit can help offenders who are not too disruptive but staff levels are often insufficient to cope with the very disruptive. Because of the growing awareness of this, a number of hospitals have begun to set up small units with appropriate policies and staffing levels aimed at taking on this clinical problem[10]. Treatment is based on practice training, token economy, other behavioural therapy strategies and counselling. Medication for aggressive behaviour (see Chapter 10) and for unwanted sexual behaviour (see Chapter 11) may be useful where psychological approaches are insufficient[11].

Special hospitals

The special hospitals, particularly Rampton and Ashworth (south), have specialized in the care of the mentally retarded. The problem for these hospitals has been overcrowding, slow turnover and relatively low staffing levels, particularly amongst specialized therapists. In a set-up such as these, constant vigilance is required to maintain staff morale and good practices in order to prevent the institutionalization of staff behaviour as well as patients. Allegations of bad practice led to the Review of Rampton Hospital[12] which resulted in 205 recommendations. Further allegation led to the Report of the Committee of Inquiry into Complaints about Ashworth Hospital[13] which concluded that the special hospitals should be closed.

Regional secure units

The regional secure units do seem to accept some mildly mentally retarded offenders – although, in general, they tend to be somewhat shy of this group[14] finding that there is work enough amongst the mentally ill. It is also true that the training of staff in a regional secure unit is usually orientated towards the mentally ill and not to the mentally retarded. At the time of the Butler Committee, there seemed little need for regional secure units for this group because many subnormality hospitals had their own locked wards. The Butler Committee (and Glancy Committee), therefore, seemed to give little thought to the mentally retarded. The need for some special provision was originally identified by the Oxford Regional Health Authority survey[15] which recommended that a special regional secure unit for the mentally retarded offender be provided. Ideas and developments are now occurring[16,17] with new proposals for the mentally impaired[18]. A number of units have shown that they can successfully look after 'medium secure' impaired patients without the panoply of physical security which accompanies many of the regional secure units. The emphasis is on high intensive staffing and good programmes aimed at returning the patient to the community, e.g. Chestnut Drive Unit at Calderstones Hospital; Leander Unit at Langdon Hospital[19].

Penal services

The penal services for adult males makes no special arrangements for the mentally retarded. Ad hoc arrangements may be made as in Case A above and, of course, educational facilities and medical help is widespread in the penal service. In the younger age group (17–21 years) there are young offender institutions which may take a disordered offender who cannot cope with ordinary regimes, e.g. Feltham and Glen Parva Young Offender Institutions have a tradition of psychiatric care for the psychiatrically disordered. The decision to refer a youth to any particular young offender institution would rest with the prison authorities. In summary, the services for the mentally retarded offender are not very good overall at present but there are now signs, after the recent upheaval in the subnormality services, that new and better services will evolve.

References

(1) Parker, E. (1974) *Survey of Incapacity Associated with Mental Handicap at Rampton and Moss Side Special Hospitals.* Special Hospital Research Unit Publication 11, London.

(2) Jones, R. (1985) *Mental Health Act Manual.* Sweet and Maxwell, London.

(3) West, D.J. (1982) *Delinquency, its roots, careers and prospects.* Heinemann, London.

(4) Hirschi, T. & Hindelang, M.J. (1977) Intelligence and delinquency: a revisionist review. *American Sociological Review* **42**, 571–87.

(5) Coid, J. (1984) How many psychiatric patients in prison? *British Journal of Psychiatry* **145**, 78–86.

(6) Craft, M. (1983) Low intelligence, mental handicap and criminality. In Craft, M. and Craft, A. (eds) *Mentally Abnormal Offenders.* Ballière Tindall, Eastbourne.

(7) Rutter, M. & Giller, H. (1983) *Juvenile Delinquency: Trends and Perspectives.* Penguin Books Ltd, Harmondsworth.

(8) Prins, H. (1980) *Offenders, Deviants or Patients? An Introduction to the Study of Socio Forensic Problems.* Tavistock Publications, London.

(9) Hucker, S.J., Day, K.A., George, S. & Roth, M. (1979) Psychosis in mentally handicapped adults. In James, F.E. and Snaith, R.P. (eds) *Psychiatric Illness and Mental Handicap.* Gaskell Press, London.

(10) Day, K. (1988) A hospital-based treatment programme of male mentally handicapped offenders. *British Journal of Psychiatry* **153**, 635–44.

(11) Clarke, D.J. (1989) Antilibidinal drugs and mental retardation: a review. *Medicine, Science and the Law* **29**, 136–46.

(12) Report of the Review of Rampton Hospital (1980). Cmnd. 8073. HMSO, London.

(13) Report of the Committee of Inquiry into Complaints about Ashworth Hospital (1992). Cmnd. 2028. HMSO, London.

(14) Treasaden, I. (1985) Current practice in regional secure units. In Gostin, L. (ed.) *Secure Provision.* Tavistock, London.

(15) Department of Psychiatry, University of Oxford (1976) *A Survey of the Need for Secure Psychiatric Facilities in the Oxford Region.* Oxford Regional Health Authority, Oxford.

(16) Isweran, M.S. & Bardsley, E.M. (1987) Secure facilities for mentally impaired patients. *Bulletin of the Royal College of Psychiatrists* **11**, 52–4.

(17) Major, J., Bhate, M., Firth, H., Graham, A., Knox, P. & Tyrer, S. (1990) Facilities for mentally impaired patients: three years experience of a semi-secure unit. *Psychiatric Bulletin* **14**, 333–35.
(18) Department of Health and Home Office (1992) Review of Health and Social Services for Mentally Disordered Offenders and Others Requiring Similar Services. (Chairman, Dr. J. Reed). HMSO, London.
(19) Johnson, C., Smith, J., Stainer, G. & Donovan, M. (1993) Mildly mentally handicapped offenders: an alternative to custody. *Psychiatric Bulletin* **17**, 199–201.

Chapter 12

Sexual Disorders and Forensic Psychiatry

Introduction

This chapter deals with disorders of sexual preference and gender disturbance. Sexual offences and sexual disorders overlap but are not the same. Rape – perhaps the gravest sexual offence – may be committed in the absence of a sexual disorder, whereas a person with a sexual disorder might not breach the law.

It is specifically stated in the Mental Health Act 1983 (section 1.3) that sexual deviancy (disorder) shall not be recognized as a mental disorder within the meaning of the Act and it cannot be used therefore as the basis for a recommendation for detention under the Act. If the sexual deviancy occurs in conjunction with a disorder which *is* recognized, such as psychopathic disorder, then that disorder can form grounds for detention. Most offenders requiring psychiatric or psychological treatment for a sexual disorder will be dealt with either on a voluntary basis (in prison or in the community) or as a condition of probation.

Normal sexuality

The term 'normal' is used to mean:

(1) Overtly approved by society, or
(2) Statistically common, or
(3) Biologically desirable – in the sense of leading to procreation.

Social and anthropological studies[1,2] indicate clearly that it is statistically common to indulge in a far greater scope of sexual activity than is socially approved. It also shows that the social tolerance of different activities is linked to culture and social level. Homosexuality amongst adults, for example, was against the law in the UK until 1967, and was categorized by psychiatrists as a sexual deviation in the ICD until removed in the ICD 10 in 1992.

Disorders of sexual preference and problems with sexual orientation

The term is applied to a well-defined group of anomalies of sexual inclination and behaviour. Essential features of a true disorder include persistence in time and preference over normal sexual behaviour.

A number of situations may lead to similar behaviour. In these cases the behaviour is transient (termed facultative) and is not the preferred form. For example:

(1) Transient disorder occurring in susceptible people in situations of loneliness.
(2) After disinhibition due to intoxication by alcohol.
(3) As a result of a severe mental illness.
(4) In non-pathological experimentation in the sexually curious. It should be noted that a sexually deviant person may have the capacity to take part in heterosexual activities although preferring the deviant activity, and in some cases a person may pass through a 'deviant' phase until establishing a mature sexual identity.

Classification of sexual disorders and gender identity disorders

Classification is usually by the form of behaviour. The ICD 10 lists the following forms:

(1) Gender identity disorders (F 64)
    F 64.0 Transexualism
    F 64.1 Dual role transvestism (wearing clothes of the opposite sex temporarily for enjoyment without the wish for a sex change and without sexual excitement)
    F 64.2 Gender disorders of childhood
(2) Disorders of sexual preference (F 65)
    F 65.0 Fetishism
    F 65.1 Fetishistic transvestism (wearing articles of the opposite sex to create the appearance of the opposite sex and for sexual arousal)
    F 65.2 Exhibitionism
    F 65.3 Voyeurism
    F 65.4 Paedophilia
    F 65.5 Sadomasochism
    F 65.6 Multiple disorders of sexual preference (having more than one disorder)
    F 65.8 Other disorders of sexual preference (e.g. making obscene phone calls, frotteurism (rubbing up against others in public

places), sexual activity with animals, use of strangulation or anoxia to intensify sexual experience, preference for a partner with an anatomical abnormality).

(3) Psychological and behavioural disorders associated with sexual development and orientation (F 66)

Sexual orientation alone is not to be regarded as a disorder though particular sexual orientations may be problematical for the individual and thus cause distress

F 66.0 Sexual maturation disorder: uncertainty about sexual orientation leading to anxiety and depression

F 66.1 Egodystonic sexual orientation: distress arising because the subject wishes to be of a different orientation

F 66.2 Sexual relationship disorder: distress arises because of difficulties in forming relationships due to the gender identity or sexual preferences

F 66.9 Disorders of sexual preference unspecified.

The DSM IIIR divides the psychosexual disorders into:

(1) Gender identity disorders:
  (302.5) Transexualism
  (302.6) Gender identity disorder of childhood
  (302.85) Gender disorders of adolescence or adulthood – non-transsexual
(2) Paraphilias (sexual disorders)
  (302.81) Fetishism (sexual arousal by objects)
  (302.3) Transvestic fetishism
  (302.2) Paedophilia
  (302.4) Exhibitionism
  (302.83) Sexual masochism (sexual pleasure from receiving pain)
  (302.84) Sexual sadism (sexual pleasure from causing pain)
  (302.89) Psychosexual disorder not otherwise specified e.g. marked feelings of inadequacy in sexuality, confusion about preferred sexual orientation (including egodystonic homo sexuality); distress over repeated sexual conquests involving using people as things to be used.
  (302.9) Atypical paraphilia, e.g. coprophilia (faeces), frotteurism (rubbing), telephone scatologia (lewdness), necrophilia (corpse), zoophilia (animals), urolagnia (enjoying urinating or being urinated on), arousal to odours.

Aetiology of sexual orientation and disorders

The observations and hypotheses about aetiology may be grouped into physiological hypotheses and psychological hypotheses. The whole area of sexuality and deviancy has been reviewed by Bancroft[3]

Physiological hypotheses

The genetic hypothesis
Support for this hypothesis come from twin studies which show higher concordance for homosexuality in monozygotic (40–60%) compared with dizygotic twins, which, in turn, have higher concordance than have ordinary siblings[4]. Monozygotic twins reared apart have some concordance for male homosexuality though not for female[5]. Very recently a region of the X-chromosome has been linked to male homosexuality[6] though some of the homosexual men (7 out of 40) did not have the gene marker. This suggests either that other genes are involved, or that environmental factors or life experiences are formative influences.

Some workers claim to have found abnormalities (smallness) in some hypothalamic nuclei in the anterior hypothalamus of male homosexuals which presumably could be genetically controlled[7]. The size of similar nuclei in rats is dependent on gender.

Prenatal influence
If fetal or newborn animals are given injections of hormones of the opposite sex at certain critical periods in their development then the adult sexual behaviour of those animals may show characteristics of the opposite sex. Giving androgens to female newborn rats causes them to show male mounting behaviour as adults[8]. Giving androgens to fetal female monkeys results in some male-like adult sexual behaviour[8]. It has been hypothesized that a similar mechanism might occur in humans when there is a failure to develop a sexual attraction to the opposite sex. On the other hand, in the more highly evolved humans it seems more likely that psychological mechanisms influence adult sexual behaviour rather than neurological ones.

Abnormal hormone levels in the adult
Failure to be attracted to females has been thought to reflect abnormalities of testosterone[9], such as the finding of a relative excess of etiocholanolone compared to androsterone in the urine of homosexuals. Evidence of such abnormalities is as yet unconvincing with little agreement between studies[3]. The problem may be complicated by the psychological effect of status and assertiveness on testosterone levels. It has been shown[10] that testosterone levels rise in monkeys promoted (artificially) to a position of increased status in the group, i.e. the testosterone level follows the change in social status rather than causing it.

Psychological hypotheses

Unsatisfactory father/close-binding mother
The evidence for an association between homosexuality and the absent or

unsatisfactory father or over protective or close-binding mother has been reviewed by Wakeling[11]. This association has received support from a number of studies on clinic populations and crops up in many of the disorders apart from homosexuality. The psychodynamics were postulated to arise from the absence of a satisfactory father for modelling in combination with an over-protective or close-binding mother. This results in:

(1) Failure to encourage independent, masculine assertiveness.
(2) The encouragement of effeminate behaviour.
(3) Perceiving all females as fear-inducing (the *dentate vagina*).

These theories have not been supported. Controlled studies of non-clinical populations showed that when men had difficulties with their parents the result was neurosis (hence the visit to the clinic) not homosexuality[12,13].

Analytical theory
Classical theory postulates that each child passes through a phase of possessive love for the parent of the opposite sex in rivalry with the parent of the same sex. The male child fears the wrath of his father, the fear of castration. Sexuality is therefore repressed during the latency period. The situation is resolved by coming to terms with the parental 'threat' and developing appropriate attachments outside the family. It is postulated that failure to reach a successful resolution will lead to a distortion of sexual development. The male, fearing the wrath of his rival the father, turns away from women, symbolic of mother, and diverts his sexual drive elsewhere. In chimpanzee colonies young male chimpanzees appease threatening older males by adopting a submissive position by presenting themselves in a sexually receptive posture. It has been postulated that in the same way homosexuality may sometimes be an appeasement of the symbolic threatening male.

Behaviour theory
The core of this hypothesis is that sexual development can be explained by modelling and conditioning. It is known that children brought up assigned to the wrong genetic sex (because of a failure to develop normal sex organs) adopt the gender assigned to them. Green[14], for example, believes that normal male children can similarly develop transvestite tendencies or other disorders as a result of parental conditioning. It has also been postulated that a disorder might arise by sexual arousal coinciding with comforting behaviour. Transvestites often give a history of cross-dressing for pleasure before puberty. The cross-dressing later acquires an erotic quality, possibly by coincidental association with sexual arousal, i.e. by conditioning.

Masculine insecurity

West[15] has argued that feelings of masculine insecurity and tortured relationships with women are problems common to all types of sexual disorders. There is a profound lack of confidence in approaching adult women, and the sexual drive is diverted elsewhere, e.g. to children, males, objects. In his own study, these features are linked to bad parenting and subsequent unsuccessful contacts with females. Rooth[16] arrived at a similar point of view in his account of exhibitionists.

The late Dr P. Scott had a picturesque way of explaining the role of anxiety. He taught that anxiety between a man and a woman could be understood as a barrier, or wall. Normally, this wall is non-existent or so small that normal friendship and sexual contact is possible. When it is too big to allow this the male may deal with the wall by:

(1) Turning away from it and choosing instead males, children or fetish objects
(2) Trying to peep over it (voyeurism) or standing on it to command the female's attention (exhibitionism)
(3) Reaching over and touching (assault or frotteurism)
(4) Crashing through it by force (rape).

Summary of aetiology of variants or disorders

Bancroft[17] has shown how these various aetiological factors might be regarded either as factors preventing adult heterosexuality or as factors promoting alternatives.

(1) Factors which are negative to adult heterosexuality:
    (a) family taboos and inhibitions about sex;
    (b) incestuous feelings about the mother leading to castration anxiety;
    (c) lack of confidence in one's sexual potency or masculinity.
(2) Factors positively leading to alternative variants or disorder:
    (a) sexual drive requiring satisfaction;
    (b) the need for one-to-one relationship;
    (c) repairing of a low self-esteem by being liked or wanted;
    (d) material gain as a rationalization (e.g. homosexual prostitution);
    (e) the possible association of erotic feelings with a particular act, e.g. the association of cross-dressing and sexual arousal;
    (f) possible genetic factors;
    (g) possible uterine factors;
    (h) possible adult hormonal factors.

The direction of the drive may be decided by the degree of impairment of relationships with others (perhaps so severe that sexual relationships can only be formed with objects) and chance associations (e.g. first sexual experience whilst handling objects of comfort, such as certain fabrics). In this way, explanations may be sought for all disorders, although they remain hypotheses – ways of understanding rather than scientific explanations.

Disorders of gender identity

Transsexualism

Definition
Transsexualism is the compulsive conviction that the subject is in fact assigned to the wrong gender, accompanied by the persistent desire to function as a member of the opposite sex and to be altered anatomically. The condition has to be distinguished from psychotic states with delusions of sex change, transvestism, histrionic claims of the severely personality disordered, and effeminate homosexuals.

Transsexualism and the law
There is no reason to stop a person adopting the lifestyle of the opposite sex. People do change their name to support this change and live a life as though of the opposite sex. However, for the purposes of marriage and other legal matters, the subjects – despite any 'corrective' surgery and having a female passport – retain their original gender.

Incidence
The incidence is estimated at between 1 in 28 000 and 1 in 40 000. It appears to be more common in men than in women.

Clinical pattern
The subject is convinced[18] from childhood, in the classical core trans-sexualism, that he is of the wrong gender. This conviction grows stronger in young adulthood. The subject may make several attempts to cope with his unnatural feelings by such actions as marrying or deliberately selecting friends of the opposite sex, or adopting hobbies to emphasize masculinity, but despite this, the conviction grows. There then follows a period of intense anxiety and disturbance until the new role is adopted. Some individuals after being transvestite become transsexual and later may reverse. Clinical experience indicates that the two conditions are not separated by as hard a dividing line as was classically thought. The subjects have a distaste for their physical sexual characteristics and press for operations and hormones to 'convert' them to their 'true' identity.

Dual-role transvestism
Here the subject gains considerable pleasure and a feeling of relaxation by

cross-dressing – 'being' of the opposite sex for a little while. In this condition there is no belief of being the wrong sex, no search for gender re-assignment, and no sexual arousal by the cross-dressing.

Disorders of sexual preference

Fetishism

Definition
Fetishists are sexually aroused and satisfied by handling and collecting inanimate objects – this being preferred to a real person. Fetishism has to be distinguished from non-pathological sexual experimentation with objects and the very rare association of fetishism with temporal lobe tumours (see Chapter 9).

Fetishism and the law
Fetishism itself is not an offence. Subjects may get into trouble with the law through the way they obtain their fetish object.

> A patient with a history of many offences also had a fetish for women's hair. He would take snips of women's hair whilst standing next to them in public places, e.g. a bus queue. He derived sexual arousal and satisfaction from placing the hair in his own underclothes. He was charged with assault after one such incident.

Patterns of fetishism
Two patterns (which may overlap) are seen:

(1) The subject has a craving for the fetish, e.g. shoes, female clothes, locks of hair. The object is used to assist the development of sexual fantasy during masturbation and the real person is not required.
(2) The subject uses the object to increase potency during a sexual relationship, e.g. requiring the partner to wear special clothes.

The fetish comes to the attention of a psychiatrist usually because the subject has been arrested (as above) or a sexual partner complains.

Fetishistic transvestism

Definition
The wearing of clothes appropriate to the opposite sex associated with sexual gratification and sexual arousal. This condition is to be distinguished from:

(1) Cross-dressing to reduce tension – e.g. some men will return home from work in the evening and dress in female clothes with a great feeling of relief and loss of tension (dual-role transvestism).
(2) Facultative transvestism – some inadequate or mentally handicapped young men steal female underclothes and cross-dress in them at times of loneliness in lieu of having a girlfriend. This behaviour stops when they have a girlfriend.
(3) Transsexualists.

Transvestism and the law
It is not illegal to cross-dress. People break the law by stealing female clothes or by behaving in an offensive or bizarre manner in public which may be considered a breach of the peace.

Incidence
The incidence is unknown. One estimate is that there are 30 000 transvestites in the British Isles and that it may be one of the commonest sexual disorders. Only a very small proportion of this group will reach the psychiatrist and, generally, they will be male.

Pattern of development of transvestism
The impulse generally arises during childhood and cross-dressing is practised at all convenient opportunities. The young boy will first steal clothes from his mother or other female members of the family. At first there is considerable pleasure from the feeling of the clothes, from the texture of the fabrics. The condition becomes very persistent and after puberty becomes associated with sexual arousal.

The cross-dressing is usually carried out in private, the clothes are often stolen from the family or from washing lines, and only occasionally are they bought. Cross-dressing is used to engender sexual arousal with fantasies of being a woman or of being with the woman. This behaviour often runs in parallel with heterosexual relationships although the cross-dressing is the preferred relationship. Some subjects will wear the female underwear in public whilst others may dress completely in female clothes.

The majority of subjects do not request or wish to be cured. Some are brought forward by their relatives or their spouse when they have been discovered cross-dressing. A spouse is likely to find this behaviour unacceptable. The cross-dressing, apart from its bizarre quality, offends because it excludes the spouse and puts her second in priority to the cross-dressing. Other subjects may present because of legal pressures, e.g. after arrest for stealing clothes, typically from washing lines. The theft is necessary in order to obtain clothes which have the quality of having belonged to a female. This assists the sexual fantasy.

Exhibitionism

Definition
Exhibitionism is the psychiatric term referring to the repeated deliberate exposing of the genitals to a member of the opposite sex for sexual excitement.

Incidence
The actual incidence is unknown but it is the commonest sexual offence with some 3 000 convictions per year in England and Wales. Some 80% of first offenders do not re-offend within five years and therefore the majority do not require treatment. The interest of the psychiatrist is in the small minority who become persistent offenders.

Classification
The classifications of true exhibitionists are inadequate and the patients often have features of several groups[19,20] – for example:

(1) Inhibited, often timid men of relatively normal personality and good character who struggle against the impulse but find it irresistible. After the event they may feel anxious, guilty and humiliated. Nevertheless the pressure to expose themselves again recurs and the subject gives way. The exposing may be with flaccid or erect penis and although there will be a reduction of tension the sexual pleasure may be slight.
(2) Less inhibited, more sociopathic subjects who expose in a state of great excitement with erect penis, masturbating with great pleasure and little guilt. This may be associated with other sexual disorders and other types of offences and, in rare cases, there may be a marked aggressive element with a potential to escalate the behaviour to a violent assault.
(3) Subjects who expose as a reaction to stress. They often ordinarily enjoy normal relationships but expose when under personal stress or in a state of depression. The exposing seems to relieve feelings of tension or despair.

Exhibitionists should be distinguished from people who expose whilst suffering from severe mental illness (schizophrenia or an organic disorder) or those who suffer from mental retardation and expose as a crude sexual invitation.

Psychopathology
Generally, the exposing can be understood as a method by which the offender can assert himself in a relationship with a woman. At the moment of exposing he is the dominant member in the 'dialogue'. The woman's reaction is, in a sense, irrelevant. Most exhibitionists do not

actually want contact. There is a small minority, usually within group (2) above, though not entirely, for whom the exposing is actually an invitation or preliminary to further contact – including, in a few cases, violence. The assessment of the patient and the predilection to violence will be based on objective accounts of the offender's behaviour and the subject's account of his own wishes and fantasies when interviewed[21].

Voyeurism

Definition
Voyeurism is the repetitive spying on people undressing or indulging in sexual activity in order to become sexually aroused and this being the preferred form of sexual activity.

Voyeurism and the law
Voyeurism is an offence. The offender may be referred to a psychiatrist for assessment.

Clinical features
The voyeur is often an inadequate person, similar to an exhibitionist, and his behaviour may be associated with exhibitionism. Very rarely it may be associated with aggressive fantasies and be a preliminary to an assault. Questioning in interview must be directed at clarifying this.

Paedophilia

Definition
A paedophile is an adult whose preferred sexual object is a child. The disorder is to be distinguished from isolated sexual acts with children by people under stress, and those who are mentally disordered or handicapped. It may also be that occasional fantasies about children are commonplace. Of 193 male students, 25% reported some sexual attraction to children including 7% who would have sex with children if they could get away with it[22].

Clinical description
There is a wide range of clinical pictures from men of otherwise good personality who despite their own good sense give way to paedophilic temptation from time to time, to psychopathic paedophiles who seize and rape children. A true paedophile will probably have had persistent paedophilic fantasies from puberty. A number will report that they were themselves victims of paedophilic assaults though it is unknown whether this is an aetiological factor. Two major groups are recognized clinically:

(1) Subjects who like children. This group will get on very well with children and will be known in the neighbourhood as being very good with them. The children will come to them readily and enjoy their company. Such men tend to be rather timid and feel rather intimidated by adult women. Some such men will very easily and repeatedly form sexual relationships with the children whom they befriend. Others will suppress the sexual aspects of their relationships with children but these may emerge at times of temptation (e.g. with a very seductive child) or at times of stress (e.g. occupational stresses or domestic problems).

(2) Subjects who use the child as a source of sexual gratification with no sympathy or affection for the child. These men are the ones most likely to report having experienced unpleasant or violent sexual assaults when they themselves were children and they seem to be passing on the act. They often have had very disturbed early lives. They do not form good relationships with their victims but obtain 'co-operation' either by:
(a) bribing with money or sweets, or
(b) progressive intimidation, or rape.

Paedophiles classically have a particular type of child who attracts them. Some are attracted to pre-pubertal boys only, others to pubertal boys. Others will be attracted principally to pre-pubertal girls and yet others to girls in early puberty. The more psychopathic will tend to be more indiscriminate. Any type of paedophile may enjoy obscene photographs of children and may commit the offences of distributing, possessing, or advertising such photographs. Some paedophiles have induced children to draw others into groups for unlawful activity. Several such groups have been discovered.

The true paedophile has to be distinguished from what might be called symptomatic paedophilia in which sexual behaviour with children occurs in special situations, for example:

(1) Psychopathic opportunism – psychopaths who are so promiscuous they take sexual pleasure from any opportunity.
(2) Mentally handicapped men who are unable to relate to adults and may be experimenting with children, although adults would be preferred.
(3) Sexual involvement with children following organic brain damage leading to disinhibition.
(4) Secondary to mental illness, e.g. depression or serious psychoses like schizophrenia.

Follow-up results[23] have shown that unlike other criminals, who tend to stop offending as they get older, each year 2–3% of paedophiles are re-arrested so that after 20 years approximately 50% will have been re-arrested. The number of previous offences indicates the chances of being re-arrested. It seems likely from questioning offenders and known paedophiles[24] that there are many more offences committed than are ever brought to light.

Victims of paedophilia
Bancroft[3] has summarized the literature. Girls are reported as victims twice as often as boys but it may be that boys report offences less often. Kinsey *et al.*[25] found that 24% of females had a pre-pubertal sexual experience with a post-pubertal male varying from indecent exposure (45%) to attempted intercourse (5%) [see also Chapter 7]. Generally the experience was frightening though usually it had no long-term effect. However, the effect does seem to reflect the reaction of adults around them, a highly emotional, alarmist reaction coupled with court proceedings will be the least help. A matter-of-fact, calming approach seems the most helpful. There is evidence that whereas some children are the unwilling and innocent victims of a sexual assault, many others who become involved with a paedophile do so out of a search for affection. Such children often come from disturbed homes, deprived of love and affection, and may easily enter into a sexual relationship though later become frightened of the result.

Masochism

Definition
Masochism is the obtaining of sexual satisfaction from being hurt or humiliated by a sexual partner and this being the preferred method of sexual arousal.

Masochism and the law
Masochistic activities in themselves are not illegal.

Clinical features
The subjects enjoy pain and humiliation which they arrange in order to control the type and degree of discomfort. The act has a tension-reducing effect as well as a sexual-releasing component. Three overlapping subtypes can be recognized[26]. The subjects may be homosexual or heterosexual.

(1) Compulsive neurotic masochist: the act is mainly to reduce tension/guilt. The subject may feel shame or guilt afterwards and try to control the impulses in the future, but, inevitably, as new tension and guilt build up in other aspects of his life he will give way to the impulse once more.
(2) Psychopathic masochist: the subject is solely concerned with sexual

arousal as a result of pain or life-threatening procedures. He then may go on to seek orgasm. This is often associated with sadistic tendencies as well.

(3) Female masochists who include:
   (a) those who use masochism (e.g. bondage) to reduce feelings of guilt about sex; the act makes her a helpless victim,
   (b) those who seek out violent partners because a violent sexual relationship confirms a self-image and a life view which has been derived from a very disturbed, violent childhood.

Sadism

Definition
The preferred method of sexual pleasure in sadism is by hurting, humiliating and tormenting others.

Sadism and the law
Sadists breach the law when their actions are with unwilling partners or constitute assaults of varying degrees. At worse, they will result in severe attacks resulting in mutilation and death.

Clinical features
The subject may be a cold and obsessional personality, unable to form warm relationships with adults. Two sub-types have been recognized[26]:

(1) Neurotic sadists: Subjects who act out their fantasies theatrically with prostitutes as a tension reducing activity as well as a sexual one.
(2) Sadistic psychopaths: These subjects have no guilt, little self-control and may show violence in other aspects of their behaviour. The sadistic behaviour seems linked to highly disturbed early relationships, a displacement of anger from mother to other females. At worst, there will be unprovoked attacks going on to severe mutilation and homicide. The attacks may well be preceded by a long period of increasingly strong sadistic fantasy[27]. Brittain[28] described a syndrome of sadistic murderers characterized by a history of fantasized sadistic scenes, social isolation and interest and admiration of Nazism and weapons used in personal violence.

Sometimes patients voluntarily present complaining of unwanted sadistic thoughts and even of pursuing potential victims whilst armed. They differ from the guilt-free sadist in that they have a desire to lose their unwanted sexual fantasies. They may be helped by counselling and support[29] possibly incorporating cognitive approaches.

Other disorders of sexual preference

There are several of these and they are listed above. They have to be distinguished from non-pathological and sexual experimentation. They lead to offending either by causing assaults on others e.g. frotteurism or by the nature of the act itself e.g. bestiality (sexual or anal intercourse with animals).

Problems associated with sexual orientation (homo or heterosexuality)

Although sexual orientation differences are not to be regarded as disorders, problems do arise for individuals – especially when their sexual orientation is at odds with what is/was expected.

Homosexuality and the law
Female homosexuality has never been recognized as an offence. Male homosexual behaviour, which used to be a crime, is no longer so (Sexual Offences Act 1967) if both partners are over 21 (the age limit is currently under discussion), consenting and the behaviour is carried out in private. Homosexual behaviour which now comes to the attention of the law includes behaviour with minors, homosexual behaviour in public places, e.g. public toilets, and soliciting by homosexuals.

Incidence
Some 10% of American males have been estimated, in the past, as having had at least one homosexual experience and 6% occasionally or fairly often. The prevalence in England is thought to be less with only 3% admitting to experience of homosexual intercourse[1]. Of 77 primitive societies studied, 48 accepted homosexual male behaviour as normal or socially acceptable[2]. Animal studies show homosexual behaviour to be common though exclusive homosexuality in the presence of the opposite sex is unusual.

Clinical aspects
Homosexuality occurs in all social levels and in all levels of social competence. It is to be regarded as a variant of human sexual behaviour and not a disorder. Comparisons[30,3] of criminal, neurotic, and normal socially integrated homosexuals with suitable control groups revealed that the homosexuals had the same range of personalities as the control group. Schofield[30] described three groups for which later studies show some support. These are:

(1) Well-adjusted homosexuals: From childhood they feel themselves different from boys, i.e. more feminine in that they enjoy playing with girls and girls' toys. They begin their sexual life by making heterosexual approaches but find little interest in this. They become dimly aware of homosexual feelings in late adolescence leading to a period of considerable anxiety and a search for a solution. They may present to a psychiatrist at that period because of their anxiety. The outcome may be identification with homosexuals and resolution of anxiety.

(2) Antisocial personalities and homosexuality: When there was association between homosexuality and antisocial behaviour there was a tendency to homosexual prostitution and homosexual offending in public. This group of people tended to come from very disturbed backgrounds, to have drifted down the social scale and to have identified with criminal subcultures.

(3) Neurotic personality and homosexuality: This combination was associated with a high incidence of a disturbed home background and a tendency not to accept their homosexual orientation. They were socially more competent than the antisocial group though there was some minor criminal activity and a susceptibility to neurotic breakdown. This group present to the psychiatrist most commonly because of neurosis and an inability to resolve sexual identification.

Treatment of sexual disorders

Introduction

A number of conditions require only counselling to help the person come to terms with his disturbing discovery of himself. This will be important in conditions such as anxiety associated with homosexuality where a young man may be helped to decide his sexual orientation and if it is homosexual, then to come to terms with it. In disorders, such as paedophilia, counselling may provide support and help for subjects anxious to control their unwanted impulses but with no expectation of a change in sexual preference. In transsexualism no treatment is likely to change the subject's conviction about himself. The psychiatrist can help in diagnosis and help clarify the subject's feelings about himself so that he can make a decision about how he wishes to run his life. If he decides to pursue a transsexual lifestyle he will be assisted by being put in touch with self-help groups for transsexuals. Some clinics have specialized in this problem and have attempted to teach the subject how to adopt their chosen lifestyle successfully by giving assistance in and advice on clothing and legal matters. Male transsexualists will often seek oestrogens to feminize their body. Surgical alteration of the genitals will be sought, though there are technical and ethical problems with this irreversible step. Conditions for operative change include having a persistent desire for change, no marital ties, a stable personality, being reasonably intelligent, and having adopted the chosen role and lived it successfully for at least one to two years. In some cases re-assignment surgery has led to considerable improvement in social and psychological adjustment[31].

Where an alteration in sexual disordered behaviour is sought then counselling is unlikely to be sufficient on its own. Psychological treatments and antilibidinal treatments may also be required.

Psychological treatments in sexual disorders

Interpretative psychotherapies

Psychoanalysis
Disorders are seen as having a defensive function in warding off the anxiety arising from infantile attachments to parents and the 'rivalries' this engenders. Although optimistic case histories have been presented, success has not been demonstrated by controlled scientific studies. Because of this there has been plenty of criticism, especially from behaviour-orientated psychologists.

Individual psychotherapy
The disorders may be understood in terms of distorted relationships. It is hoped that change will occur if these are understood. Although many have become pessimistic about the effectiveness of this approach, some people, nevertheless, seem to benefit. It may be most useful in those who have the intelligence and ability to take part in such psychotherapy. It may be used as an adjunct to behaviour therapy.

Supportive psychotherapy
This is most helpful with the inadequate, neurotic, anxious subject of low self-esteem who seems to gain esteem and a reduction in tension from regular counselling and support from a trusted and friendly professional. It forms the backbone of outpatient clinic or probation work and its aim is to reduce the acting out of fantasies rather than to expect to change them.

Group psychotherapy
This is currently a very popular approach with the aim of revealing feelings and social behaviour. Such groups have been run by psychologists, probation officers and lay therapists. Subjects living in the community seem to be very good at spotting when a fellow group member is being less than frank. Although there is no comparative scientific evidence of success, groups certainly seem helpful to those who use them. Clinically they seem good at keeping people out of trouble at least during the time they attend the group. Clinical experience suggests

that a community setting can work particularly well for shy, inadequate, unassertive people.

Behaviour therapies

Behaviour therapists[32] treat the problem at a more symptomatic level. They aim both to change the direction of the subject's sexual preferences (re-orientation training), as well as to decrease disordered sexual arousal. They also attempt to improve general social skills so that the subject can approach adult women satisfactorily and be more at ease in an adult world; and finally, they try and improve self-control. The techniques are very specialized and often require the use of psychological laboratories with equipment to measure physiological functions and penile reactions as well as equipment for showing slides, videos and films under laboratory conditions.

(1) Re-orientation training This may be attempted by a number of techniques:
  (a) orgasmic re-conditioning by teaching the subject to:
      (i)   switch fantasies from an unwanted one to a preferred one just prior to orgasm during masturbation;
      (ii) gradually change the disordered fantasy, e.g. encourage paedophiles to gradually increase the age of the fantasy-subjects during masturbation;
      (iii) alternate disordered fantasies with normal fantasies during sexual stimulation.
  (b) exposure to explicit stimuli Sexually stimulating heterosexual films can be shown to increase heterosexual interest. This has been done with homosexuals and has led to increased heterosexual arousal.
  (c) Classical conditioning – shaping Various attempts have been made to reward normal sexual responses when a subject is shown adult heterosexual stimuli, e.g. water-deprived patients were given drinks of iced water when they had a normal heterosexual response to heterosexual stimuli.
  (d) operant condition – fading This technique involves showing a sexually stimulating heterosexual slide on top of a deviant slide. The deviant slide is gradually faded out and the heterosexual picture is increased in intensity as the patient becomes aroused.
  (e) biofeedback with enforcement This approach involves making the subject aware of the physiological measures of his sexual responses and rewarding appropriate sexual arousal.
  (f) systematic desensitization If there is excessive anxiety about normal heterosexual stimuli then systematic desensitization can be offered.
(2) Decreasing deviant arousal

(a) aversion therapy   Faradic, drug-induced or olfactory methods of aversion have been used. The subject is shown the deviant situation or is involved in it. The aversive stimulus is applied as the patient begins to respond to the deviant stimulus. Used on its own (without re-orientation training) this produces only temporary results. There may be difficulties in getting real consent, particularly for offenders, i.e. the consent may be given only because of the threat of penal measures.

(b) covert sensitization   Here an unpleasant stimulus, e.g. the fantasy of being sick, is brought into a deviant fantasy scene which is rehearsed with the subject. There is some evidence of success and it avoids ethical problems as the patient is not being assaulted and can control the fantasy.

(c) biofeedback   In this method the subject is taught first to detect early signs of sexual arousal to deviant stimuli and second to suppress them. The idea is that if he can detect the signs of arousal early enough he will be in a better position to control them.

(d) masturbatory satiation   In this approach the patient is isolated in a private room and instructed to masturbate whilst verbalizing his disordered sexual fantasies for an hour and continuing to masturbate after achieving orgasm. There have been some reports of successful outcome in some case studies.

Cognitive restructuring
The aim is to improve the subjects' understanding of their own psychology and to expose the various cognitive self-deceptions which the subjects employ to maintain their offending to which they have become 'addicted'. The subjects are made aware of the way they 'organized' the offending (e.g. deliberately going to a particular wood at a particular time). Similarly, they are made aware of the way they deny the impact on the victim. In groups, subjects are made aware through discussion, of the various denials and rationalizations which they employ. This approach appears effective at altering awareness which is believed to be essential to any real change. It is claimed to be the best approach to reduce sexual re-offending in many offenders (though not in rapists) especially when combined with anti-androgen medication[33]. The approach has been adopted nationally by psychologists in the prison system in England and Wales in a national scheme to treat sentenced sex offenders.

Skills training
The aim here is to improve the general social functioning of the subject so that he will cope better in the adult role – the theory being that deviancy is a reflection of an inability to cope with adult situations. Skills training includes:

(1) Social skills training: In individual and group approaches, with a trained therapist, the patient is encouraged to express his feelings, take part in interviews, deal with aggression, approach women, etc. The therapist, perhaps using techniques like psychodrama or family sculpting, will try to help the subject deal with family interactions and his own feelings of aggression or inadequacy.

(2) Sexual education: This is often inadequate in sexually disordered patients, especially in those of dull intelligence. Their ignorance increases their anxiety and is a complicating factor in their dealings with others. Sexual education is given individually or in groups using didactic methods, books and discussion. A useful start is to show pictures or use anatomically correct dolls and ask the subject to name the parts and give their function.

(3) Sensate focus therapy: Techniques devised by Masters and Johnson employed in the treatment of sexually dysfunctional couples have been applied to homosexuals with some evidence of success[34]. This treatment, which involves the direct sexual arousal of the patient by the female, surrogate partner, has met with considerable ethical problems in the United Kingdom.

(4) Gender role behaviour: This approach is particularly appropriate for transsexual subjects wishing to adopt a new gender role. Training will cover practical matters such as clothes, make-up and the legal aspects of having one's name changed.

(5) Self-control training: In this approach the subject is taught self-monitoring to recognize potentially dangerous situations or situations of particular temptation. Men with a paedophilic tendency have to accept that being alone with children will place them in temptation. The subject is also taught how to recognize the early signs in himself of being aroused or at risk of giving way to his unwanted behaviour and he should be taught how to take evasive action. He is encouraged in self-motivation by self-reinforcement with intention statements and inter-personal contracting (agreements between patient and therapist).

(6) Violence control: Learning anger management through role play and relaxation with cognitive and behavioural modification methods may be helpful where violence is part of the offender's response.

Effectiveness of psychological treatments
The effectiveness of the treatment is said to be increased in people of stable personality with high motivation and some adult heterosexual adult fantasies. The worst prognosis seems to be with those who have no normal sexual fantasies, e.g. men who have never had heterosexual fantasies and have little desire to change. Motivation is always very difficult to assess especially under the stress of court appearances. One would feel most optimistic with a subject who made the approach before

arrest and least optimistic with a person who has been referred to a therapist several times in the past but has failed to take up the offer of therapy or on whom the therapy had previously been ineffective. Proving the long-term value of these therapies has been difficult. There are single case studies to demonstrate improvement in all the psychological methods. Trials of treatment with behaviour therapy have shown improvement, at least in the short term, but there are no good controlled trials to demonstrate long-term efficacy[32].

Antilibidinal treatment in sexual disorder

Definition
Antilibidinal treatment is treatment aimed at reducing the strength of sexual drive. It does not concern itself with the direction of the drive. It is usually used as a way of reducing sexual offending. It is most effective where the sexual activity is carried out in order to obtain an orgasm. It will be less effective where the activity is carried out in order to form a relationship as in some paedophiles. The treatment should only be used with the full co-operation of the patient who must have all its effects explained to him. Many authorities recommend that the patient sign a consent form. It is particularly useful as an emergency measure to help motivated patients who are experiencing a temporary exacerbation of an unwanted and undesirable sexual drive. Other treatment measures (e.g. psychotherapy, group work) can be instituted at the same time. The principal problem with medication from the court's point of view is that there is no way of checking whether the patient is taking the prescription.

Types of antilibidinal treatment

(1) Castration
Castration has been used in the past on the Continent but never in the United Kingdom. There have been claims for its effectiveness on recidivist sexual offenders. Sturrup[35] in Denmark considered it most effective as an operation in that the majority, though not all, of his recidivist offenders stopped offending – a view supported by other studies[3]. The usual operation was to remove the testes from the scrotum and replace them with a prosthesis. There are obviously ethical problems due to the irreversibility of the operation and the uncertainty of obtaining real consent. It was generally only offered in situations where the alternative might be prolonged incarceration, either in prison or hospital. It should be noted that, from the public safety point of view, although there appears to be a substantial reduction in recidivism, the reduction is not 100%.

(2) Oestrogen therapy
Oestrogen has a marked antilibidinal effect. Two preparations have been used:

(a) Oral stilboestrol 5mg daily up to three times daily.
(b) Parental oestrogen pellets (100mg) implanted subcutaneously. (If parental oestrogens are used then consent from the Mental Health Act Commission would be required, even if the patient consented. The treatment is regarded as grave and with irreversible effects, in the same category as leucotomy.)

Pharmacology – Oestrogens inhibit the secretions of gonadotrophins by action on the anterior pituitary. There is some possibility that there may be some enlargement of the pituitary with congestion and haemorrhaging. Oestrogens produce atrophic changes in the testicles and impotence and loss of ejaculation accompanying loss of sexual drive.

Wanted effects – Bancroft et al.[36] showed by controlled trial that oestrogens definitely reduced the production of sexual thought and behaviour.

Unwanted effects – Oral oestrogens produce gastrointestinal discomfort (nausea and dizziness). All the oestrogens produce venous thrombosis, breast enlargements with proliferation of the alveoli and ducts and growth of the epithelium of the nipple, such that plastic surgery may be required. They also cause a reduction in beard growth.

It is generally said that the effects of oestrogen treatment are reversible. This certainly seems to be so after treatment of up to a few months, though there may be a lag before a return to normal. The long-term effect for prolonged treatment is less certain. In certain cases large doses of oestrogens may be given yet the patient retains the ability to have erections and sexual thoughts even though he may lose the ability to ejaculate.

(3) Benperidol (Anquil)
A synthetic neuroleptic in the butyrophenyl series, it has chemical and pharmacological properties similar to haloperidol and shares the anti-libidinal effects which are seen in many neuroleptics. It is used initially in doses of 1–1.5 mg per day. Its maintenance dose is 0.5–1.0 mg per day used either continuously or periodically as the patient has symptoms.

Wanted effects – Benperidol is said to produce a suppression of sexual desire. It was claimed in early trials that it would reduce unwanted behaviour in demented or mentally abnormal patients. In one controlled trial it only reduced sexual fantasy through impairing concentration[37]. In clinical use it seems much less potent than oestrogens or cyproterone acetate.

Unwanted effects – These include the effects of butyrophenones, especially drowsiness, weakness of the lower limbs, akathisia and extrapyramidal symptoms.

(4) Cyproterone acetate (Androcur)
Cyproterone acetate (usual starting dose 50 mg bd) is an antiandrogen preparation. It has in fact been used in smaller doses as a male contraceptive. It is claimed to be useful in hypersexuality, indecent exposure, reducing unwanted sexual fantasies and reducing sexual misbehaviour in the severely subnormal or demented.

Pharmacology – Cyproterone acetate inhibits the production of testosterone by enzyme block, acts as a competitive antagonist to testosterone, has an action on the hypothalamic centre and is progestogenic.

Wanted effects – It causes a reduction in sexual drive after 10 to 14 days but some effect will be obtained often in 48 hours. It reduces sexual thoughts and behaviour, though its effect is only weak in terms of reducing arousal to erotic stimuli[36].

Unwanted effects – Cyproterone acetate causes a reduction in spermatogenesis giving oligospermia and loss of ejaculation. Gynaecomastia occurs in 10–15% of subjects and is said to remit when treatment stops. Other effects include dizziness, depression in the third week, habituation after some weeks requiring larger dose and loss of body hair on prolonged treatment.

Reversibility – The manufacturers claim no case has failed to revert to the patient's normal fertility and sexual response after ceasing medication although there may be a lag of several months. Some patients seem to retain the ability to have erections and sexual drive despite high doses. It is also said not to work with sexual offending associated with alcohol abuse.

> A patient with severe personality difficulties had a history of paedophilic urges and indecent exposure. He was finally convicted of seriously sexually attacking a child. He was sent to special hospital on a hospital order with a diagnosis of psychopathic disorder. There he received social skills training, sexual education and individual and group psychotherapy. After some years he lost his paedophilic fantasies and developed adult heterosexual fantasies. He was transferred to a regional secure unit and the psychological treatment continued. He then returned to the community maintaining regular contacts with his therapist at the regional secure unit. Some 18 months later he encountered some difficulties socially. He became anxious and despondent. There was a return of his paedophilic thoughts and he gave way to the impulse to expose. He admitted the return of his symptoms to his therapist. Psychological support

was intensified and he was re-admitted to the unit for a short period. Because of the resurgence of his paedophilic urges he was given a course of cyproterone acetate which quickly reduced them. Consideration was also given to giving him an anxiolytic but it was not required. His 'relapse' came under control in some weeks and he returned to the community. The cyproterone acetate was tailed off when it was clear that he had settled. He then continued to make progress, growing in confidence and social competence.

The management of this case illustrates the use of security and interaction of different treatments in the eclectic way proposed by Rooth[16] and Bancroft[3].

(5) Goserelin acetate (Zoladex)
This depot preparation (used in the treatment of prostate cancer) is a luteinizing hormone-releasing hormone agonist and blocker. It initially acts like luteinizing hormone then blocks the effects of luteinizing hormone with a subsequent fall in testosterone. It is therefore a potent antilibidinal agent (though not yet licensed as such) which is just starting to be used. It has been characterized as a non-hormonal preparation[38] given by non-surgical means in terms of the Mental Health Act 1983.

(6) Medroxyprogesterone acetate (Depo-Provera)
This is a progesterone which can be given in a depot form. It is used primarily for dysfunctional uterine bleeding, secondary amenorrhoea and certain neoplasms. In men it lowers testosterone levels by inhibiting luteinizing hormone. It has been used as an antilibidinal in North America but not much in the UK where cyproterone acetate is preferred.

References

(1) Forman, D. & Chilvers, C. (1989) Sexual behaviour of young and middle aged men in England and Wales. *British Medical Journal* **298**, 1137–42.
(2) Ford, C.S. & Beach, F.A. (1952) *Patterns of Sexual Behaviour.* Eyre and Spottiswoode, London.
(3) Bancroft, J. (1989) *Human Sexuality and its Problems* (second edn). Churchill Livingstone, Edinburgh.
(4) Heston, L.L. & Shields, J. (1968) Homosexuality in twins: a family study and registry study. *Archives of General Psychiatry* **18**, 149–60.
(5) Echert, E.D. Bouchard, T.J., Bohlen, J. & Heston, L.L. (1986) Homosexuality in monozygotic twins reared apart. *British Journal of Psychiatry* **148**, 421–5.
(6) Editorial (1993) Marker on X-chromosome linked to being gay. *British Medical Journal* **307**, 220.
(7) Editorial (1991) Homosexuality and the hypothalamus. *Lancet* **338**, 688–9.
(8) Baum, M.J. (1979) Differentiation of coital behaviour in mammals: a comparative study. *Neuroscience and Behavioural Reviews* **3**, 265–84.

(9) Margolese, M.S. & Janiger, O. (1973) Androsterone/etiocholanolone ratios in male homosexuals. *British Medical Journal* **3**, 207–10.

(10) Rose, R.M., Gordon, T.P. & Bernstein, I.S. (1972) Plasma testosterone levels in the male rhesus: influence of sexual and social stimuli. *Science* **178**, 643–5.

(11) Wakeling, A. (1979) A general psychiatric approach to sexual deviation. In Rosen, I. (ed.) *Sexual Deviation*. Oxford University Press, Oxford.

(12) Siegelman, M. (1974) Parental background of male homosexuals and heterosexuals. *Archives of Sexual Behaviour* **3**, 3–18.

(13) Siegelman, M. (1978) Psychological adjustment of homosexual and heterosexual men: a cross national replication. *Archives of Sexual Behaviour* **7**, 1–12.

(14) Green, R. (1987) *The Sissy Boy Syndrome and the Development of Homosexuality*. Yale University Press, New Haven and London.

(15) West, D.J., Roy, C. & Nichols, F.L. (1978) *Understanding Sexual Attacks*. Heinemann Educational Books, London.

(16) Rooth, G. (1980) Exhibitionism: an eclectic approach to its management. *British Journal of Hospital Medicine* **23**, 366–70.

(17) Bancroft, J. (1970) Homosexuality in the male. *British Journal of Hospital Medicine* **3**, 168–81.

(18) Christie Brown, J.R.W. (1983) Paraphilias: sadomasochism, fetishism, transvestism and transsexuality. *British Journal of Psychiatry* **143**, 227–31.

(19) Rooth, F.G. (1971) Indecent exposure and exhibitionism. *British Journal of Hospital Medicine* **5**, 521–33.

(20) Gayford, J.J. (1981) Indecent exposure: a review of the literature. *Medicine, Science and the Law* **21**, 233–41.

(21) Rooth, G. (1973) Exhibitionism, sexual violence and paedophilia. *British Journal of Psychiatry* **122**, 705–10.

(22) Brière, J. & Runtz, M. (1989) University males' sexual interest in children: predicting potential indices of paedophilia in a non-forensic sample. *Child Abuse and Neglect* **13**, 65–75.

(23) Soothill, K.L. & Gibbens, T.C.N. (1978) Recidivism and sexual offenders: a reappraisal. *British Journal of Criminology* **18**, 267–77.

(24) Abel, G.G., Becker, J.V., Mittelman, M., Cunningham-Rathner, J., Rouleau, J.L. & Murphy, W.D. (1987) Self-reported sex crimes of nonincarcerated paraphiliacs. *Journal of Interpersonal Violence* **2**, 3–25.

(25) Kinsey, A.C., Pomeroy, W.B., Martin, C.E. & Gebhard, P.H. (1953) *Sexual Behaviour in the Human Female*. Saunders, Philadelphia.

(26) Trick, K.L.K. & Tennant, T.G. (1981) *Forensic Psychiatry, An Introductory Text*. Pitman Book Ltd, London.

(27) MacCulloch, M.J., Snowden, P.R., Wood, P.J.W. & Mills, H.E. Sadistic fantasy, sadistic behaviour and offending. *British Journal of Psychiatry* **143**, 20–9.

(28) Brittain, R.P. (1970) The sadistic murderer. *Medicine, Science and the Law* **10**, 198–207.

(29) Langton, J. & Torpy, D. (1988) Confidentiality and a future sadistic sex offender. *Medicine, Science and the Law* **28**, 195–99.

(30) Schofield, M. (1965) *Sociological aspects of homosexuality: A Comparative Study of Three Types of Homosexuals*. Longman, London.

(31) Mate-Kole, C., Freschi, M. & Robin, A. (1990) A controlled study of psychological and social change after surgical gender reassignment in selected male transexuals. *British Journal of Psychiatry* **157**, 261–4.

(32) Crawford, D.A. (1981) Treatment approaches in paedophiles. In Cook, M. and Howells, K. (eds.) *Adult Sexual Interest in Children*. Academic Press, London.

(33) Marshall, W.L., Jones, R., Ward, T., Johnston, P. & Barbaree, H.E. (1991) Treatment outcome with sex offenders. *Criminal Psychology Review* **11**, 465–85.

(34) Green, J. & Miller, D. (1985) Male homosexuality and sexual problems. *British Journal of Hospital Medicine* **33**, 353–5.

(35) Sturrup, G.K. (1972) Castration, the total treatment. In Resnick, H. and Wolfgang, M. (eds) *Sexual Behaviour*. Little, Brown, Boston.

(36) Bancroft, J.H.J., Tennant, G., Loncas, K. & Cass, J. (1974) Control of deviant sexual behaviour by drugs: behavioural effects of oestrogens and anti-androgens. *British Journal of Psychiatry* **125**, 310–15.

(37) Tenn ant, G., Bancroft, J. & Cass, J. (1974) The control of deviant sexual behaviour by drugs: a double-blind controlled study of benperidol, chlorpromazine and placebo. *Archives of Sexual Behaviour* **3**, 261–71.

(38) Dyer, C. (1988) Mental Health Act Commission defeated over paedophile. *British Medical Journal* **296**, 1660–1.

Chapter 13

Women and Juvenile Offenders

Women offenders

Introduction

The purpose of this section is to:

(1) Describe the incidence of criminal behaviour in women and of mental abnormality amongst female offenders.
(2) Describe relevant aetiological factors associated with criminality in women.
(3) Describe any special types of offences seen in women and any particular medicolegal problems they present.

Incidence of criminal behaviour

The incidence of crime in females, as in males, rises throughout childhood to a peak in adolescence (around 16 years) and then rapidly falls. However, unlike males, who maintain this falling rate throughout their life, there is a small secondary hump in the curve around the mid-forties and mid-fifties, coinciding with the menopausal period. The pattern of criminal behaviour, as measured by official statistics, shows that females offend much less than males. Self-report studies support the official figures. The extent of the difference varies with age and the extent has also varied over the years. In recent times, the female rate has increased so that there is now less difference between male and female rates than there used to be. The overall male to female ratio for offenders convicted or cautioned for indictable offences was 4.8:1 in 1991[1] having been 11:1 in 1949. This varies between 3.1:1 for 15 year old offenders to 5.9:1 for 17–20 year-olds. There are thirty times as many males in prison as females which reflects partly the quality of the offending (females tending to commit lesser offences), and possibly the courts being less punitive to women[2]. However, a study[3] of convicted women in Cambridge showed that the apparent leniency of the courts to women merely reflected the fact that women commit less serious offences and have fewer previous convictions. When this was taken into account there was no sex difference in sentencing.

The pattern of misbehaviour in the two sexes is different. Boys are likely to present primarily with property offences, whereas girls are more likely to come to the attention of the authorities because of being in 'moral danger' from sexual behaviour. This may not result in an official offence but may lead to a care order. At a later age, men have a greater chance of being involved in violent offences and major property offences (burglary, robbery). It was said that the most typical adult female offence was shoplifting (though there are reports that males have caught up with females in this area) and offences linked to prostitution[4]. However, it is said that women are increasingly imitating their male counterparts and becoming more violent and criminal as the pattern of offending is changing reflecting, perhaps, female emancipation and social upheaval.

Aetiological factors in female offending

In the case of recidivist female offenders, as in males, there is a strong association with childhood factors, such as bad parenting, criminal fathers, alcoholic parents, large family and lower IQ. Subsidiary factors include physical abnormalities, brain damage, mental illness, bad school records, poverty and mesomorphic build. Cloninger and Guze[5] demonstrated that recidivist female prisoners had a strong family history of psychiatric disorder (as do male offenders). The principal disorders were alcoholism (61%), sociopathy (36%) and drug dependency (14%) in the male relatives and hysteria (34%) in the female relatives. As girls, they showed behaviour disorder at school with a high level of truancy (30%), and expulsion or suspension (30%). They had poor work records with unemployment or frequent changes of jobs and they formed unsatisfactory marriages. The impression was gained, as in other studies[6], that these factors, though similar to those in the case of boys, were worse in the case of girls. It is as though the girls needed greater stress before they became delinquent and when they did so they were much more likely to be disturbed in other aspects of their life which coincides with the findings that girls may be more resilient in the face of family discord than boys[7]. The possible reasons for girls being less criminal than boys have been summarized by Rutter and Giller[7]. Differences in behavioural disorder between the sexes are culturally linked, e.g. the differences between girls and boys in West Indian cultures is less than in Asian cultures (where girls are particularly well behaved). Differences between the sexes have not remained steady with the years, as already noted above; girls are becoming more like boys in their delinquency.

It has been argued that girls are more likely to be better behaved than boys because:

(1) Males are more aggressive in their interactions than girls, though there is considerable overlap. Differences for aggression are apparent from early childhood and are seen between the sexes in subhuman primates. It may be linked to the effect of male hormones on the fetus.
(2) Parents and society train and expect girls to be better behaved, they are subject to closer supervision and are given conforming, passive models rather than striving, assertive models.
(3) As noted above, girls seem more resilient to stress than boys.

On the other hand, it has been argued that female hormonal changes cause periods of stress which may be associated with offending. The *premenstrual syndrome* has been defined as the occurrence of symptoms in the premenstruum with absence of symptoms in the postmenstruum. Numerous symptoms have been described including the psychiatric ones of irritability, anxiety, tension, depression, hostility, mood swings, impulsive behaviour and difficulty in concentrating. Dalton[8] claimed that 50% of women prisoners offended in the premenstrual week. Dalton asserted that this coincided with other disturbed behaviour, e.g. infraction of prison rules, poor examination results and motoring offences, as well as with symptoms of premenstrual tension. Epps, in Gibbens' study[9] failed to find a link between shoplifting and the menstrual period. However, Hands *et al.*[10] found a regular link between disturbed behaviour and the menstrual period in a small group of women who were showing behaviour disorder in special hospital.

d'Orban and Dalton[11] concluded from a study of women prisoners convicted of violent offences, that the violent behaviour was more likely to occur in the three days before and the two days into the menstrual period rather than in the rest of the cycle. They also found that the women's awareness of premenstrual symptoms (such as depression or tension) did not correlate with the cyclical violent behaviour, i.e. the women might be quite unaware that they had a cyclical behaviour pattern because they did not have the expected symptoms of the premenstrual syndrome at the same time.

It has been asserted that the change in hormone levels during the menopause period was responsible for the increased rate of offending in women aged 45 55. However, closer examination has not always supported this idea, e.g. Gibbens did not find menopausal problems to be more common in the shoplifters of that age group. It has been shown[12] in population studies that there is a vulnerable group who have a history of psychiatric complaints in the past for whom the menopausal period is an additional and significant stress. To what extent physiological factors are responsible rather than the psychological stresses which occur at this time is unclear and presumably vary from case to case. The psychological factors which might be significant include the movement of children away from the home, coming to terms with ageing, marital stresses and changes in the role of the woman in the household in the absence of her children.

Women in prison

There are some 1600 women in prison on any one day in England and Wales (3% of the prison population). They are held in a variety of prisons covering different security requirements. Studies (see below) reveal higher levels of psychiatric disorder than in male prisons. In the sentenced population this will be due to personality disorder, neurosis, and substance abuse. Psychiatric care is provided in the prison hospitals or on the ordinary wings depending on the severity of the disturbance. There is, however, no equivalent to Grendon Prison for female prisoners.

Arrangements are made for pregnant prisoners to receive antenatal care and for the baby to be delivered in a NHS hospital. Two secure prisons and one open one provide basic facilities and allow the mother to keep the baby up to 9 months (secure) and 18 months (open). The policy of then separating mother and child has been criticized (and hostel provision proposed). At any time there are some 30 women with children in prison.

Psychiatric disorder in female offenders

Cloninger and Guze[5], in their study of convicted American adult female prisoners, found that the incidence of serious mental illness (e.g. psychosis) was not significantly raised compared to the general population (a credit perhaps to their psychiatric services). They found, however, that only 12% had no psychiatric disorder. The principal diagnoses (26% of the women had both) were sociopathy (65%) and hysteria (41%). Sociopathy is equated with antisocial personality and hysteria (Briquet's syndrome) with somatization disorder (DSM IIIR) characterized by chronic complaints of multiple body disorders due to neurotic difficulties. These two groups would be covered in the ICD 10 by the dissocial personality disorder (F 60.2) and somatization disorder (F 45.0). Alcoholism occurred in 47% and drug dependence in 26%. Other diagnoses included homosexuality (6%), anxiety neurosis (11%), depression (6%), mental deficiency with an IQ less than 60 (6%) and schizophrenia (1.5%).

Other findings are in line with this study. Cowie *et al.*[6] studied adolescent girls detained in a classifying centre. This group was less delinquent than the adult prisoners and the level of disturbance less. Nevertheless, 51% of the girls had a psychiatric disorder varying from neurotic symptoms in 20% to seriously disturbed personalities and some serious mental illness in 31%. Staff from Holloway Prison for women stated in evidence to the Butler Committee that there was a much higher ratio of disturbed offenders in a female prison compared to a male prison, the majority of the disturbance being due to severe personality disorder, behaviour disorder or psychopathic disorder.

In a study at Holloway Prison[13] every fourth reception (remand and convicted) was studied to include 638 women. Physical ill health was a major problem in 17% mainly due to genitourinary diseases. Major psychosis occurred in 5%, neurosis in 5%, psychopathy or personality disorder in 21%, alcoholism in 8% and drug dependence in 5%. Thus 44% had some form of psychiatric disorder. One quarter had a history of psychiatric hospital admissions. A later study of 708 women in Holloway produced similar results[14].

These studies do illustrate the common finding of a high incidence of psychiatric disorder in serious female offenders. However, the bulk of this disorder is unlikely to lead to a transfer to a psychiatric hospital. Dell and Gibbens[15] found, for example, that only 6% of women remanded for medical reports to Holloway Prison were placed on hospital orders. Of the remainder 80% were released to the community and only 14% imprisoned.

Less serious offenders might be expected to have a lower incidence of psychiatric disorder. This was demonstrated in Gibbens' survey[9] of female shoplifters and the 10-year-follow-up[16]. The majority of the shoplifters (80%) were first offenders and most of them would not re-offend. Some 20% of first offenders and 30% of recidivists had psychiatric disorder at the time of the offence. In the follow-up (which was incomplete) 8.5% became inpatients in a mental hospital which is some three times the expected rate. The chance of becoming an inpatient increased with the number of previous offences so that 20% who had both offended before and after the index offence went into hospital. The commonest reason for admission was depression and suicide attempts.

Mediocolegal aspects of psychiatric disorder

Psychiatric disorder is used in mitigation or as a defence in exactly the same way as in males. There are nevertheless two situations specific to females:

(1) A defence of infanticide following the killing by the mother of her baby (see below and Chapters 3 and 7).
(2) Defences associated with hormone changes particularly the premenstrual syndrome, a subject reviewed fully by d'Orban[17].

There is a long history of women being excused their crime in the belief that disordered menstruation caused a disordered state of mind, e.g. Aurelia Snoswell (1851) was acquitted of the murder of her baby niece on the grounds of insanity due to disordered menstruation. Ann Shepherd

(1845) was acquitted of theft on the grounds of 'temporary insanity of the menses'. In a modern court the effect of the premenstrual syndrome was used as the basis for an acquittal against a charge of shoplifting where it was shown that the accused had cyclical episodes of confusion associated with menstruation. The theft was said to have occurred during such an episode. In that case there was clear evidence from the defendant's diary and her husband of the cyclical pattern.

There have, in the English Courts, been at least two cases of defendants using the effects of premenstrual tension successfully to plead diminished responsibility to a charge of murder.

> Craddock had 30 previous convictions, many for impulsive offences. In 1979 she quarrelled with and lethally stabbed a fellow barmaid. Premenstrual syndrome with tension and impulsivity was diagnosed. She was found guilty of manslaughter on the grounds of diminished responsibility. She was placed on probation with a condition of treatment (injections of progesterone). Later she missed two injections and subsequently threw a brick through a window. She was convicted and conditionally discharged. She later appealed against conviction on the grounds that she had had a temporary loss of criminal responsibility, a temporary derangement and inability to control herself. Her appeal was unsuccessful.

d'Orban concludes that the effects of the premenstrual syndrome may be used in mitigation only in the ways described, i.e. it has to be shown that the syndrome has caused a disturbance of mind of sufficient severity to be a mitigating factor. It would be too simplistic to regard the syndrome as accounting for all the disturbed behaviour shown by the offender. It is usually the final straw in a situation of women with a personality disorder already under a lot of stress. Whether or not a plea will be successful will depend in part on the proof that there is a cyclical disorder recognized by the doctors as premenstrual syndrome and the severity of the symptoms.

In making the diagnosis care has to be taken as histories may be falsified (consciously or unconsciously). On the other hand, the cyclical behavioural changes which occur may not coincide with subjective symptoms of depression, tension, etc. as discussed above.

It has been difficult to demonstrate scientifically the success of treatment for premenstrual syndrome though there are plenty of case histories asserting the value of intramuscular progesterone, pyridoxine or oral duphaston.

Offences especially associated with women

Prostitution

Although prostitution *per se* is not an offence, there are offences related to it, e.g. soliciting or keeping a brothel. Some 6% of women in prison are serving sentences directly related to prostitution and 25–30% of women remanded to prison are or have been a prostitute. Some 15% of the prostitutes had a history of signs of a mental breakdown[13], 25% had attempted suicide, 25% were alcoholic, 25% were dependent on drugs and 25% had physical disorders and deformities. There was a very high incidence of sociopathic personality and 16% were lesbian or bisexual. A number had a sadomasochistic relationship with their male ponces. Temporary prostitution, particularly in adolescents, may be a depressive act or a psychologically suicidal gesture though economic motives are a common rationalization.

Child stealing

Child stealing is an offence under the Offences Against The Person Act 1961. It applies to the stealing of any child under the age of 14 years with the intent to deprive the parent or guardian. It excludes the abduction of the child by a natural parent which may occur in arguments over access and possession.

Child stealing is a relatively rare offence and is actually committed more often by males when the motive is usually a sexual one. In the case of women, there is a high incidence of psychiatric disorder. Among 24 such female offenders d'Orban[18] found 8 cases of schizophrenia, 6 cases of mental retardation (including 2 with a transient psychosis) and 10 cases of personality disorder. Three main motivations were found:

(1) Comfort
    This group included girls from all the diagnostic groups. They tended to be young girls from large sibships with a history of parental neglect, a broken home and a delinquent milieu. The child-stealing was related to feelings of loneliness and deprivation. Many had had children of their own taken into care or had become separated from them. The common pattern was to take a child they already knew, perhaps through baby-sitting, alleging perhaps that the child was being badly looked after or was unwanted. It seemed that this allegation was largely a projection of their own feelings of rejection.
(2) Manipulation
    The four subjects in this group were of hysterical personality. Only one had a delinquent history and one had a psychiatric history. The child was stolen (often after considerable planning) in order to control a particular situation and to manipulate their partners. Typically, they might steal a baby and claim it was theirs in order to deceive their partner – 'you must stay because this baby is yours'. Most of this group receive penal sentences.
(3) Psychotic impulsivity
    This contained a schizophrenic patient and transiently psychotic

subnormal patients. All had a history of previous psychiatric treatment. The offences seemed bizarre and impulsive. Sometimes the act was understandable in terms of their delusional ideas, in some the act was inexplicable and in others the stealing seemed to be a comforting action to a psychotic subject whose own children had been taken into care.

A 35-year-old separated from her husband and child developed the delusion that people were talking about her and spreading unpleasant rumours. She saw a baby and 'knew' that it had been put there by the police to tempt her. She determined to take it to 'show them'. The court placed her on a hospital order with a restriction order to ensure that aftercare would be adequate.

In such cases the courts, whilst sympathetic to the mentally ill or subnormal offender, are very concerned for the safety of the public. d'Orban reported a repetition of child stealing in 3 of his 24 cases. The children stolen in d'Orban's series were well cared for except for one who was killed by a psychotic offender.

Homicide by women

Women commit homicide five times less than men. When they do, the victim is, in 80–90% of cases, a family member (50% a child, 34% a spouse) whereas only 40% of victims of males are family members. In two-thirds of cases the women are found to be mentally disturbed compared to one third of men[19].

Spouse murder

In most cases the women kill in retaliation for years of abuse, physical violence and emotional stress. The killing is often precipitated by the victim starting the physical confrontation, the violence commonly occurring in the kitchen. The charge is generally manslaughter (due to lack of intent) though a defence of self-defence is sometimes successful. The courts generally deal sympathetically with the case.

In a minority of cases the killing will arise from criminal motives such as revenge or greed (for financial gain) and occasionally a third party may be hired to do the killing.

Parricide (murder of parents)

This seems to be rare[20] i.e. 3.5% of all killing. Daughters commit parricide much less often than sons. Of 17 parricides by women, gathered from prison and psychiatric hospital, 14 were matricides and 3 were patricides. The matricides were committed by middle-aged women with psychoses

(11 cases), personality disorder (2 cases) or alcoholism (1 case). The women were living in a hostile, dependant relationship with their mothers and the killing was precipitated by mother's deteriorating physical and mental condition. Two patricides were committed by younger women in retaliation for chronic abuse and violence by the father.

Infanticide and child killing

Incidence
25% of all homicide victims are under 16 years and 80% of these children are killed by their parents. In children under 1 year, 60% are killed by their mother.

Classification
It is useful to consider three groups:

(1) Neonaticide: Killing the child within 24 hours.
(2) Fillicide: Killing the child within the first year for which the defence of infanticide (see Chapter 3) is possible as it is for neonaticide.
(3) Killing of the child after the first year.

The same motives for killing[21] occur in all groups and include:

(1) Parents who eliminate an unwanted child.
(2) Mercy killing (e.g. altruistic killing of a deformed child).
(3) Aggression attributable to gross mental pathology such as severe mental illness (killing for delusional reasons).
(4) Killing as a result of displaced hostile feelings, provoked by situations outside the victim, e.g. anger felt towards the spouse being directed onto the child as Medea killed Jason's sons.
(5) Killing as a result of a hostile feeling in the offender provoked by the victim, e.g. persistently crying babies provoking hostility in inadequate parents.

Consecutive filicide

This is thought to be rare but cases are described of mothers killing babies serially. They are usually found to be of psychopathic personality[22].

Neonaticide

The commonest reason (80%) is to get rid of an unwanted child at the time of its birth. Methods of killing include suffocation, strangulation, head trauma, drowning, exposure and stabbing, though other more bizarre methods occur. Drowning is commonly in toilets where the child may be born. Suffocation usually occurs after the first cry. After the death an attempt is often made to hide the body. The offender is almost always an unmarried mother who is usually under the age of 25 years. The majority of the offenders are passive young women who have become pregnant and wish to get rid of the unwanted child because of shame and fear. Most are otherwise totally law-abiding and indeed it is their degree of conformity which inhibits their seeking an abortion or coming to terms with the pregnancy. They usually ignore the pregnancy and carry on their life as if nothing had happened. They often manage to hide the fact of their pregnancy completely from the family. Whilst there are a very small number of women with little ethical restraint who may repeat the offence, the majority of the group will not. Whilst this accounts for the majority of cases Resnick[23] and others have also described neonaticide as a result of:

(1) An acute psychosis where the motive was delusional.
(2) Altruistic killing for the child's sake in cases of deformed children.
(3) Child battering.

Killing within the first year

D'Orban's series[24] showed the two causes which were equally common were 'battering' (see Chapter 7) and mental illness which between them account for 80% of the deaths. The mental illnesses included psychotic illness, acute reactive depression associated with a suicide attempt and severe depressive symptoms in mothers with marked personality disorders. Some two-thirds of women who kill their child commit suicide before trial. The battering cases were sudden impulsive acts with loss of temper precipitated by the baby's behaviour. There were also some cases of killing to get rid of an unwanted child, one case of a mercy killing of a deformed child and cases of women killing the child to make the spouse suffer (the Medea complex: Medea killed her children, when her spouse Jason left her, in order to punish him).

It has been suggested that some killings by suffocation escape detection and are mistaken for 'sudden infant death syndrome'[25].

Killing after the first year

As the children get older the chances of being killed by the mother decrease markedly – largely due to the fact that battering, as the cause of death, falls rapidly by the fourth year. By this time, the children are mobile and are able to recognize their parents' tension and avoid provoking parental wrath. It is also found that mercy killing did not occur after the first year. Mental illness remained an important cause.

Legal outcome after child killing

Neonaticide

The courts are sympathetic to this group of offenders. Generally, a plea of infanticide is successful despite the infrequency of gross psychiatric illness in this group. The Infanticide Act 1938 required only that there should be a disturbance of the balance of mind. There is no doubt that at the time of the killing the women are in a disturbed emotional state. In actual practice the degree of disturbance acceptable to the court seems much less than that required had the defence been one of diminished responsibility. In these cases the sentence after the finding has usually been a probation order with or without psychiatric supervision.

Killing within and after the first year

A verdict of murder is rare. In d'Orban's series there were only two cases of murder and in both, older children had been killed in retaliation against a spouse. There seems to have been little connection otherwise between the motivations of the homicides and the verdicts and sentences of the court. In the cases of homicide by battering, for example, the main verdicts were: manslaughter due to lack of intent to kill, manslaughter due to diminished responsibility, and infanticide. The sentences varied from hospital orders, probation and imprisonment. A similar variety of verdicts and sentences occurred in each group. This great variety reflects how any particular motivation may occur with any mental states for which there are a variety of appropriate disposals.

Munchausen's syndrome by proxy

The term covers the syndrome of mothers deliberately creating an impression that their child is ill[26]. Information may be falsified (tampering with charts, heating the thermometer) or the child may be repeatedly suffocated (to resemble blackouts), poisoned or gassed. The child is repeatedly brought before the medical staff. Diagnosis may require admission and secret observation of the mother with the child (e.g. using video). The false illness may start within the first two years and the child may be taught to lie and cheat doctors. Excess investigations may be carried out, the child may be kept from school and treatments may be given. Death may result where abuse occurs. Mothers seem to be inadequate people who enjoy the status and contact with hospital staff, perhaps escaping from domestic problems. There may also be considerable hostility towards the child particularly where there is physical abuse.

Management (involvement of social services and police) will depend on the extent of the danger to the child.

Young offenders

Introduction

The purpose of this section is to complete the information about young offenders. The incidence and aetiology of juvenile delinquency is discussed in Chapter 4. The courts and law in relation to young offenders is discussed in Chapter 2. This section will be used to list the facilities made available for young offenders. Rutter and Giller[7] discuss in detail the interventions which have been tried with juvenile delinquents.

Modern surveys have resulted in pessimistic conclusions about the efficacy of such interventions. At best, there is some evidence that some treatment programmes can be effective with some subpopulations, at least in the short term. The problems involved in research in this field are immense. The main ones may be listed as follows:

(1) Ascertaining exactly what intervention was carried out and whether it was done competently and persistently (e.g. was the group therapy given by trained and sensitive personnel or by untrained, poorly motivated staff?).
(2) Being sure that other interventions (not measured by the research) were not also being used, e.g. punitive measures or greater supervision as well as the 'psychotherapy' being studied.
(3) Being sure that the treatment group is as expected (and not altered during the course of the study) and that the matching group is truly like the treatment group. This is often extremely difficult to do, particularly when dealing with small numbers.
(4) Being sure of the validity and sensitivity of outcome measures (e.g. being a member of a treatment group may bias whether official action is taken after an offence and thus the treatment group may appear to have a different outcome to the comparison group. Simple offence counting may ignore a change in quality of the offending).
(5) Being sure that the follow-up period was long enough. It is frequently found that the improvement obtained in the institution is gradually dissipated over the next three years.

The principal interventions which have been tried include:

(1) Behavioural modification programmes (in the community and the family): These clearly produce changes in behaviour in the short term whilst treatment is being carried out, but there is uncertainty about the longer-term benefits.

(2) Counselling and psychotherapy: Overall studies have not demon-strated improved outcome results but there is evidence that some (the neurotic or willing) may do better with psychotherapy whereas others (the aggressive or non-amenable) do worse. Similarly, it seems that matching the supervising officer to the personality of the offender may affect the results.

(3) Therapeutic institutional regimes: These have not been shown to be convincingly superior to traditional institutional regimes in terms of re-conviction rates – both traditional and therapeutic regimes having re-conviction rates about 60–70%. However, studies of individual institutions show that in some institutions the delinquents improve while they are there and in others they get worse[27]. This seems to reflect the quality of the 'parenting' by the staff, with good staff–pupil relationships, firm expectations, discipline, higher standards and a harmonious, warm atmosphere producing the best result. Unfortu-nately, the beneficial effects of the institutions do not persist beyond three years' follow-up. What is not clear is whether a custodial approach is better or worse than a non-custodial one. There are a number of studies suggesting, overall, that a non-custodial is, at least, as effective as a custodial approach but there may be some delin-quents who do better after a period of custody.

Facilities available for the management of young offenders

Introduction

In recent years there has been an increasing emphasis on keeping young offenders out of the legal system and in the community because of the failure to demonstrate the efficacy of interventions. There is a fear of doing harm to the young people in institutions either by their picking up criminal ways or being subject to brutalization which is so often a feature of such places. Thus police are encouraged to caution first offenders rather than prosecute (depending on the offence) though it remains to be conclusively proven that this is a more effective way of dealing with delinquents. McCord[28] reviewed the legal actions taken against the children in the Cambridge Somerville study (see Chapter 5) and showed that the children who had been cautioned did less well, in the long run, than those who were actually taken to court, in terms of re-offending, everything else being equal. On the other hand, once taken to court, the least punitive sentences were followed by the least re-offending. For those who are prosecuted, various non-custodial alternatives are officially available and there is considerable experimentation with other non-custodial approaches on a voluntary basis, e.g. bringing offenders and victims together to allow the offender to realize the damage he has caused and to make amends.

Increasingly social services, probation, police and courts are successfully working together to divert the young offender away from custodial care using cautioning and non-custodial sentences (see Chapter 2), coupled with counselling and family work. This has led to a marked reduction in the number of juveniles sent into custody by the court (some 8000 in 1980 reduced to 3100 in 1989). However, the activities of some persistent young delinquents (who persist in offending on bail and afterwards) has aroused public demand for more control. It is likely therefore that there will be some modification of this more liberal policy, and the re-introduction of very secure units for this group (age 12–14).

This section will describe custodial facilities.

Custodial facilities

These facilities fall into those organized by the local authority or Department of Health and those organized by the Home Office.

Local authority and Department of Health facilities

(1) *Observation and assessment centres*
These are places in which juveniles can be detained while observations are made on the offender and background information collected. They may be single- or mixed-sexed institutions. They provide facilities for education, exercise and hobbies. They may have a secure wing or access to such security in another centre. The secure wings are physically secure areas designed to prevent absconding. Children cannot be held in them, however, for more than 72 hours without a juvenile court's permission. In the observation and assessment centres psychiatrists will be involved in providing psychiatric reports in relevant cases.

(2) *Community homes*
This term covers a variety of local authority-run homes for juveniles who are usually on care orders. They may also be used where a residence requirement has been placed on a juvenile offender who is on a supervision order. The homes may provide education on the premises or make use of local schools. The degree of security varies considerably but most are not secure establishments. The home, besides providing care and training, can provide counselling through its own staff and social workers. Psychological and psychiatric expertise may also be available. Within the same system are a few secure establishments which are able to look after those juveniles who have shown dangerous behaviour. The secure

establishments are otherwise run on the same principles as the open ones.

(3) *Youth treatment centres*

At the time of writing there are two such centres serving the country: Glenthorne, near Birmingham and St Charles at Brentwood, Essex[29]. They are Department of Health-run secure treatment units. The staff are drawn from social work, nursing and education. Psychologists and psychiatrists attend on a sessional basis. The clients are a heterogenous group of psychologically disordered juveniles of both sexes between the age of 12 and 18 years, though the younger ones are preferred as having a greater chance of benefitting. They will have behaved very dangerously or have been very difficult or persistent absconders elsewhere. An account of the Glenthorne Youth Treatment Centre is given by Reid[30], where a behavioural approach is adopted. A psychotherapeutic community approach is adopted at St Charles.

> A youth of 13 with a history of a series of increasingly violent serious sexual assaults on females was charged with an attempt to stab his female social worker. Psychiatric assessment showed him to have mild mental retardation but not to be mentally ill. The local subnormality services did not feel they could manage him safely. He was too young for special hospital. A place was obtained for him in a youth treatment centre through the Department of Health. He was sent there on a care order, though he might well have been dealt with by section 53(2) of the Children and Young Persons' Act 1933, a sentence made by a crown court which is the equivalent of a long sentence for adults or by section 53(1) of that Act, the equivalent of a life sentence.

(4) *Psychiatric services*

Juvenile offenders may be referred to the psychiatric services when it is suspected that they have a mental disorder which is treatable by the services. In most cases the referral will be to the child guidance clinic for assessment and treatment, though some assessments will be in the observation and assessment centres. Inpatient care can be offered in children's psychiatric wards or an adolescent unit. Such units show an increasing wish to concentrate on those with mental illness or psychoneurotic disorders – having failed to demonstrate any particular efficacy with conduct disordered children[31]. Secure psychiatric adolescent facilities are very rare as are units specializing in conduct disordered juveniles.

Moyes *et al.*[32] describe a hospital-based behaviour modification programme for adolescents referred for treatment because of severe conduct disorder due to behaviour or personality disorders. They were characterized by antisocial behaviour, aggression, truancy, absconding and self-mutilation. The results were compared with an appropriate comparison group who had been managed conventionally. They found that the improvement in behaviour which they obtained in the hospital appeared to persist to a greater extent than would have been expected from previous published results. These had given negative reports about the lasting efficacy of institutional behaviour modification programmes. It remains to be seen whether these results can be confirmed by further study.

Age is no bar to the use of hospital orders, and therefore, where appropriate, juveniles can be admitted on all the sections of the Mental Health Act. Special hospitals have, in the past, accepted juveniles but as far as possible they are not now admitted.

Home Office facilities

(1) *Remand centres*

These centres take young adults on remand. Although these centres may be geographically adjacent to adult prisons they are designed to keep these offenders away from adult offenders. The remand centre should provide appropriate work and recreation. Whereas the age group is normally 18–21 years, in rare cases very difficult boys of 15 years or more can be admitted if a certificate of unruliness can be obtained from the court. This practice is discouraged and it is expected that the secure facilities in observation and assessment centres should contain these boys. Remand centres will make use of prison medical staff and visiting psychiatrists to prepare psychiatric reports for the courts and to provide treatment for the mentally disordered offenders as appropriate.

(2) *Young offender institutions*

This term, from the Criminal Justice Act 1988, covers a variety of institutions set up under the 1988 Criminal Justice Act. It encompasses the old detention centres and youth custody centres (previously borstals). The aim is to develop a positive regime through activities and staff relationships in order to encourage self-discipline, a sense of responsibility, and personal development. Each offender has an individual officer who takes a special interest. Links with families are encouraged as is through-care with probation.

The institutions vary in security and are divided into those for juvenile males (15–17 years), those for short-term young adult males (18–20 years), those for long term young adults (18–20 years) and those for females. The regime for the juvenile and short-term older males is brisk and busy with a very structured day and an emphasis on education. The longer-term inmate will have an emphasis on work skills and education. Some contain on the same campus a remand centre alongside the areas for the convicted.

Psychiatrists are attached to a number of young offender institutes to offer an assessment and treatment service as required. Feltham Young Offender Institution and Glen Parva Young Offender Institution have both full-time medical staff specializing in the care of offenders with psychiatric problems.

The institutions have been criticized for sometimes failing to separate satisfactorily the different categories of offender, and for failing to provide satisfactory regimes or single accommodation.

Children as witnesses

Children may give evidence in court. If the court judges that a child does not understand the oath, evidence may be received anyway if the court judges that the child is sufficiently intelligent and understands the duty of speaking the truth (s.38(i) Children and Young Persons' Act 1933). Furthermore, since 1988 this evidence does not have to be supported by independent evidence. There has been a recent innovation in that video connection with the court and the child is permitted to save the child having to appear in court. Arrangements can also be made for a child in court to be shielded from seeing the offender in appropriate cases (e.g. sexual assault). At the time of writing it is unclear whether courts will accept as evidence a video-taped recording of an interview with a child (e.g. an interview between a psychiatrist and an abused child). It is not resolved whether the lack of opportunity to cross-examine the child would bar the use of such evidence. The jury would be expected to bear in mind the child's age and maturity in making a decision about the evidence.

References

(1) Home Office (1992) *Criminal Statistics*. England and Wales 1991. Cm. 2134. HMSO, London.
(2) Walker, N. (1965) *Crime and Punishment in Britain*. University Press, Edinburgh.
(3) Farrington, D.P. & Morris, A.M. (1983) Sex, sentencing and reconviction. *British Journal of Criminology* **23**, 229–47.
(4) d'Orban, P.T. (1971) Social and psychiatric aspects of female crime. *Medicine, Science and the Law* **11**, 275–81.
(5) Cloninger, R.C. & Guze, S.B. (1970) Female criminals: their personal, familial and social backgrounds. *Archives of General Psychiatry* **23**, 554–8.
(6) Cowie, J., Cowie, V. & Slater, E. (1968) *Delinquency in Girls*. Heinemann, London.
(7) Rutter, M. & Giller, H. (1983) *Juvenile Delinquency, Trends and Perspectives*. Penguin Books, Harmondsworth.
(8) Dalton, K. (1961) Menstruation and crime. *British Medical Journal* **2**, 1752–3.
(9) Gibbens, T.C.N. & Prince, J. (1962) *Shoplifting*. Institute for the Study and Treatment of Delinquency, London.
(10) Hands, J., Herbert, V. & Tennant, G. (1974) Menstruation and behaviour in a special hospital. *Medicine, Science and the Law* **14**, 32–5.

(11) d'Orban, P.T. & Dalton, J. (1980) Violent crime and the menstrual cycle. *Psychological Medicine* **10**, 353–9.

(12) Ballinger, C.B. (1976) Psychiatric morbidity and the menopause: clinical features. *British Medical Journal* **2**, 1183–5.

(13) Gibbens, T.C.N. (1971) Female offenders. *British Journal of Hospital Medicine* **6**, 279–86.

(14) Turner, T.H. & Tofler, D.S. (1986) Indicators of psychiatric disorder among women admitted to prison. *British Medical Journal* **292**, 651–3.

(15) Dell, S. & Gibbens, T.C.N. (1971) Remands of women offenders for medical reports. *Medicine, Science and the Law* **11**, 117–27.

(16) Gibbens, T.C.N., Palmer, C. & Prince, J. (1971) Mental health aspects of shoplifting. *British Medical Journal* **3**, 113–30.

(17) d'Orban, P.T. (1983) Medicolegal aspects of the premenstrual syndrome. *British Journal of Hospital Medicine* **30**, 404–9.

(18) d'Orban, P.T. (1976) Child stealing: a typology of female offenders. *British Journal of Criminology* **16**, 275–81.

(19) d'Orban, P.T. (1990) Female homicide. *Irish Journal of Psychological Medicine* **7**, 64–70.

(20) d'Orban, P.T. & O'Connor, A. (1989) Women who kill their parents. *British Journal of Psychiatry* **154**, 27–33.

(21) Scott, P.D. (1973) Parents who kill their children. *Medicine, Science and the Law* **13**, 120–6.

(22) d'Orban, P.T. (1990) A commentary on consecutive filicide. *Journal of Forensic Psychiatry* **1**, 260–5.

(23) Resnick, P.J. (1970) Murder of the newborn: a psychiatric review of neonaticide. *American Journal of Psychiatry* **126**, 1414–19.

(24) d'Orban, P.T. (1979) Women who kill their children. *British Journal of Psychiatry* **134**, 560–71.

(25) Meadows, R. (1989) Suffocation. *British Medical Journal* **298**, 1572–3.

(26) Meadows, R. (1989) Munchausen syndrome by proxy. *British Medical Journal* **299**, 248.

(27) Sinclair, I. & Clarke, R. (1982) Predicting, treating and explaining delinquency: the lessons from research on institutions. In Feldman, P. (ed.) *Developments in the Study of Criminal Behaviour, Vol. 1., The Prevention and Control of Offending.* John Wiley and Sons Ltd, Chichester.

(28) McCord, J. (1985) Deference and the light touch of the law. In Farrington, D.P. and Gunn, J. (eds). *Reactions to Crime: The Public, The Police, The Courts and Prisons.* John Wiley and Sons Ltd, Chichester.

(29) Parker, E. (1985) The development of secure provision. In Gostin, L. (ed.) *Secure Provision.* Tavistock Publications, London and New York.

(30) Reid, I. (1982) The development and maintenance of a behavioural regime in a secure youth treatment centre. In Feldman, P. (ed.) *Developments in the Study of Criminal Behaviour. Vol. 1., The Prevention and Control of Offending.* John Wiley and Sons Ltd, Chichester.

(31) Steinberg, D. (1982) Treatment, training, care or control. *British Journal of Psychiatry* **141**, 306–9.

(32) Moyes, T., Tennant, T.G. & Bedford, A.P. (1985) Long term follow-up study of a ward-based behaviour modification programme for adolescents with acting-out and conduct problems. *British Journal of Psychiatry* **147**, 300–5.

Chapter 14

Dangerousness

Introduction

The forensic psychiatrist is frequently expected to comment on the 'dangerousness' of subjects. The request for this opinion will come from the court in relation to the sentencing of mentally disordered offenders; from the Mental Health Review Tribunal in relation to patients being released into the community; the Home Office in relation to patients detained under restriction orders being considered for discharge into the community; and from the managers of a hospital in relation to the detention of a patient under the Mental Health Act 1983. In addition, within the prison service, an opinion on dangerousness may be requested by the parole board for inmates serving long or life sentences. Furthermore, the dangerousness of a patient is forefront in the mind of a psychiatrist on a day-to-day basis in relation to management, degree of security and observation required, progress of the underlying disorder, the reaction of the offender to stress and various possible provoking situations.

This chapter will deal with:

(1) What is meant by dangerousness.
(2) The estimation of dangerousness.
(3) The relationship of dangerousness to mental abnormality.

Definition of dangerousness

There is no agreed definition of dangerousness. The Butler Committee[1] equated 'dangerousness' '... with a propensity to cause serious physical injury or lasting psychological harm'. Scott[2] defined dangerousness as 'an unpredictable and untreatable tendency to inflict or risk irreversible injury or destruction'. Others have objected to 'unpredictable and untreatable' feeling that the recognition of risk or the treatability of the patient does not reduce the danger[3] although it does allow protective steps to be taken.

The dangerousness of a subject refers to dangerousness in a particular situation or in a particular state of mind. It may well be that whilst the patient is suffering from a paranoid delusion about his mother he represents a severe danger to her whilst he lives at home, judging by his previous assaults and his emotional reactions. The danger of harm to the mother is decreased by admitting the patient to hospital, and substantially decreased by admitting him to a secure unit. The danger will similarly diminish if the illness is treated successfully with loss of the delusions.

Nevertheless, one of the problems which remains in the concepts of dangerousness is the lack of precision in the terms such as 'serious' injury or 'lasting' psychological harm. There is always a risk of a gradual extension of the meaning so that it ends up encompassing minor offenders. The other major problem is the questionable ability of professionals to gauge future dangerousness.

Reconviction prediction score

It might be expected that a careful evaluation of all the factors known to be associated with repeated offending would allow a checklist to be prepared by which any single case could be judged. There have been various attempts at what might be called an 'actuarial system'. In the UK, the parole board system is probably the best. This computerized system, which was used by the parole board, gives a *'parole score'* according to the presence or absence of relevant factors in a particular case, e.g. age of onset of convictions, number of previous convictions, behaviour in institutions. By careful refining, it has become clear which factors are the most helpful and what weight can be attached to them.[4]

The Reconviction Prediction Score Table with the conversion table is reproduced in Table 14.1. A number is obtained for a subject by adding up the relevant subscores. The number is then converted to the Reconviction Prediction Score (using the conversion table, see Table 14.2). This score is the percentage chance of re-offending within two years for the group the subject falls into. Of those with a high score (25 or above), 90% or more will re-offend. Of those with a very low score (minus 25 or less), 10% or less will re-offend. The problem remaining for the parole board (and any one else making a prediction) is, of course, to interpret a particular score for a particular individual. The score can only be a guide in an individual case. The score is validated for prisoners and not for psychiatric patients. Allowance would have to be made for the influence of the illness on the individual's behaviour. At the extremes, a low re-offending rate would be expected where the abnormal mental state was controlled and the parole score was a low one. The reverse would be true when the mental state was not improved and the score was a high one.

Table 14.1 Calculation of the reconviction prediction score

The raw score is obtained by adding together the relevant subscores.

Main offence		Number of previous convictions	
Burglary	+2	None	−9
Theft	+1	1 or 2	−5
Robbery	−1	3 to 5	nil
Homosexual offences	−1	6 to 14	+1
Taking and driving away	−2	15 or more	+5
Criminal damage	−2		
Living on immoral earnings	−2	**Age at first conviction**	
Drug offences	−2	Under 14	+2
Drunken driving	−2	14 to 20	+1
Other indictable offences	−2	21 to 29	−2
Immigration offences	−2	30 to 39	−5
Arson	−2	40 to 49	−8
Fraud and Forgery	−3	50 and over	−9
Receiving and handling	−3		
Heterosexual offences	−4	**Number of previous imprisonments**	
Homicide	−8	15 or more	+5
Other offences	nil	6 to 14	+3
		5	+1
Age at offence		1 to 4	nil
Under 21	+5	0	−4
21 to 24	+1		
25 to 39	nil	**Interval at risk since last release**	
40 to 49	−1	Less than 6 months	+3
50 and over	−2	6 months but less than 1 year	+1
		1 year but less than 2 years	nil
Value of property stolen		2 years but less than 5 years	−2
None	nil	5 years or more	−5
Less than £50	+3		
£50 but less than £1000	nil	**Juvenile custodial treatment**	
£1000 or more	−2	None	nil
Not applicable	nil	Approved school only	+1
		Borstal/detention centre	+2
Number of associates			
3 or fewer	nil	**Probation history**	
4 or more	+4	None	−3
		More than once, never breached	−3
Offences during current sentence		Once only, not breached	nil
1 or more escapes	+4	Once only under 17, with breach	+1
No escapes	nil	Once only 17 or over, with breach	+2
		More than once, with breach	+3

Reconviction prediction score

Prison offences		Time in last job	
1 or more escapes	+4	Short or casual	+3
No escapes	nil	No job for 5 years since release	+2
		Less than 1 month	+3
Occupation (Registrar-General's Class)		1 but less than 6 months	nil
Non-manual I or II	−4	6 months but less than 1 year	1
Non-manual III	−3	1 but less than 3 years	−4
Non-manual IV	nil	3 but less than 5 years	−5
Manual II, III or IV	−1	5 years or more	−6
Manual V	+1		
		Living arrangements at time of offence	
Employment at time of offence		No fixed abode	+3
Unemployed	+1	Sibling or friend	+1
Employed part time	nil	Cohabiting	−1
Employed full time	−2	Wife	−2
Self-employed	−1	Relatives/in-laws	−3
		Other	nil
		Current marital status	
		Single	+2
		Divorced	+1
		Married/widowed	−2

Reproduced with the permission of the Controller of HMSO.

Table 14.2   Conversion to reconviction prediction score

Raw score	RPS	Raw score	RPS
−31 or less	0	+1	52
−30	2	+2	53
−29	4	+3	55
−28	5	+4	56
−27	7	+5	58
−26	8	+6	60
−25	10	+7	61
−24	12	+8	63
−23	13	+9	64
−22	15	+10	66
−21	16	+11	68
−20	18	+12	69
−19	20	+13	71
−18	21	+14	72
−17	23	+15	74
−16	24	+16	76
−15	26	+17	77
−14	28	+18	79
−13	29	+19	80
−12	31	+20	82
−11	32	+21	84
−10	34	+22	85
−9	36	+23	87
−8	37	+24	88
−7	39	+25	90
−6	40	+26	92
−5	42	+27	93
−4	44	+28	95
−3	45	+29	96
−2	47	+30	98
−1	48	+31 or more	100
0	50		

The estimation of dangerousness

There is some evidence that some doctors may be able to predict dangerousness in the very short term. Two-thirds of patients, admitted on section as emergencies because of dangerousness, were assaultive within the first 72 hours compared to one third of voluntary patients[5].

Nevertheless it is often asserted that clinicians have, in fact, very little ability to assess dangerousness in the longer term and that doctors grossly overpredict it. The belief that clinicians have a special ability to gauge the dangerousness of mentally disordered offenders was shaken by the findings in the 1970s by Steadman *et al.*[6] on the follow-up of patients released from the Dannemora State Hospital for Insane Criminals in the USA. Baxstrom, a prisoner, was declared insane and dangerous by psychiatrists and detained in the above hospital for treatment. His appeal, based on the lack of treatment, was successful and his detention was declared unconstitutional. He and 969 patients were therefore transferred to a civil hospital although all were thought to be dangerous. At four years follow-up 20% of the men and 26% of the women had assaulted someone though the majority of these assaults were minor. On the other hand, some 50% of the original 969 survived in the community. The others stayed in or were returned to ordinary psychiatric hospital. In short, over 75% of the original 969 patients appear to have been detained unnecessarily in the secure hospital on the grounds of 'dangerousness'. Similar findings occurred in other hospitals in the United States.

So, although it seems that dangerousness was overpredicted, is it the case that doctors are really no better than anyone else at gauging dangerousness? Kozol et al.[7] studied a group of sexual offenders who they believed were dangerous and had been detained. A subgroup of these patients were released as 'safe' by a tribunal against the doctor's advice. Another group was released after treatment when the doctors considered them to be safe. The doctor's group had a recidivism rate of 6.1% whilst the tribunal's group had a recidivism rate of 34.7% – strongly suggesting that the doctors were better at estimating dangerousness than the tribunal. This finding was echoed by Acres[8] in his study of patients discharged from Broadmoor hospital by doctors or by tribunals. Nevertheless, it is also clear that whilst one-third of the tribunal group re-offended, two-thirds would nevertheless have been detained unnecessarily. It does seem therefore that it is probably impossible at the present time to identify future dangerousness amongst a group of offenders with a successful prediction rate greater than 45%.

On the other hand, whilst Kozol et al. showed that doctors were better than the tribunal at assessing dangerousness, Harding et al.[9] found, in an experimental situation, that doctors did not achieve a high level of agreement about dangerousness and psychiatrists tended to rate patients as more dangerous than did non-psychiatrists. They concluded that there should be better training for psychiatrists based on operational definitions of dangerousness in order to get better inter-rater reliability but the problem of predictive accuracy would remain.

There are two reactions to this dilemma. The libertarian view, outlined by Bottoms[10], argues that because of the poor prediction rate, and the tendency of the psychiatrist to be cautious, only those offenders with a history of, say, three previous offences should be subject to this judgement. In such a subgroup of offenders, the chances of a successful prediction would be about 66%, much higher than in a general population. Bottoms argues that the current system of locking up three people in order to prevent one offending is unjust. The protectionist view is outlined by Walker[11, 12]. He argues that the detention of three offenders to prevent one offending is justified to prevent harm to the innocent victim.

Simply because we cannot prevent the majority of cases of violence, does not mean we should give up trying to prevent a few cases. At the present time, the protectionist view is the one adopted by society and the courts, and is the one most psychiatrists are identified with.

Dangerousness and mentally disordered offenders

Some patients are seen who have shown no delinquent or violent behaviour until the development of mental illness. For that particular patient, undoubtedly the mental illness made the patient more dangerous than he would otherwise have been. What is not known is what percentage of people becoming mentally ill become dangerous. It appears that different psychiatric conditions contribute differently to the violence figures (see Chapter 7). Taylor and Gunn[13] found a higher percentage of schizophrenic and other psychotic subjects amongst serious violent offenders than expected. Similarly, Hafner and Boker[14] showed in a 10-year-review of violent offenders in Germany that schizophrenics were more likely to be amongst violent offenders than would be expected, whilst depressives, organic brain syndrome, and the mentally handicapped were less. It was calculated that the rate of violent offending was 5 in 10 000 schizophrenics and 6 in 100 000 with affective psychosis. Many studies have also shown that there is a high percentage of people with a psychopathic disorder amongst violent offenders.

In earlier years, patients discharged from conventional large psychiatric hospitals had rates of criminality and violence which were lower or the same as the rates for the community at large. However, in recent years – perhaps coinciding with a policy of rapid discharge coupled with an intolerance of difficult patients – there has been a raised rate of violence in ex-hospital patients (see Chapter 8). Penrose[15] showed in 1936, in a study of criminality rates and psychiatric facilities in different European countries, that a higher national homicide rate correlated with a lower number of hospital beds. The current situation may reflect 'Penrose's Law'.

Particular interest has been aroused about the dangerousness of ex-special hospital patients in view of the publicity attached to certain cases. Tidmarsh[3] and Bowden[16] have reviewed relevant studies of patients discharged from Broadmoor and other special hospitals. In general terms over a five-year-follow-up, 50% of the patients will have committed an offence, most of which will have been minor. However, some 1% will have committed homicide and some 10% will have committed a serious violent offence. Tidmarsh also found that there seemed to be a greater incidence of violent re-offending in patients discharged in 1971 compared to those discharged in 1960–65 – perhaps reflecting the changes (mentioned above) in ordinary psychiatric hospitals. Home Office figures[17] for mentally disordered offenders discharged from all hospitals on restriction orders show that at five years, 28% will have committed a standard list offence (this ignores a number of very minor offences) and 5% will have committed a grave offence (murder, rape, arson, etc). The Home Office figures are lower because they also include restricted patients sent to ordinary psychiatric hospitals (less dangerous and less recidivistic). Interestingly, their figures show that patients referred from special hospital to ordinary hospital before conditional discharge have nearly 30% less convictions than those conditionally discharged directly from a special hospital.

The Home Office figures on patients are very similar to the figures on the re-conviction rate of life-sentenced offenders released on licence. Both groups had an approximately 28% re-offending rate including 5% committing grave offences. These rates of re-conviction are much lower than the average re-conviction rate for persons released from prison. Of violent men released from prison, 52% will have been re-convicted of an offence in two years compared to the 2 year rate in lifers of 9% and 14% in restricted patients. The public reaction to re-offending of ex-hospital patients is not to question the ability of the psychiatrist to label someone dangerous but to question the ability to label someone as 'safe'.

It must be concluded therefore that some mental disorders will increase the chances of dangerous behaviour in an individual although only a small portion of the mentally abnormal will be violent (violence is after all a relatively rare offence) and only a very small proportion of all violent offenders will require psychiatric treatment for serious mental illness. It must also be the case that re-offending will be affected by the quality of care and follow up given to the patient.

The clinical assessment of dangerousness

The clinician will be concerned, broadly, with two situations where dangerousness has to be considered.

First, possible dangerous behaviour in the very near future, e.g. when considering admission after an incident or on parole. The factors which will be most important here will be current mental state, the state of arousal, hostility and the expressed (overt or covert) intention of the patient plus recent behaviour and past dangerous behaviour (violence, threats, collection of weapons), as well as the social tensions playing on the patient. Unco-operativeness with treatment, the presence of substance abuse and any relevant neurological or other medical disorder will also be indications of instability.

Second, in estimating the long-term dangerousness of a patient where there is no evidence to suggest an immediate short term danger. Here actuarial factors (previous offences, etc) will be more important (see parole score above) coupled with an assessment of the chances of a return to the clinical state in which the dangerousness is likely. A detailed knowledge of the clinical pattern of the past and the overall pattern of behaviour, as shown by a detailed history, will help in this judgement. Undoubtedly the best predictive factors remain the number (and type) of previous offences, sex and age. The clinician attempts to gauge how the patient's particular clinical features colour the assessment.

The key to the clinical approach has been outlined by Scott[2]. An understanding of the case is built up from a study of the development of the subject, patterns of behaviour in the past and current mental state. The relevant questions are:

(1) Is there a recurrent pattern in the past which will help estimate the future?
(2) Are any alarming new patterns emerging of, say, escalating violence?
(3) Are there new circumstances (alterations in states of mind, changes in domestic situations) which make a previous equilibrium unstable?

In making this assessment, there is no substitute for including a painstaking appraisal of all previous medical notes, social reports and relevant statements.

Personal data

Childhood

Poor parenting, violent parents, an alcoholic father and a dominant mother are all features which correlate with later violent behaviour. The loss of a parent sensitizes the subject to loss at a later age which may result in an over-reaction to loss or the threat of it. A triad of firesetting enuresis and cruelty to animals has been said to be linked to later violent behaviour, though it may be difficult to prove[18]. Early signs of persistent antisocial behaviour may be detected from behaviour at home or at school (persistent stealing, lying, running away, fire raising, truanting, suspension or expulsion from school or fighting). Isolation from peers, inability to sustain relationships, deep hostility to authority may all presage adult difficulties. Certain features have not been proven to be significantly linked to violence although formerly suspected to be so. These include minimal brain damage, temporal lobe disorders, the presence of an extra Y-chromosome and a raised serum testosterone level.

Sexual history

The sexual history of the subject will reveal his ability to form and sustain mature relationships. It is common to find among violent sexual offenders a history of fantasies of violence which have progressed gradually to acting out of lesser assaults and then the actual offence. Tactful enquiries should be made about the subject's experience of sadistic fantasies. On direct questioning, a subject may admit to beginning to act out fantasies, first thinking about an attack, later going into a park and watching potential victims, initially lacking courage and then making the first tentative attack. Where a subject can relate such a development, i.e. when a subject can speak frankly of his feelings and actions and at the same time express a wish to rid himself of these impulses then there can be a hope for a therapeutic rapport. The future seems bleaker when the subject is obviously refusing to talk about fantasies or behaviour which, from all the evidence, must be there. Similarly, there is little optimism for the subject who has failed to co-operate with therapy in the past and only asks for help after a further arrest.

A degree of jealousy in sexual relationships is normal. Excessive jealousy which arises independently of the partner's behaviour (sometimes called pathological or morbid jealousy) may well be associated with extreme violence (see Chapter 8).

Occupational history

The work record of the subject may throw light on the characteristics of the subject. A careful history should be obtained of the number of jobs, the reasons for changing, a history of any dismissals and the reasons for them. The subject's relationship to authority and his peers, his ability to cope with stressful situations at work (criticism and conflicting orders), and his ability to work in harmony with others (avoiding arguments and fights) reflects his personality. It is important to determine if any periods of unemployment were due to periods of illness, particularly mental illness, the inability to cope with work and its stresses, or due to the effects of alcohol or drug abuse. While such factors may not correlate specifically with dangerousness in themselves, they may, in conjunction with other factors, give information about the subject which may contribute to an understanding of the offence and hence the future.

Personality

An understanding of the personality of the subject will be built up partly from the information so far obtained but it can be expanded by specific questions about his ability to relate to others. Enquiries should be made as to whether the subject is isolated and friendless or sociable and outgoing. Is he placid or tense with a tendency to overreact? Does the subject take offence easily, suspect people are talking about him in public places and if so, does he ever confront them? Is he known as a man with a chip on his shoulder? Is the subject considerate and empathic or egocentric and lacking in sympathy? Is he of normal or low self-esteem? Does he react badly, perhaps with aggression, to situations which threaten this self-esteem? Is this a factor in his offence? What is his attitude to authority as measured by previous offending? In the case of violence, one previous violent offence is associated with a 14% chance of re-conviction. Four previous convictions for violence is associated with a 60% chance of re-conviction[11]. When studying previous convictions details should be sought to elicit what actually has happened. A charge of actual bodily harm (ABH) may hide the fact that an attempt to do serious harm was aborted.

Alcohol or drugs are both disinhibiting factors and their abuse, in conjunction with other factors predisposing to violence, is likely to increase the chance of violence recurring. Attention should therefore be paid to assessing carefully the amount taken at any one time, how often, in what situations and with what untoward effects, e.g. fights, assaults, arguments, loss of temper or precipitation of abnormal mental states such as hallucinosis or paranoia.

Psychiatric history

Where there is a history of psychiatric illness or other mental disorder then a very thorough history of previous contacts with psychiatric agencies is required. The time of onset of the illness should be carefully ascertained. It may become clear that the onset corresponds to the onset of antisocial or violent behaviour and thus light may be thrown on the aetiology of the disturbance. The nature of the illness, its symptoms and response to treatment should be noted in detail for each previous admission or period of care. Note should also be made of the extent to which the patient co-operated with treatment and the times, if any, when he failed to co-operate and the effects of this. Care should be taken to note the extent to which the patient sought help as he became ill or the extent to which compulsory measures had to be employed. An estimate can be made about the extent to which the patient is likely to co-operate with treatment in the future. This is helpful in organizing aftercare and in commenting on the need for restriction orders or probation orders in order to ensure adequate community supervision.

Details of previous violent episodes in hospital and in the community should be recorded. A note should be made of the person hurt, the extent of the injury, the precipitant and the motivation for the attack looking for the links between the disturbed mental state and the violence. Was the relationship a direct one due to delusions and hallucinations, an indirect one due to the general decline brought about by the illness or was it quite independent of the illness? Are there any particular people placed at risk by the disturbed mental state and is violence increasing or decreasing? These questions will lead to a body of information which will contribute towards the prognosis and recommendations about management.

One of the commonest complaints of relatives of schizophrenics is that doctors fail to react quickly enough to relatives' reports that a patient is becoming ill. A week or two may elapse before action is taken. This delay is particularly worrying where violence or threats of it are features of the case. Cases are regularly seen where tragedy has occurred within that period of delay. What percentage of all such cases end badly is not known but there must be room for improvement. Situations which should alert the doctor to the need for rapid action include any of the following:

(1) Recurrence of a mental state which in the past has been associated with violent behaviour, including suicidal attempts.
(2) A mentally disordered patient making threats that he will do harm, particularly where there has been previous violence.
(3) A relative (or other person) reporting that a mentally disordered patient is behaving threateningly or dangerously, even if the patient denies it (as will occur with some patients).
(4) A mentally disordered patient with a history of violent behaviour being reported to have a deteriorating mental state, e.g. increased irritability, tension, isolation.
(5) A patient, with a history of violence and instability, refusing to continue taking medication.

Behaviour in hospital or prison

The patient's behaviour in the institution in which he is detained has to be examined when release is being considered. In the case of *mental illness* the most desirable improvements are:

(1) Loss of the anger and tension present at the time of the offence.
(2) Control or reduction in the psychotic or neurotic phenomena which were present at the time of the offence. Persecutory delusions and command hallucinations are said to be particularly associated with violence. The patient should no longer hold the old belief with the same intensity and his emotional reactions to the original stimuli should now be normal. The hallucinatory experiences should stop or be substantially reduced. The patient may not gain full insight into the illness but can still be safe if the current phenomena are sufficiently suppressed by treatment.

In the case of the *mentally impaired*, there should be:

(1) Improvement in behaviour with the loss of the aggressive or irresponsible responses originally seen, and a loss of antisocial attitudes.
(2) Improvement in social functioning with increased ability to cooperate with others, and improved social skills.

In the case of *psychopathic disorder* there should be:

(1) Improvement in behaviour and in emotional reactions to others;

consideration where previously there was egocentricity and no consideration.
(2) Acceptance of authority, toleration of frustration and other stresses without reacting badly.
(3) Appropriate and sufficient change in sex offenders – as measured by psychological and psychophysiological tests. In interview, they should be able to discuss their sexuality frankly and form a good therapeutic rapport. The unwanted fantasies should have been lost and, ideally, replaced by acceptable ones or, at least, impulse control be in place.

Making the assessment of a subject in an institution involves the very careful reading of all the records of his stay and particularly the notes of the staff who look after him on a day-to-day basis. A detailed record should be made of any relevant incidents, violence, aggression, episodes of mental disturbance, improvements in relationships, etc. In this way a detailed account of the patient's development in the institution will be made. This can be checked by discussion with staff and with the patient. The patient, when interviewed, will naturally attempt to make a good impression and this must be balanced against the actual record. An attempt must be made to assess whether any apparent progress is due to genuine improvement or whether it merely reflects the ability of the subject to conform. The latter may be revealed by the careful combing of the notes and discussion with staff. However, it will be impossible to assess certain weaknesses of the subject for he will not be exposed to them in the institution, e.g. alcohol, drugs, access to gambling, access to children or women. It may be possible to transfer the subject to a less restricted situation where these things can be tested relatively safely, e.g. from special hospital to a regional secure unit, from prison to a hostel, from regional secure unit to local psychiatric hospital.

The offence

The legal category will not help, e.g. theft or assault. What is required is a detailed account of the behaviour at the time. This is best obtained by seeing the witness statements or interviewing relatives, as well as the subject. Gross misjudgements can occur where the doctor has not been appraised of the facts:

> A schizophrenic patient was charged with assault against his wife. He was admitted to a hospital on a treatment order. He seemed to improve and was given home leave. During the leave he killed his wife and children. Only then did it become known to the hospital staff that the original assault was not, as had been assumed, a single blow. It had, in fact, been an aborted serious attempt to stab the wife arising from a delusional idea.

From the information about the offence and information relating to the subject's mental state at the time of the offence various questions may be answered. Was the behaviour impulsive or prepared? If impulsive, was it provoked or spontaneous? What was the nature of the provocation? Does it arise from the victim or from a distorted perception by the offender? Is it such that the offender is likely to meet it again and how is he likely to cope with it in future? What is the relation of the victim to the offender? Are there others who may in the future have a similar relationship and therefore be at risk?

The degree of violence seems to increase according to the defence-lessness of the victim, especially where the offender has no fear of retaliation. It seems greater in family killings, multiple killings, where the offender has a mental illness, where women are killed and where the offender is intoxicated with alcohol. What is not known is whether it has any prognostic value. A bizarre quality (mutilation or ritual) associated with the violence may indicate mental illness but more often a grossly disturbed personality. The bizarre quality is assumed to indicate a poor prognosis in the absence of effective treatment. Disinhibiting factors which should be looked for include:

(1) Alcohol and drugs.
(2) Companions.
(3) Fatigue leading to irritability.

Were these common features in the past and are they likely to be present in the future?

Emphasis is often placed on the behaviour of the offender after the offence – the extent to which he shows remorse or not, either by word or deed. However, this is often a very difficult thing to estimate and it is easy to be misled either way.

A particular offence may be understandable only in terms of a sudden regression to a primitive rage reaction in the face of stress. In such a case how easily did the offender regress – is this a rare event or a frequent one in his life? How resistant normally is he to stress and how much stress is required before such a reaction would occur again? What were the roles of such variables as provocation, the presence of disinhibiting factors, etc.? A view will then be obtained which will allow the balancing of all the factors past and present and contribute to an assessment of the chances of recurrence.

Mental state of the subject at the time of interview

It is a good practice to have examined the medical notes and the statements before interviewing the subject. This has the advantage of clarifying the issues beforehand. There will be a natural tendency for the subject to gloss over embarrassing points, to tone down the more unpleasant aspects, to hide motivations and deceive the interviewer about his true mental state. The interviewer will have a better chance of eliciting the true state of affairs if he has already seen independent accounts, then, should he find a difference between the subject's account and the independent one, he can direct the interview to clarify this.

In assessing dangerousness the psychiatrist undoubtedly has to be sceptical and to be prepared to be interrogative, though always tactful and sensitive. One cannot assume that the subject will give a full account. He may be too embarrassed, or, in the case of the mentally ill, he may wish to hide his delusions. All this will therefore have to be gently and tactfully elicited. One has to try and match the independent account with the subject's account so that the whole incident makes psychological sense. When it does not do so it is usually because something has been hidden from the psychiatrist and this is often by the subject.

The interview should be used to clarify and fill out the information already gained about the subject's background and development. During this process the interviewer will gain an impression of the frankness of the subject and his willingness to examine and treat any problems he may have.

The subject's current emotional state will be apparent from his demeanour in interview but special questioning should also be directed to his state at the time of the offence and at the time leading up to the offence. The violent outburst may be the culmination of a long build-up of emotional disturbance such as depression, anger or anxiety. Care must be taken to check if this is now improved. Has the state of tension resolved? Does the subject now feel he is safe? Homicides, like suicides, are often preceded by warnings and, like suicide, intention can be uncovered by careful interview. Ask about current violent fantasies: Is there still an urge to do harm? Ask if weapons are still being carried or are easily available. Ask what is the worst thing he has done and whether he feels safe from others and himself. Homicidal intention should be treated with the utmost gravity.

It will become apparent also during the interview whether or not there is any gross disturbance of memory or orientation. Any disturbance of consciousness will also become apparent as will any disturbance of ability to concentrate.

In the formal taking of the current mental state it is imperative to check for all psychotic symptoms where mental illness is suspected. The subject must be asked if he has experienced now, at the time of the offence, or in the distant past, such symptoms as hearing voices, having experience of the television or radio speaking to him, etc. Failure to examine the mental state in detail will lead to failure to detect the illness. It seems to be a not uncommon error to miss psychotic symptoms or dismiss them as 'learned' and therefore misclassify someone as 'personality disordered' when in fact they are actually suffering from a psychosis.

Putting the whole picture together

At the end of this examination a psychiatrist should be in a position to give a historical account of the development of the subject in which his current behaviour becomes understandable. It is on this basis, in conjunction with a knowledge of the statistics of re-offending, that predictions are made about the future as well as recommendations for treatment and management.

References

(1) Home Office and DHSS (1975) Report of the Committee on Mentally Abnormal Offenders (Butler Committee). Cmnd 6244. HMSO, London.
(2) Scott, P.D. (1977) Assessing dangerousness in criminals. *British Journal of Psychiatry* **131**, 127–42.
(3) Tidmarsh, D. (1982) Implications from research studies. In Hamilton, J.R. and Freeman, H. (eds) *Dangerousness: Psychiatric Assessment and Management.* Gaskell, for The Royal College of Psychiatrists, London.
(4) Ward, D. (1987) *The Validity of the Reconviction Prediction Score.* Home Office Research Study No. 94. HMSO, London.
(5) McNiel, D.E. & Binder, R.L. (1987) Predictive validity of judgements of dangerousness in emergency civil commitments. *American Journal of Psychiatry* **144**, 197–280.
(6) Steadman, H.J. and Keveles, G. (1972) The community adjustment and criminal activity of the Baxstrom patients 1966–1970. *American Journal of Psychiatry* **129**, 304–10.
(7) Kozol, H.L., Boucher, R.J. and Garofalo, R.F. (1972) The diagnosis and treatment of dangerousness. *Journal of Crime and Delinquency* **18**, 371–92.
(8) Acres, D.I. (1975) The after care of special hospital patients. In *Home Office and DHSS Report of the Committee on Mentally Abnormal Offenders.* Appendix 30 Cmnd 6244. HMSO, London.
(9) Harding, T. & Montandon, C. (1982) Does dangerousness travel well? In Hamilton, J.R. and Freeman, H. (eds) *Dangerousness: Psychiatric Assessment and Management.* Gaskell for the Royal College of Psychiatrists, London.
(10) Bottoms, A.E. (1982). Selected issues in the dangerousness debate. In Hamilton, J.R. and Freeman, H. (eds) *Dangerousness: Psychiatric Assessment and Management.* Gaskell for The Royal College of Psychiatrists, London.
(11) Walker, N. (1982) Ethical aspects of detaining dangerous people. In Hamilton, J.R. and Freeman, H. (eds) *Dangerousness: Psychiatric Assessment and Management.* Gaskell for The Royal College of Psychiatrists, London.
(12) Walker, N. (1991) Dangerous mistakes. *British Journal of Psychiatry* **158**, 752–7.
(13) Taylor, P.J. & Gunn, J. (1984) Violence and psychosis I – risk of violence amongst psychotic men. *British Medical Journal* **288**, 1945–9.
(14) Hafner, H. & Boker, W. (1973) Mentally disordered violent offenders. *Social Psychiatry* **8**, 220–9.
(15) Penrose, L.S. (1939) Mental disease and crime: outline of a comparative study of European statistics. *British Journal of Medical Psychology* **18**, 1–15.

(16) Bowden, P. (1985) The special hospitals. In Gostin, L. (ed.) *Secure Provision*. Tavistock Publications, London.

(17) Home Office (1988) 1. Reconvictions and recalls of life licences, England and Wales 1986. 2. Reconvictions and recalls of mentally disordered offenders, England and Wales 1986. *Home Office Statistical Bulletin* **9/88**. Government Statistical Service, Croydon.

(18) Festhouse, A.R. & Kellert, S.R. (1987) Childhood cruelty to animals and later aggression against people. *American Journal of Psychiatry* **144**, 710–17.

Chapter 15

Writing a Report

Introduction

Reports on offenders suspected of having an abnormal mental state will
be requested from:

(1) Courts and solicitors.
(2) The Mental Health Review Tribunal.
(3) Managers of hospitals in relation to detention in hospital.
(4) The Home Office in relation to restricted offenders.
(5) The Home Office in relation to the transfer of mentally abnormal
    offenders from prison to hospital.
(6) The Department of Health in relation to applications for a patient to be
    admitted to a special hospital.
(7) Prison doctors for
    (a) advice on diagnosis and treatment
    (b) advice to the parole board on the mental state of offenders
        suspected of having an abnormality.
(8) Consultant psychiatrists in ordinary psychiatric settings for advice on
    subjects with a 'forensic' or management problem.
(9) The Mental Health Act Commission when requesting a second
    opinion.

This chapter will deal with each type of report and the specific problems
attached to it. However, the paradigm for all reports is the report to court
on mentally abnormal offenders. Bluglass[1] has given an excellent guide
to this.

A psychiatric report may have far-reaching effects as Scott[2] has
pointed out. It may play a large part in the decision to deprive a patient of
his liberty for years in hospital, or it may delay his return to the community. As well as doing good, a report can do harm. As will become
apparent, the relationship of a psychiatrist to a patient whom he is
assessing as an expert witness is not the same as that which normally
exists between a doctor and a patient. The psychiatrist considers not only
the patient's needs and wishes but is obliged to balance this against the

estimated dangerousness of the patient. The psychiatrist's opinion may be primarily for a third party with the public safety in mind.

In order to retain credibility, the psychiatrist must prepare a report which is as accurate, independent and as fair as possible. It must be free of emotion and prejudice, moral judgements and exasperation. At the same time, the report should be one which appears to be prepared by a doctor, one who is impartial yet genuinely concerned with the welfare of the offender[2].

(1) *The report on a subject appearing in court*

The request for the report

Requests for psychiatric reports on offenders are made relatively rarely. The request may come from the court, or from the prosecuting or defending solicitor. Gibbens[3] found that the rate of requests for reports varied in different parts of the country. In London, for example, the rate was 8.8% for indictable offences and only 4.5% in Wessex. The proportion for non-indictable offences was 1.2% in London and 0.3% in Wessex. Mackay[4] looked at all cases going through Leicester Crown Court over two years (3523 cases); 153 (4.34%) were subject to psychiatric assessment. The reports were used mainly in relation to mitigation or to obtain an acquittal on the basis of lack of *mens rea* (e.g. confusion in a shoplifter). Only 19 received a medical disposal (0.539%) of the 3523. Mackay calculated that the overall national figure for crown courts was 0.18%.

The reasons for asking for a report include:

(1) Disturbed behaviour in court.
(2) A bizarre offence.
(3) A history of mental disorder.
(4) Information from the probation officer.
(5) Requests from the defence solicitor or prosecution.
(6) An offence which is out of character.
(7) The nature of the offence, e.g. homicide or repetitive sexual offences.

The *magistrate or judge* requests a psychiatric report, for the above reasons, after finding the subject guilty but before sentencing in order to assist sentencing. Very occasionally a court may request a report before conviction if the patient is clearly very disturbed and the question of fitness to plead or a need for immediate psychiatric treatment has been raised. The *Crown Prosecutor* may directly request a report before the final trial in the case of homicide as the psychiatrist's finding may affect the charge (murder or manslaughter). They may also request it in the case of a very disturbed offender who may not be fit to plead, otherwise the prosecution leaves the requests to the court or defence. The *defence solicitor* usually requests a report before trial in order to see if:

(1) His client is fit to plead.
(2) There are grounds to consider absence of intent at the time of the offence.
(3) There are any psychiatric mitigating factors or special defences (e.g. automatism, infanticide).

Before submitting the report, it is good practice to discuss the contents with any relevant professionals such as probation officers or psychiatrists in order to check its accuracy. A copy of the report requested by the court should be sent to the probation officer. When the report is requested by the solicitor it is proper to obtain permission before sending copies elsewhere. It is not uncommon for the doctors employed by the defence and prosecution to be in contact and make their opinions known to each other before the court case. This does have the advantage that there is an opportunity for a sharing of information.

The crucial questions

The psychiatrist generally considers the following questions:

(1) Whether the defendant is fit to plead and stand trial.
(2) Whether he was capable of forming intent at the time of the offence.
(3) Whether the defendant suffered or suffers from any form of mental disorder – particularly a form subject to a treatment order. If so,
(4) Whether he is in need of treatment. If so,
(5) Where and by whom should this treatment be given.
(6) Whether it should be as an inpatient or outpatient, and which category, (see Chapter 3).
(7) The prognosis.

Background information

Before seeing the defendant it is good practice to obtain and study background information. The court itself, in making the request, should under the Magistrates' Courts' Rules (1968) supply:

(1) The reasons which led the court to request the report.
(2) Previous medical and family history.
(3) Circumstances of the offence.
(4) Where the offence took place.
(5) Previous conduct including previous convictions.
(6) The home address and circumstances.
(7) The name and police station of the relevant police officer.
(8) The name and telephone number of the relevant probation officer.

In practice, the background information supplied by the court is extremely sparse and it is usually necessary, and always desirable, to make direct contact with the probation officer (for past and present reports), and the police if details of the offence are required. Solicitors may supply more background information but contact with other agencies will still be needed. A list of previous offences may be obtained from the court or solicitors. It is increasingly common practice for typed witness statements to be presented in magistrates' courts as well as in the crown court, and copies of these should be obtained through the solicitor or court. Other relevant papers may include social service reports, school reports, medical and psychiatric notes. If the defendant is in prison or a hostel enquiries should be made about treatment and his behaviour. This information should all be studied thoroughly before interviewing the defendant.

The interview

The interview in a remand prison is held in the prison hospital. It is necessary to contact the hospital beforehand to arrange the interview. The times available will normally be on weekdays between 9 AM–11.45 AM and 2 PM–4 PM, though prisons are trying to be more helpful and allowing interviewing out of these hours. If the subject is on bail, the interview can be arranged at a suitable outpatient clinic. If the subject is in a hostel (e.g. a bail hostel) it may be more useful to go there to obtain the staff's observations.

At the interview the psychiatrist should first check that the person before him is the man he wants to see. There are several Smiths in a prison! After normal introductions the psychiatrist should explain who requested the report and for what reason, and who will see the report and the inevitable lack of confidentiality (see Chapter 16 on the ethics of reports and confidentiality). A report requested by the court will be disclosed in open court to both defence and prosecution. A defence report, on the other hand, may be retained by the solicitor if it does not help his client. It is proper to explain to the subject what information the psychiatrist has already had.

An explanation to the subject of the way the interview will be conducted is often very helpful. For example: 'I understand you are charged with theft. It seems to me that my best chance of understanding how this came about is to take a history of your life and see what has led up to this event.' Then obtain basic information, date of birth, address, GP, probation officer (if not already known) and, if known, the date of the court appearance. The procedure can then be that of a standard psychiatric interview covering family history, development, sexual history, occupational history, personality development, medical and psychiatric history, and the events and mental state associated with the offence. Any symptoms of illness at the time of interview should be recorded as part of the assessment made of his current mental state. Physical examination should be carried out if indicated.

From the history it may become clear that further interviews or clinical investigations may be needed. If more time is required to obtain any information then this can be explained to the court or solicitor and the subject can be remanded for a further period. Some investigations may be difficult to arrange if the subject is in custody and it will be necessary to liaise with the prison medical officer. On the other hand, it may be that it would be a suitable case for observation and investigation in hospital under section 35 and this can be recommended to the court.

The subject may refuse to co-operate with the interview even though it is requested by his solicitor or ordered by the court. In the case of a subject remanded on bail he may simply refuse or fail to attend. In that case, the referring agent should be informed. In the case of a court request the subject may then be remanded in custody for the report. When an offender attends but proves hostile and difficult this too can be reported as well as any other observations. The subject's hostility may arise from a mental abnormality such as paranoid delusions which involve the court and the psychiatrist. Where such an abnormality is suspected it may be appropriate to recommend further observation in hospital under section 35 but enough information may have been gathered to allow a diagnosis to be made.

The arrangements

When a diagnosis has been made the following arrangements must be considered:

(1) Treatment order (section 37): A psychiatrist should assure himself that there is a hospital willing to take the patient within 28 days of the order being made. He must ensure that a second doctor has interviewed the patient and prepared a report in accordance with the Mental Health Act (see Chapter 3). Both psychiatrists will submit full written reports and it is also common to complete and submit a form 1303, which covers the legal points, with whom the court is concerned. Where there is no hospital bed available for the patient, then the psychiatrist should contact the appropriate District Health Authority with details of the case and his recommendations. The authority is then in a position to discharge its responsibilities.
(2) Guardianship order (section 37): Here the psychiatrist must be sure that the local social services are willing to receive the patient into guardianship. Again a second doctor is required (see Chapter 3).
(3) Probation order: The psychiatrist must be sure that the probation officer agrees to the order and that the subject is willing to accept it. If

psychiatric care is to be recommended then specific provisions for such care must be made.
(4) Sections 35/38/36: In these cases the psychiatrist who accepts the patient is likely to be the one who prepares the report. He must be sure that facilities are available to allow the court to make the orders within the legally prescribed times (see Chapter 3). If facilities cannot be made available within the appropriate time a request for a further remand should be made.

Style of the report

The report to the court will be read by laymen and must be given in non-technical language. Very recently a local solicitor puzzled for hours over the meaning of 'bilateral periorbital haematoma', much simpler to say 'two black eyes'. If a technical term is used, then a phrase explaining it should be added: 'he experiences auditory hallucinations (hears voices) saying insulting things and he has delusions (false beliefs unamenable to reason) that he is being persecuted by bodies such as the CIA'.

Psychodynamic and psychoanalytical terms are notoriously difficult for the laymen. Repression, dissociation, etc. should be expressed in ordinary language: 'he pushed the memory to the back of his mind', 'he ignored the reality of the situation'. Other words which give trouble are: 'personality disorder', 'EEG', 'schizoid', etc. Terms like 'immature' or 'unstable' should be qualified to explain their meaning. Intelligence expressed in terms of mental age or IQ can be very misleading without explanation to put the figures into perspective.

Form and length of report

In England reports are usually 4–6 sides long, though some favour longer reports, especially in complex cases. Very brief reports (one or two paragraphs) are unlikely on their own to have sufficient information in them to win the court's confidence. There are various ways of writing a report. The following is an example on which reports may be based. The main part of the report must be factual and opinions restricted to the final paragraph. The legal terms for mental disorder must be used where appropriate. Some find it useful to use sub-headings.

Heading and Introduction

Psychiatric Report
John SMITH (dob: 20.3.66)
Charge: Actual Bodily Harm
Court of appearance: Barchester Magistrates' Court

The introductory paragraph should include where and when the patient was seen, what papers were examined, which people were spoken to.

I interviewed Smith at Barchester Prison on 8.8.86 at the request of the ... court. I examined witness statements relating to his case, his previous psychiatric notes from Barchester Psychiatric Hospital and a report from his probation officer, Mr Jones. I have also interviewed his mother. I have discussed his recent behaviour on remand with Dr MacKenzie, prison medical officer.

Family history

This should draw out the main positive and negative events which help in the understanding of the case. Tact is required if facts turn up of which the subject was unaware, e.g. illegitimacy. The court can be warned in the report that the subject does not know it or it should be left out if not relevant. The nature of the family relationships, and a history of mental disorder or delinquency in the family is relevant. Beware of apportioning blame, particularly beware of attacking parents. The events usually happened many years before and time will have distorted the history. The offender may have learned what makes an interesting tale for a psychiatrist or may be a person who is very willing to blame others for his own failings.

> Smith is the third of four brothers. His parents were happily married. Their relationship with Smith was good during his childhood and adolescence. However, in recent years their relationship with Smith has become increasingly strained. This period coincides with his showing disturbed behaviour and developing symptoms of severe mental illness. Smith's brothers are well. The only family history of mental disorder is that of an aunt who died in a psychiatric hospital. The exact nature of her disorder is unknown to me. There is no history of delinquency in the family.

Development

This section deals with birth, physical and emotional development, experiences of separation, evidence and chronology of behaviour disorder (running away, lying, stealing, fire raising, violence, school behaviour and truancy) or neurotic behaviour (phobias, nightmares, anxieties, depressions). The development of relationships with peers, teachers and school performance should also be covered. Some subjects will show disturbance in many areas from an early age and this should be documented.

> Smith's birth and early physical development was unremarkable. There was no evidence in his history of emotional disturbance. He was born and brought up in Barchester and attended school there. He got on well at primary school, making friends, getting on well with teachers and doing reasonably well at school work. This progress continued into comprehensive school until the sixth form. He had obtained three 'O' level passes at the age of 16 and decided to stay on and try to pass more. However, at that time he became increasingly withdrawn and hostile at home, spending more and more time in his bedroom, becoming increasingly isolated at school, having less and less to do with his

school friends and his performance at school declined. He stopped attending school altogether before his seventeenth birthday.

Sexual history

This section deals with sexual orientation, the onset of puberty, sexual relationships, in fact and fantasy, and any manifestation of sexual deviation. Care has to be taken that no more is described than is required for the particular case. Clearly, where sexual offending is the problem this section will be fuller. However, it is otherwise enough to assure the court that it is not an area that gives rise to public concern.

> Smith developed a normal sexual orientation. He formed friendships with girls during his mid-teens though his relationships were never long-lasting. However, since the age of 17 he has not had a girlfriend, though would like one. I found no evidence to suggest that he would be likely to be sexually violent.

Occupational history

This section recounts the subject's experience of work with particular attention to steadiness, relationships to others, ability to accept orders, criticism and conflict, the reasons for any dismissals and any evidence of inability to sustain himself in work through restlessness or psychiatric disorder. Many offenders have extremely poor work records and show inability to accept orders, poor time keeping, and an unwillingness to submit to the discipline of work. In this case the reasons were somewhat different:

> After Smith left school he failed to obtain work at all. He increasingly restricted himself to his room. Some months later he began treatment for psychiatric illness. He improved after his first course sufficiently to obtain work in a factory which he kept for some six months until his illness flared up again. He then spontaneously stopped attending work. He has not worked since.

Personality

This section covers personality features, such as ability to sustain friendships, emotional stability, tendency to violence and substance abuse.

> His personality before his illness was that of a friendly, quiet boy capable of making and sustaining friendships. He is said to have been of stable disposition. Since his illness began he has become increasingly isolated, hostile and irritable. There have been episodes of sudden and apparently unprovoked violent outbursts as well as violence when his irrational and unreasonable demands have been frustrated. There is no history of drug or alcohol abuse.

Previous medical and psychiatric history

This section deals with any physical illnesses as well as giving details of any contact with psychiatrists. Sometimes this is very brief but in this case it was quite complicated:

Smith has not suffered from any serious physical illnesses. He was first brought to the attention of psychiatrists at the age of 17 years when he was assessed at his home because of his increasing isolation and his aggressive behaviour towards his parents. A diagnosis of the mental illness of schizophrenia was made. The principal symptoms at the time were the false beliefs (delusions) that there was a conspiracy against him to which his parents were party. He was admitted to Barchester Psychiatric Hospital on a treatment order. He made a good recovery and was able to return to his home and obtain work. He attended outpatients and received necessary medication. However, after some 5 months he refused further medication because he believed it was no longer necessary, despite the advice of his doctor. His mental illness recurred some months later. He was admitted, aged 19 years, on a treatment order, after further violence at home. He improved after two months and was discharged home to attend the hospital as a day patient. On this occasion, he failed to regain his initial competence. After some months he again refused medication. His condition deteriorated once more with a return of the idea that he was being persecuted through the television and by people in the street. He believed that they spoke and laughed about him behind his back.

Time of the offence

This section deals with the subject's behaviour just before and at the time of the offence. Deciding what criminal act happened at the time is the province of the court and the subject is best avoided, particularly avoid giving the defendant's account to the court. The psychiatrist's job is to throw light on the mental state at the time. Was there a psychiatric disorder, if so what was it and how would it affect his behaviour? In this case Smith had been found guilty of approaching a group of strangers in a street, berating them and striking one of them (at which point he was overpowered):

> At the time of the offence [use the phrase 'alleged offence' if the report is written before guilt has been established] Smith was under the delusion that people were talking and laughing about him. This delusion had been present for some months. He had also come to believe that he was being poisoned. These symptoms had increased in intensity in the weeks before the time of the offence. He believed that the victims in this case were his persecutors.

Current mental state

This describes the patient when interviewed and lists the important features, both positive and negative:

> In interview, Smith was alert and co-operative, giving a clear account of his past. At the time I saw him he was receiving medication from the prison doctors. He was, nevertheless, tense and perplexed. He still believed that he was subject to persecution by the television and the general public. At the time of interview he denied hearing voices though he admitted to having done so in the past. He did not think himself ill.

Conclusions

Most people find it useful to head this last section 'Opinion' to differentiate it from the preceding part which should be an account of the facts obtained by the doctor. This section will give the doctor's opinion as to whether the patient is mentally disordered or not, the nature of the disorder, and what should be done about it. Where there is doubt about diagnosis or management this should be stated (for example: 'It is difficult to be certain in this case as the symptoms are vague, but nevertheless, on balance, I believe that the defendant has the mental illness of depression and requires psychiatric treatment').

Recommendations must be made with the problems of the court in mind. Not only will they follow logically from the early part of the report but the psychiatrist must be aware of the court's anxieties. The court may have a reasonable fear about the dangerousness of an offender and attention must be given to this even if only to reassure the court. A recommendation which might seem to be in the best interests of the subject may not be accepted if it does not take account of this sort of anxiety. However, a recommendation for psychiatric treatment is nearly always followed, though a court may wish to assure itself that the doctor's arrangements will provide protection for the public if needed. If they do not, the court may ask the psychiatrist to make other, safer arrangements.

Opinion
Smith is fit to plead and stand trial.

Smith suffers from the mental illness of schizophrenia which began at the age of 17 years. The principal symptom, in this case, is the belief that he is being persecuted. His illness has responded to treatment in the past though it has recurred when he has stopped treatment. At the time of the [alleged] offence he held these beliefs and was in such a state that he might well approach strangers in a hostile fashion believing that they were part of the persecutory plot. He has accepted treatment voluntarily during his period on remand and he is now somewhat improved but he still requires further treatment in hospital. He can be accepted by Barchester Psychiatric Hospital into Ward 3 within 28 days of the order being made under section 37 of the Mental Health Act 1983, if the court feels that this is the most appropriate disposal. On his eventual return to the community he will be offered outpatient care and he will be visited regularly by a community nurse to try and ensure that treatment is continued.

In a case where there is no disorder which could respond to treatment the opinion might be expressed as follows:

Opinion
Jones is fit to plead and stand trial.

Jones does not suffer from mental illness. He is of dull intelligence though he is not subnormal. He has, perhaps in part due to his disturbed upbringing, developed strong anti-authoritarian attitudes, and temperamental difficulties with poor control of his temper, both of which are compounded by his heavy drinking. He has no wish to alter his drinking habits or his lifestyle at the present time. I have therefore no psychiatric recommendation to make or suggestions about his management.

Had it been appropriate, the opinion could have concluded with the suggestion that the court might consider a fine or probation etc. on the basis that, in this case, such a course would be effective from a psychological point of view.

The recommendation should be expressed with proper respect for the court, realizing that the court has to find a balance. The court may be offered other opinions which are diametrically opposed to the psychiatric report and it may have before it evidence which makes the psychiatric recommendation inappropriate.

Oral evidence

In the majority of cases, the written psychiatric report to the court is sufficient. However, the psychiatrist may have to appear in court to be cross-examined on his report in several situations, including:

(1) When the defence and prosecution have reports with opposing views.
(2) When the prosecution is unwilling to accept a psychiatric defence, e.g. the Sutcliffe case. Sutcliffe, the 'Yorkshire Ripper', was charged with multiple murder. His defence of diminished responsibility rested on all the psychiatrists asserting that he suffered from the mental illness of schizophrenia. The prosecution refused to accept this and cross-examined every psychiatric witness about his examination (how carefully had the case been examined); the reliability of his findings (could the defendant be imitating illness?); and his interpretation (how certain can one be that these are signs of illness).
(3) When a judge wishes to make a restriction order he is obliged to take oral evidence from one of the psychiatrists who saw the patient, though he may disregard the psychiatrist's view. The judge may enquire about dangerousness, the prognosis, and whether the arrangements the psychiatrist has made will protect the public.
(4) Oral evidence is required for a jury to consider the question of fitness to plead.

When giving oral evidence to support his report and opinion, the psychiatrist is an expert witness. He may attend the trial from the beginning to hear all the evidence to make sure that none had escaped him. He should have his psychiatric notes with him and can consult them as needed. The psychiatrist will have little difficulty if he has followed Scott's golden rule[2] of reading his finished report and then asking himself the question: 'Could I substantiate all the facts mentioned if I were to be cross-examined upon them and is the whole report strictly fair to the offender?'

The psychiatrist, when giving oral evidence, will be asked about his findings, which he can affirm, explain or enlarge upon, if necessary, and describe how he obtained them. He will also be asked about his conclusions. He should stick to his original conclusion unless some conflicting facts (sufficient to make him change his mind) appear with which he was previously unacquainted. It is perfectly understandable to a court that two experts, seeing the same facts, will reach different opinions. The barrister may want to test the psychiatrist's views: 'Is it not the case, doctor, that the offender showed no signs of illness when seen by Dr X?' or, 'Is it not the case, doctor, that the offender may have learned the symptoms of this illness and may be deceiving you?'

The psychiatrist is well advised to admit to the possibility of such a suggestion but to assert firmly his own opinion that he believes his view to be the more probable: 'It is possible that a person can imitate mental illness and deceive a doctor but in this case, taking all the evidence, (which can be listed if necessary), it is my opinion that the offender is suffering from mental illness and is not deceiving me'. The psychiatrist's view in the end may not be accepted by the court who will have had the very difficult job of balancing conflicting and powerful arguments.

In the court the clerk of the court (a lawyer) and the usher organize the proceedings. On arriving at court, the doctor should introduce himself to them. They will show him where he can sit. When the magistrate or judge enters the court the usher orders the people in the court to stand and the magistrate or judge exchanges a bow with the body of the court before all sit. The clerk of the court, sitting below the bench, informs the bench of the case to be heard. The defendant is then called to the dock to answer the charges put to him. When the doctor is called to give evidence he will be asked to swear on the Bible to tell the truth. He may choose alternatively to affirm (without the Bible). Questions will be directed first by the barrister (or solicitor) who called him and then he may be cross-examined by the other barrister. In simple cases the questions are merely a way of getting the doctor to affirm the statements in his report. The magistrates or judge may also ask questions for clarification.

A coroner is addressed as 'Sir', a magistrate as 'Sir' or 'Madam', county court judges, recorders and circuit judges in crown courts as 'Your Honour', a senior judge from the crown court, Court of Appeal or House of Lords as 'My Lord'. Presidents of Tribunals are addressed as 'Sir' or 'Madam'.

In court speak clearly and audibly to the bench and the barrister with sufficient pauses to allow the statements to be written down. It is normal practice to dress conservatively for the court.

The opinion in court reports on special cases

The following sections deal with opinions in homicide, infanticide and automatism (see Chapter 3).

Homicide

Let us assume that Smith killed his victim and is charged with murder. In the opinion deal with this situation as follows:

(1) Fitness to plead:

Smith is fit to plead and stand trial.

(2) Insanity:

At the time of the alleged offence Smith knew what he was doing and whether or not it was wrong. Although under a delusion of persecution he did not feel immediately threatened by the victim. He was not therefore insane within the McNaughten Rules.

(3) Diminished responsibility:

At the time of the alleged offence Smith was suffering from a mental abnormality caused by the severe mental illness of schizophrenia. The main symptoms in this case are delusions of persecution. The mental abnormality is such in his case as to substantially diminish his responsibility within the meaning of the Homicide Act 1957.

(4) Need for treatment:

He continues to suffer from the mental illness of schizophrenia and he requires treatment in a psychiatric hospital.

(5) Security and restriction order (covering prognosis):

At present he could be safely managed in the regional secure unit at Barchester Hospital to which he could be admitted under section 37 of the Mental Health Act 1983 within 28 days if the court felt it appropriate. He is likely to respond rapidly to treatment. The court may feel in this case that a restriction order under section 41 would be appropriate in order to provide statutory supervision and aftercare to prevent Smith deteriorating again in the community as he has in the past.

Infanticide

A woman, White, was charged with the murder of her one-month-old baby whilst suffering from a depression coming on after the birth.

(1) Fitness to plead:

White is fit to plead and stand trial.

(2) The balance of her mind:

At the time of the alleged offence the balance of White's mind was disturbed due to the effects of lactation and giving birth so that she became severely depressed.

(3) Need for further treatment (and prognosis):

White has recovered substantially having had medical treatment during the remand period. She is no longer seriously suicidal or depressed. She still, however, becomes disturbed emotionally when recalling the birth and requires to continue medication. The court may feel that a period of probation for support and counselling with a condition of attendance at psychiatric out-patients for up to one year would be appropriate in this case. I would expect White to make a complete recovery from this illness.

Automatism
Doe has attacked a fellow drinker after a brief concussion sustained in a fight.

(1) Fitness to plead:

Doe is fit to plead and stand trial.

(2) The presence of automatism, type, and prognosis:

At the time of the alleged offence Doe was behaving automatically in that his mind was not controlling his actions. He was in a post-concussional state in which his consciousness was gravely disturbed. He would not be conscious of what he was doing. The automatic behaviour arose from an external cause (the blow on the head) and therefore was a 'sane' automatism. There is no danger of it recurring spontaneously.

(3) Disposal:

There is no need for any treatment in this case.

Who sees psychiatric reports for the court?

Psychiatric reports requested by the court or prosecution are in no sense confidential. The court will send a copy to the prosecuting and defence solicitors. It should be expected that the offender will at least be told the main points by the court or the defence solicitor and may even be given a copy of the report. The report is also likely to be given to the probation officer. If the offender is sent to prison or hospital it is quite possible that the report will be sent with him or follow him. The report will then be referred to by other psychiatrists, psychologists, nurses, Mental Health Review Tribunal doctors, prison medical doctors, parole boards, etc. Finally, the report may appear at future court appearances.

(2) *Psychiatric reports to mental health review tribunals*

The request for the report

The Tribunal will ask the responsible medical officer for an up-to-date report. In cases on restriction orders requests also come from the Home Office to the responsible medical officer who can send the Home Office a copy of his tribunal report. The Home Office, who may disagree with the responsible medical officer, will then send their comments about the report to the Tribunal. The detained patient's solicitor may ask an independent psychiatrist to provide a psychiatric report. The Act states that this doctor should be given every facility to examine the case.

The crucial questions

These are outlined in Chapter 4. They include:

(1) Is he still suffering from a mental disorder?
(2) Is it of such a nature that detention in hospital continues to be required?

Sources of information

The information will principally be in the records of the patient's treatment and progress (medical and nursing notes). Staff looking after the patient will also be a valuable source of information.

Arrangements

Where a responsible medical officer or independent doctor is recommending discharge or transfer then it clearly gives the Tribunal the maximum chance of accepting the recommendation if the necessary arrangements have been made. Applications may be for transfer to another hospital (in which case a place should be arranged, at least provisionally), conditional discharge to the community (in which case lodgings, social work and psychiatric follow-up should be arranged provisionally) or absolute discharge (in which case no arrangements are necessary, except perhaps lodgings).

The style of the report

It can be assumed that the Tribunal is relatively sophisticated in psychiatric terminology and common technical terms will be understood.

The form of the report

Some hospitals have a standard questionnaire to be filled in. There will be space for a very detailed history, similar to a psychiatric court report, and of similar length. The main differences will be that for the purposes of the Tribunal, details of the offence can be discussed and progress in hospital must be covered. The Tribunal will be interested in understanding the patient's motivation for what he did at the time (discussed under mental state at time of the offence) and his subsequent reaction to it (was there insight and remorse?). Similarly, his previous convictions can be openly discussed (usefully in the section on personality) and the bearing this has on estimating his current dangerousness. These previous convictions can be listed with, if appropriate, details to describe exactly what happened (a simple charge of actual bodily harm may conceal an abortive serious offence). The Tribunal will be interested in the treatment he has received (give details) and the patient's response with particular attention to his current mental state and prognosis. An estimate of his future danger-ousness is required (see Chapter 4). The list of questions set by the Home Office for restricted patients (see below) is a useful guide.

The opinion aims to answer the Tribunal's crucial questions. It is now good practice for the responsible medical officer to discuss his reasons and recommendations with the patient before the Tribunal. The respon-sible medical officer is normally expected to attend the whole Tribunal to be ready to be cross-examined by the patient or his solicitor or by the Tribunal members (see Chapter 4).

Who will see the report?

The Tribunal will pass the report to the client's solicitor who will show it and discuss it with the client unless the psychiatrist has convinced the Tribunal that it would do harm to do so. The report will become part of the Tribunal's file as well as part of the patient's notes and will therefore be read in the future. In restricted cases the Home Office will also keep a copy to which it will refer in future years.

(3) *Psychiatric report to the managers of a hospital*

The request for the report

The managers (see Chapter 4) request a brief report when the responsible medical officer proposes renewing the detention of a patient. It has been proposed that patients should make more use of their right to appeal to managers for release in between renewals if they wish.

The crucial questions

These are presented on the appropriate form:

(1) Does he suffer from mental illness or severe mental impairment and is his mental disorder of a nature or degree which makes it appropriate for him to receive medical treatment in a hospital, and *either*,
  (a) such treatment is likely to alleviate or prevent a deterioration in his condition, or
  (b) the patient, if discharged, is unlikely to care for himself, to obtain

the care which he needs, or to guard himself against serious exploitation.

or

(2) Does he suffer from psychopathic disorder or mental impairment, and is his mental disorder of a nature or degree which makes it appropriate for him to receive medical treatment in a hospital and such treatment is likely to alleviate or prevent deterioration in his condition?

(3) Finally is it therefore necessary,
     (a) for the patient's health or safety, and/or
     (b) for the protection of other persons that the patient should receive treatment and it cannot be provided unless he continues to be detained under the Act?

The source of information

The answers will be derived from the knowledge of the responsible medical officer, derived from all the team and contained in the medical and nursing notes.

Making arrangements

It is only necessary to be sure that the patient can be continued to be looked after in the hospital. The patient must be informed that the renewal is being considered and that he has a right to speak to the managers.

The style of the report

The report will be read by the lay managers of the hospital who will have only a very simple understanding of psychiatric terms, therefore non-technical language with an explanation of terms should be used.

The form of the report

The report is usually made on a standard form (form 30). The psychiatrist has to indicate whether other methods of treatment are available, e.g. outpatient basis, and why they are not appropriate or why informal admission is not appropriate. The reasons for this have to be stated and might be:

(1) 'Informal admission is not appropriate because the patient remains unaware that he is ill and constantly strives to leave the hospital.'

or

(2) 'The patient is frequently violent to others and has to be restrained.'

Or

(3) 'His absconding and violence make it inappropriate to treat him on a voluntary basis or as an outpatient.'

The written report is read by the managers who commonly expect to meet the doctor at the same time in order that the very brief written report can be enlarged upon, if necessary.

Who will see the report?

The report is usually held in the manager's Medical Records Department. Under current practice the patient does not see it. The report may be produced at future renewals.

(4) Psychiatric report to the Home Office in relation to restricted patients

The request

The Home Office, on behalf of the Minister responsible for restricted patients, requires:

(1) Regular, short reports on the progress of restricted patients.
(2) A further report about a patient if the responsible medical officer is proposing a change in the parole status of the patient. It will be recalled that a restricted patient can be moved within the hospital or grounds at the responsible medical officer's discretion but cannot leave the grounds or be transferred within the Minister's permission. The patient's return to the community is normally accomplished in stages. The Home Office requires a full report about each patient when an application is made by the responsible medical officer to accomplish one of these stages. It is this report which gives most trouble to psychiatrists looking after restricted patients, and is discussed below.

The crucial questions

The Home Office has recently offered a check-list of points which should be covered by the report accompanying a request for increased freedom for a restricted patient. It is sensible to ring the appropriate officer at the

Home Office to discuss the proposal and the type of letter required. The list is reproduced below:

Checklist of points considered by the Home Office in examining cases of restricted patients

(1) Has any information come to light since the last report which increases understanding of the circumstances surrounding the index offence?

(2) Is the motivation for behaviour that has put others at risk understood?

(3) Is there any evidence that the patient has a persistent preoccupation with a particular type of victim or a particular type of violent/sexual/arsonist activity?

(4) What are the chances of circumstances similar to those surrounding the offence arising again and similar offences occurring?

(5) In cases of mental illness, what effects have any prescribed drugs had? Do any symptoms remain? How important is the medication for continued stability? Has stability been maintained in differing circumstances? Does the patient have the insight into the need for medication?

(6) In the cases of mental impairment, has the patient benefitted from training? Is the patient's behaviour more socially acceptable? Is the patient explosive or impulsive?

(7) In cases of psychopathic disorder, is the patient now more mature, predictable and concerned about others? Is he more tolerant of frustration and stress? Does he now take into account the consequences of his actions? Does he learn from experience?

(8) Does the patient now have greater insight into his condition? Is he more realistic and reliable?

(9) Have alcohol or drugs affected the patient in the past? Did either contribute towards his offence?

(10) How has the patient responded to stressful situations in the hospital in the past and how does he respond now – with physical aggression or verbal aggression?

(11) If the patient is a sex offender, has he shown in the hospital an undesirable interest in the type of person he has previously been known to favour as his victim? What form has any sexual activity taken? What have been the results of any psychological tests?

(12) What views do members of the clinical team have about the patient's continuing dangerousness?

(13) Is it considered that the patient should/should not continue to be detained? For what reasons?

(14) If so, is it considered that detention in conditions of special security is necessary?

(15) What parole has the patient had so far and how has it been used?

Sources of information

Clearly the information is contained in all the documents relating to the patient – particularly the medical, nursing, psychological and social reports. A copy of the original witness statements relating to the index offence should be obtained in order that the offence is properly understood.

Making arrangements

Provisional arrangements appropriate to the stage requested should be made and described along with the request. The Home Office has to consider the safety of the public and therefore arrangements should be thorough and commensurate with the dangerousness of the patient in that situation. Whilst it might be too risky to send a particular deluded paranoid schizophrenic unaccompanied and unsupervised to live in the community, it might be perfectly safe to let him go shopping in the local village accompanied by staff. When the proposals are for the patient to live in the community and leave the hospital (either on trial leave or conditional discharge), a detailed plan or provisional arrangements should be made, a social worker identified to be the supervisor and a doctor to be the responsible medical officer. These people should be made familiar with the case and know how to elicit the crucial points from the patient, i.e. the state of his delusion, his sexual drive, etc.

The style of the report

Home Office officials may have become familiar with psychiatric terms but they have no formal training in the language, and neither does the Minister. It is better, therefore, to stick to non-technical language with explanations of technical terms.

The form of the report

The report is usually in the form of a letter which may begin (or end) with a recommendation or request by the responsible medical officer. This is then supported by a detailed report on the patient covering the relevant points required by the Home Office in order to show the request is reasonable. At the end the proposed arrangements should be explained in detail to reassure the Minister that the proposal is a safe and sensible one. The letter will therefore run to about one-and-a-half sides. A telephone call to support the letter can be useful. The Home Office currently takes some four to six weeks to reply to the letter and may require further information before giving a decision. In the end, the request may be rejected or modified arrangements proposed.

Who sees the report?

The report becomes the property of Home Office officials and the Minister. It will remain on the Home Office file and will be referred to in future and may influence later judgements. It is essential therefore to be particularly accurate, fair and moderate.

(5) *Psychiatric reports to the Home Office in relation to the transfer of subjects from prison to hospital*

The request

The prison medical officer will request the report when either (a) a remanded patient, or (b) a convicted patient requires transfer to a psychiatric hospital (section 48 or section 47, Mental Health Act 1983 – see Chapter 3). Reports by two doctors are submitted to the Home Office. A prison medical officer may prepare one report and request a psychiatrist to prepare the other.

The crucial questions

In the case of section 48 the doctor must decide if the subject is suffering from mental illness or severe mental impairment. The doctor must give the information which establishes these diagnoses, and the reason that detention in hospital is appropriate. As this is for a remanded prisoner the reasons for the conclusions that the patient needs urgent treatment must be given, and why delay is not acceptable. If a special hospital place is requested the reasons for this must also be given.

In the case of section 47 the situation is the same except the order for transfer can be made for psychopathic disorder and mental impairment as well. The questions and reasons for diagnosis and treatment remain the same but there does not have to be a case for urgent treatment. The case for a special hospital must also be given.

Source of information

This will lie principally in the prison records and medical notes. There may also be useful information in the prison officer's daily record, particularly if the prisoner has been in the prison hospital.

Style of the report

The reports appear to be handled by officials with some knowledge of ordinary psychiatric terms but it would be prudent to avoid specialized terms except with an explanation.

Form of the report

It is usual to complete the routine forms issued for such a recommendation (F1305 and F1306) in which case the bare bones of the matter are outlined. Nevertheless, it is helpful to supply a full report in the style of a court report to expand on this brief form.

Who will see the report?

The Home Office will pass the request to the Department of Health who will pass the request down the system via the appropriate Health Authority to reach the appropriate psychiatrist if he is not already involved. That psychiatrist will probably wish to interview the subject having first had a copy of the reports. The reports will become part of the prison file and part of the psychiatric file. It is unlikely that the patient will see them at that stage but they may be presented to a tribunal later.

(6) Psychiatric reports in relation to applications for a subject to be admitted to special hospital

The request for the report

The local admission panel of each special hospital (see Chapter 1) requires a psychiatric report to accompany a request for a bed within a special hospital. The report will usually be prepared by the doctor who is currently responsible for the patient, e.g. the responsible medical officer if the patient is detained in an ordinary hospital; the prison medical officer (or psychiatrist instructed by the defence) if the patient is in prison. Sometimes the responsible medical officer will ask for an opinion from a special hospital consultant before submitting a report, in which case both can write to the local admission panel. In case of difficulty, a request can be sent to the central admissions panel of the Special Hospital Service Authority.

The crucial questions

It must be shown the subject fulfils the criteria for detention under the Mental Health Act. It is also necessary to demonstrate that the subject is a grave danger to others in any setting other than a special hospital. This may be because of:

(1) Being a persistent absconding risk, even from a regional secure unit, coupled with behaviour which makes him a grave and immediate danger to the public, or
(2) That although he is not an absconder (or his absconding is controlled) his behaviour in the hospital represents a grave danger to staff and patients and cannot be controlled, even within a regional secure unit.

In short, what must be asked is whether, after all reasonable measures have been taken, is it the case that unless the patient is moved to a special hospital someone will be seriously injured.

Sources of information

The medical and nursing notes including incident sheets, witness statements (in the case of offenders), prison notes (in the case of convicted prisoners), contain the essential information. A careful search must be made to discover all the relevant incidents and the factors which surround them.

The arrangements

It is expected that alternative approaches to the patient have been excluded, e.g. transfer to an intensive care ward or regional secure unit.

The style of the report

Knowledge of psychiatric terms can be assumed. However, it is necessary to be particularly accurate, detailed, thorough and clear.

The form of the report

The report and request usually are put in a letter beginning or ending with the request. The report will follow the lines of a court report which not only shows which psychiatric disorder the patient suffers from but will give particular attention to the behaviour which is causing anxiety. A list should be included in the discussion of all violent or dangerous incidents, giving dates and a brief description of what he did, what he was trying to do and any injuries sustained. In this way a very clear picture can be built up of the development of the present situation and why it is so worrying. It is also important to report what measures have been taken and with what results. The current legal situation should be discussed. The subject may be detained in hospital already on a section or may be awaiting trial and it may be hoped to recommend to the court that a hospital order be made.

The report may be the sole basis for discussion by the admission panel who makes the decision as to whether a special hospital bed can be offered. As they may have no other information, the importance of clarity and a high level of detailed information cannot be underestimated.

Who sees the report?

The report will become part of the special hospital files if the patient is accepted, as well as remaining in the local hospital file. It will be examined by many people in the future when judgements have to be made about release. It could turn up at a Mental Health Review Tribunal at which time it could be seen by the patient.

(7) Psychiatric report to the prison doctor

The request

The prison doctor may request a report for:

(1) A second opinion, or
(2) A body such as the Parole Board or Discretionary Lifers' Panel (for which oral evidence may also be required, as in a Mental Health Review Tribunal).

The crucial questions

Where a second opinion is required the questions will be:

(1) What is the diagnosis?
(2) What treatment should be given?
(3) Where should the treatment be given?

It may be that the subject will accept treatment in prison and his psychiatric condition is such that it can be easily managed there, or it may be that psychiatric hospital care will be required. The prison doctor hopes to make use of the psychiatrist's experience, both of the disorder and of the psychiatric facilities. Where the opinion is required for a body such as a Parole Board the reason for the request must be clarified. It may be that there is a hope that the psychiatrist can contribute to the estimation of dangerousness or it may be that the Board or Panel wish to know what psychiatric facilities could be made available for supervision of the subject once he returns to the community.

Source of information

This will be derived from all the prison notes and hospital case paper. Observations of the subject's behaviour in prison and his response to treatment will be recorded in the prison medical notes. Social reports will be available in the prison file and a summary of the case and previous offences will also be listed in the file.

The arrangements

Normally, any special arrangements will be made by the prison doctor unless it is clearly more sensible for the visiting psychiatrist to do so.

The style of the report

The report for the Parole Board will be read by lay people and therefore psychiatric terms should be explained and technical terms avoided as far as possible.

Form of the report

This should be similar to that of a court report so that the opinion can be seen to follow from the history. If a return to the community is being considered then the report must describe accurately what facilities are available.

Who sees the report?

The report will go into the prison medical file and where appropriate to the Parole Board. It must be assumed, therefore, that it will have fairly general circulation and may be seen by a prisoner at a Board.

(8) Psychiatric reports for other psychiatrists in ordinary settings

The report

The consultant in a catchment area hospital may request a second opinion from a forensic psychiatrist in order to advise on a forensic problem, or a difficult or dangerous patient.

The crucial questions

These will depend on the reason for referral, which must be clarified.

Usually, the consultant wants help to manage dangerous or difficult patients and is hoping to make use of the forensic psychiatrist's experience in this field or the security facilities. The questions will then be:

(1) What is the diagnosis and can this patient be detained if necessary under the Mental Health Act, or should he be discharged from hospital?
(2) Is the optimal treatment being given already?
(3) Is it safe to leave the patient where he is or should he be transferred to a more secure unit and, if so, which one?

Sources of information

This will be contained in all the previous psychiatric and nursing notes – the latter often being the more accurate. If there has been violence or an offence then objective accounts (witness statements, incident forms) should be obtained, if possible. A full psychiatric history must be obtained, including all forensic details.

The arrangements

The referring consultant will be grateful for any help about the legal aspects with which he may be unfamiliar such as advising on how to contact a special hospital. It will often help if the forensic psychiatrist plays an active part in affecting a transfer to a more secure environment.

Style of the report

Clearly, in this case, the report can be in ordinary technical language.

Form of the report

It may be sent as a letter or as a report with a covering letter. The latter has the advantage that it can be used as a supporting report should it be required. The report will cover the history in the same way as a court report but will also deal with the questions brought up by the referring doctor. The opinion should be addressed to these questions. Clear advice is welcomed which recognizes the anxieties in the original referral.

Who will see the report?

The report will become part of the psychiatric notes of the patient. If used to apply for a transfer or for a report to the court it will be fairly generally distributed. It will be read in the future and may affect judgements. It is possible that it could turn up at the Mental Health Review Tribunal and be seen by the subject.

(9) *Plan of treatment report for the Mental Health Act Commission for second opinions*

The request

The Commission asks that, when a psychiatrist requests a second opinion when the problem of consent is being considered (see Chapter 4), the psychiatrist should write his plan of treatment in the medical notes. The plan is for the benefit of the visiting appointed practitioner.

The crucial questions

In all cases, the reasons for the treatment should be given, and why it should be given against the patient's wishes,

> ECT is required because the patient has an unremitting depression and has recently stopped eating. Her fluid intake is now down to a bare minimum, even after considerable coaxing.

When ECT is proposed the maximum total number of treatments to be given should be stated. When medication is proposed the class of medication and number, as used in the British National Formulary (BNF) (e.g. antipsychotic medication BNF_{16} 4.2) should be given. If the dose will be no greater than BNF levels then it is sufficient to put 'up to BNF levels'. If it is desired to use drugs above that level then the upper maximum dose proposed should be stated in terms of BNF levels e.g. 2 × BNF upper limit. The route of administration of drugs should also be given, i.e. oral, depot, parenteral.

Sources of information

The reasons for treating without the patient's consent will be found in the medical and nursing notes.

Arrangements

The process is set in motion by the responsible medical officer ringing the Mental Health Act Commission and requesting a second opinion. Arrangements have to be made for a nurse and another professional involved with the patient to be available to see the appointed practitioner when he visits. There should also be a written plan of treatment in the notes as already mentioned.

Style of the report

Clearly, technical language can be used in this case.

Form of the report

A brief outline of one to two paragraphs is all that is required.

Who will see the report?

The reports stays in the medical notes.

References

(1) Bluglass, R. (1979) The psychiatric court report. *Medicine, Science and the Law* **19**, 121–9.
(2) Scott, P.D. (1953) Psychiatric reports for magistrates' courts. *British Journal of Delinquency* **4**, 82–97.
(3) Gibbens, T.C.N. (1974) Preparing psychiatric reports. *British Journal of Hospital Medicine* **12**, 278–84.
(4) Mackay, R.D. (1986) Psychiatric reports in the crown court. *Criminal Law Review*, April, 217–25.

Chapter 16

Ethics and Forensic Psychiatry

Introduction

Ethics are defined in the *Oxford Dictionary* as: 'the rules of conduct recognized in certain limited departments of human life'. In the last two decades there has been an increasing interest in medical ethics, particularly in psychiatry, by many bodies interested in the rights of patients. This has led to a close examination of the relationship between the patient, the psychiatrist and the State. In this country, such a debate contributed substantially to the Mental Health Act 1983 and affected the advice given to the Secretary of State. This is now reflected in the Secretary of State's Code of Practice for psychiatry[1]. The ethics of working with prisoners and other detained people have been addressed in a United Nations declaration in 1981, the World Medical Association 1975 'Declaration of Tokyo', and the World Psychiatric Association 1977, 1983 'Declaration of Hawaii' – as well as in the Royal College of Psychiatry's ethical guidelines specifically concerning psychiatric care in prison[2].

Essentially, a doctor must offer in prison (or other place where people are detained) the same standard of care as he would offer if the person were not in detention. The doctor must not partake in any activities involving torture or inhuman and degrading treatment or punishment. Medical skills should not be used for non-medical purposes. Where they are used for investigative purposes such as in forensic psychiatry, the situation must be fully explained to the prisoner. The prisoner's rights and dignity must not be over-ridden.

The British Medical Association (BMA) in their handbook of medical ethics[3] draws together the ethical position of doctors in the United Kingdom. The handbook deals with many situations met generally in medicine, as well as certain specific situations in psychiatry. It recognises that a doctor may have either a therapeutic collaborative relationship with a patient or a relationship where the doctor acts as an impartial examiner (in order to provide a report at the request of a third party). In a traditional therapeutic relationship the patient is free to choose his doctor, the patient gives informed, free consent to any treatment and the doctor is responsible to the patient.

It will be immediately obvious that this traditional relationship is rarely obtained in forensic psychiatry where patients do not have a right to choose their doctor when in prison or detained in hospital and where the doctor may feel a duty to the institution. This chapter will deal with the ethics of the following:

(1) The psychiatric report.
(2) Predicting dangerousness.
(3) Assessing the defendant's responsibility.
(4) Treatment and management of detained patients.

The ethics of the expert psychiatric report

The Royal College of Psychiatrists considers it unethical for a psychiatric report to be done by doctors other than by consultant psychiatrists or trainees under their supervision. The present arrangements in England and Wales, however, do not always meet this standard.

When the defence or Crown Prosecution Service require a psychiatric report a psychiatrist should be asked to provide one. Ideally, such an expert would not be professionally connected with the case but would give an opinion or interpret facts, using specialized knowledge and experience. In practice, the defendant's own psychiatrist is also usually asked to give an expert opinion. Sometimes in the case of a defence report, defendants occasionally ask that the report be obtained from a totally independent psychiatrist because the defendant has lost confidence in their own psychiatrist.

The court commonly refers a request for a report to a collection of doctors, e.g. the team of prison medical officers or the team of forensic psychiatrists who decide amongst themselves who will do the report. This may mean that the report is prepared by a prison doctor who does not have a consultant psychiatrist's training though there is a move to correct this.

When the court orders a report, the defendant is expected to co-operate with the doctor. If he refuses to co-operate or fails to attend whilst on bail, for example, the court may order a remand in custody for an examination by the prison doctors. Generally, if the defence is asking for a report the defendant will have been consulted. However, it is possible (e.g. when a patient is so disordered as to be unfit to plead) for the defence to ask for a report without being able to obtain consent from the defendant. Nevertheless, whatever the court orders, nothing can force the defendant to give either a frank or a full history.

The psychiatrist will obtain information from the documents in the case and from the defendant which he will incorporate into the report which may lead to conclusions which the defendant may prefer to avoid. The opinion of the psychiatrist will be primarily addressed to the questions raised by the person or body who requested the report. It is now regarded as proper that the psychiatrist makes all this clear to the subject at the start of the interview. It is good practice after normal introductions to tell the subject:

(1) Who invited the doctor to see him.
(2) What the doctor does professionally (i.e. that he is a psychiatrist).
(3) The purpose of the examination (e.g. to prepare a report for the court or the solicitor on the mental state of the defendant with particular attention to its relationship to the offence).
(4) What information the doctor has already been given (e.g. statements, social report).
(5) That this is not a normal medical interview and what is learned and is relevant to the report may not be regarded as confidential between patient and doctor.
(6) How the report may be used in the sentencing (e.g. to allow the court to consider the possibility of making a hospital order).
(7) What rights he has to refuse to co-operate.
(8) That a report will be sent on the basis of available information – even in the absence of the subject's co-operation.

Sometimes an ill defendant will refuse or be unable to co-operate. The reasons for this vary from the effect of a paranoid psychosis which renders the defendant hostile and suspicious, to an inability to concentrate or think logically due to severe mental illness. In these situations the psychiatrist will report the unwillingness or inability of the subject to co-operate. The demeanour of the defendant coupled with other information derived from the observations of those around him (family or prison staff) plus information from documents (social report, previous medical report, previous psychiatric notes, witness statements) may often be sufficient to allow the psychiatrist to make a diagnosis. There is here a possible ethical dilemma for the BMA advises that a doctor may properly choose to refuse to examine a subject who does not wish to be examined. However, in the case of an obviously seriously mentally disordered offender it is normal practice to submit a report and opinion about the subject's refusal to co-operate. This situation has clear affinities to making a recommendation for detention for treatment, though in this case the court is acting as the 'applicant'.

Although ideally an expert witness is not professionally involved with the patient, as mentioned above the situation often arises that the psychiatrist making the report already knows the defendant and may actually be treating him. Should the report then be based only on what the defendant is willing to reveal at that particular time or should it be based both on the interview and what the doctor has learned to date when acting as the defendant's doctor?

The BMA firmly advises that the doctor must distinguish between his two roles and clarify this with the subject. It advises that he should report to the third party only what the subject wishes to reveal in the interview. The BMA gives no guidance as to whether the third party should be advised that the subject has in fact placed inhibitions on what the doctor can report. Fortunately, this problem is a rare one, as defendants are generally anxious (or can be persuaded) to allow past medical information to be used as it increases the chances of mitigation in court. However, the situation could lead to a psychiatrist giving a report which he knew to be misleading, e.g. a deluded subject may be anxious and able to hide delusions in an interview although they influenced his behaviour at the time of the offence. The interviewing psychiatrist may be aware of the hidden delusions from his past knowledge of looking after the patient but may feel he cannot report it if the patient does not reveal it in interview. It would seem proper, therefore, in such a case to tell the court that the information is based solely on the interview and not on previous knowledge which he is not allowed to reveal. In practice, however, in such a situation many psychiatrists would override the defendant's wishes and incorporate in the report their previous knowledge of the patient if it was felt to be in the public or patient's interest.

In approaching the defendant, the psychiatrist must always maintain that consideration for the defendant which is part of the medical ethic and his report should be clearly seen to be the report of a doctor brought in to give an objective account. In the report, care must be taken to distinguish between those things which are supported by objective evidence and those which are not. The psychiatrist's opinion must be clearly separated from his findings (see Chapter 15). The report, once completed, is sent to the party requesting it. The party may be willing to allow copies of the report to be sent by the psychiatrist to other interested people, e.g. a probation officer or the prison doctor. This permission is usually assumed if the court requests the report as it is normally in everyone's interest that this be done. On the other hand once the report is sent to a third person the psychiatrist has no control on who else will see it.

The ethics of the prediction of dangerousness

A psychiatrist will inevitably be caught up in the process of giving an opinion on the degree of dangerousness of a subject (see Chapter 14). He will be asked directly about dangerousness in the following instances:

(1) Application of a restriction order by a court.
(2) Applications to the hospital managers for the renewal of detention.
(3) The Mental Health Review Tribunal request when discharge is being considered.

(4) Reports to the Home Office on patients detained on a restriction order.
(5) When commenting about the degree of hospital security required.
(6) When making a recommendation for an order for detention in hospital under sections 2, 3, 4 and 5.
(9) When reporting to the parole board and lifers' board.

The imperfections in the psychiatrist's ability to make accurate predictions have already been noted (Chapter 14). A situation in the USA has particularly highlighted the problem[4]. In certain States the death penalty can be pronounced after certain homicide offences if the offender is believed to represent a continuing threat to society. Psychiatrists have been involved in assessing this and some have made a substantial reputation in pronouncing the subjects dangerous. This has led to considerable unease in the psychiatric profession. It has been argued that psychiatrists should dissociate themselves from this particular activity because they are both inaccurate and, more importantly, advising that someone is so dangerous as to require execution is inconsistent with the medical profession's traditional ethical code.

A psychiatrist's comments on dangerousness may lead to the prolonged detention of a defendant. This, too, has been subject to criticism and declared unethical because of the lack of data confirming the psychiatrist's alleged skills as a predictor of dangerousness[5]. Nevertheless, despite these criticisms it remains normal practice to continue to give such advice. The BMA does not comment on this specialized area. Currently, the Mental Health Act requires psychiatrists to continue to take on the task and it is clearly still regarded as ethical to do so by the profession as a whole.

The ethics of assessing responsibility

Psychiatrists, in providing a psychiatric report dealing with the question of responsibility (intent, disordered mental states, diminished responsibility, insanity, etc.) enter an area in which – it may be argued – the psychiatrist is being taken beyond the boundaries of his expertise. In the case of diminished responsibility, for example, the psychiatrist will be asked not only to describe the defendant's mental state at the time of the offence – (a reasonable question to be asked of an expert) but also the extent to which this impaired his responsibility – a question really for the jury. The complaint has been made[6] that the court uses the psychiatrist to enable it to avoid severe sentences in those cases which evoke sympathy. The court's decision as to whether a milder degree of disorder (e.g. depression) combined, say, with a disorder of personality constitutes substantially diminished responsibility may depend more on the circumstances of the offence than on the defendant's mental state. Despite the difficulties it is still regarded, generally, as ethical to give an opinion about responsibility.

The ethics of the care of the detained patient

The ethics of detaining patients

The decision about which categories of mental disorder allow detention, and under what conditions, is made by Parliament and incorporated into the Mental Health Act 1983. There was considerable criticism before the Act that patients were detained for too long by doctors without enough rights of appeal[7]. This criticism was met by reducing the length of time detention orders last before renewal becomes necessary, and by introducing compulsory regular reviews by a Mental Health Review Tribunal – as well as allowing more frequent access to a tribunal. It is regarded as good practice to use compulsory detention as little as possible, and to use the order which detains the patient for the shortest time – though this presents considerable problems when looking after patients with chronic illness who fail to comply with treatment. There is a school of thought which would abolish compulsory detention procedures involving doctors on the ethical ground that a forced admission is not what the patient wants though there is an equally strong argument that say, that the mentally ill have a right to be treated even if it be against their will[8].

In certain States in America, e.g. California, detention procedures have become difficult. It is reported that the effects of this are that many seriously mentally ill people are not treated but live a disordered life in urban squalor and find themselves sooner or later transferred to the criminal justice system. There is a growing feeling that the pendulum has swung too far in such cases[9].

The ethics of consent

Normally, it is illegal to give treatment without the patient's consent – except in certain special circumstances, e.g. emergencies when capacity to consent is affected (e.g. by unconsciousness, confusion or the undue influence of others) and when the conditions in Part IV of the Mental Health Act 1983 are met (see Chapter 4). In the case of detained patients, consent should be sought if at all possible. For consent to be genuine, it should be uninfluenced by coercion or by fraud or by misdirection, and it must be based on sufficient information. The doctor must decide what a reasonable doctor would give as information, as well as providing information about alternative treatments[10]. The Department of Health recommend (following Court of Appeal rulings) that where treatment carries substantial or unusual risks, the patient should be so advised. The doctor should give reasons for his own choice. The doctor has a duty to use reasonable care and skill in this matter.

Children under 16 can give consent if they have sufficient under-standing, otherwise parental consent is required. Parental consent may be required for 16–18 year-olds if they cannot understand.

The problem arises of the patient, detained or not detained, who is permanently unable to consent (e.g. a severely subnormal patient) to treatments not covered by the Mental Health Act. The House of Lords has ruled[11] that the doctors have a common law duty to act in the best possible interests of the patient. This would cover routinely accepted physical treatments.

> F, a severely subnormal woman, was cohabiting with a severely subnormal man. The question of her sterilization was raised. It was ruled that in such a case, not only should a second opinion be sought, but also application should be made for a court order from the Family Division of the High Court with the patient represented by the Official Solicitor. For a less serious operation a second opinion and consultation with the relatives may be enough.

It can be argued that no patient detained against his will can give free consent because he is always aware that the doctor in charge of his detention will be influenced by whether or not he complies with treat-ment. He may feel that he will only get out if he takes the treatment! The normal practice before the present Mental Health Act was for the doctor to order any treatment he felt appropriate once a treatment order had been made – even including psychosurgery. This situation came under heavy criticism: it was felt that the patients' own views should not so easily be overridden. But there was considerable argument about the solution to this ethical problem. At one pole was a proposal that a multidisciplinary committee should officiate. On the other, was the assertion by many psychiatrists that the old system worked and abuse was minimal. The outcome, incorporated into the Mental Health Act, was the setting down of clear guidance of what to do when consent was not obtained (see Chapter 4). The setting up of the Mental Health Act Com-mission ensured that the rights of detained patients would be protected. A further complication in the case of the detained mentally disordered patient is the impaired capacity of the patient to understand the situation. The Code of Practice[1] gives guidance on recognizing whether a patient has the mental capacity to give consent. The problem usually (though not always) is associated with mental impairment, organic brain syndrome, severe psychoses or serious emotional disturbances. The matter is one for clinical judgement in the light of the law and the Code's guidelines. To be capable of giving consent the patient should be able to understand what medical treatment is and that someone thinks they should have it, and why. The patient should also be able to understand the nature of the proposed treatment, its consequences (and the consequence of not having it) and its risks (expressed in broad terms). The patient has a right to be given all relevant information and the right to choose if possible. When it is necessary to obtain consent then the psychiatrist has to judge if real consent has been given, if not then he must seek a formal second opinion from the Mental Health Act Commission.

Confidentiality and the detained patient

The ideal ethical position for all patients is that a doctor must protect information acquired in the course of a doctor–patient relationship. The BMA and Royal College of Psychiatrists[12] set high value on medical confidentiality. There are, however, a number of exceptions when information is not kept confidential:

(1) The patient gives consent.
(2) The information is given to a relative or carer where, on medical grounds it is undesirable to seek the patient's consent (where this would reveal damaging medical facts to the patient) or the patient is unable to give consent and the carer needs to know (e.g. a psychotic patient).
(3) The information is required to be revealed through due legal process.
(4) Where the doctor has an overriding duty to society to reveal the confidence, e.g. in relation to an incapacity to drive, knowledge of a serious crime, terrorism.
(5) For medical research which has been approved by a recognized ethical committee.

However, in the case of detained patients there are further situations where information is disclosed without the patient's consent. These are:

(6) For a Mental Health Review Tribunal.
(7) To the hospital managers on recommending renewal of detention.
(8) To the Home Office who require information on restricted patients.
(9) Information to the Advisory Board to the Home Office.
(10) To the Mental Health Act Commission.

These situations are discussed below. The first five follow advice in the BMA guidelines.

(1) Consent to disclosure
Information that a patient gives to a doctor remains the property of the patient and should not be disclosed without permission, with the exception of the necessary sharing of information with other persons concerned with the clinical care of the patient. Permission to disclose is valid only if the patient fully understands the nature and consequences of the disclosure.

(2) Information to a relative or carer
It is regarded as ethical to disclose relevant information to a relative or other appropriate persons when it is thought undesirable for the patient to be told the full implications of his condition or the patient is incapable

of giving consent. A difficult situation can arise when an abused person asks that information about the abuse be kept confidential. Sometimes disclosure is justified in the victims interest particularly in the case of children or the incapacitated.

(3) Information required by due legal processes
This may happen either because:

(1) There is a statute requiring certain information to be given to particular bodies, e.g. the reporting of certain infectious diseases.
(2) An order is made by a court of law that the doctor disclose information. In this country, unlike some, information given by a patient is not regarded as privileged in law, i.e. protected from disclosure in all circumstances. A refusal by the doctor to comply may be regarded as contempt of court. Such a court order is likely to be issued in cases of personal litigation. Legal advice should be sought if there are doubts. The court may order the medical records to be disclosed to:
    (a) the subject,
    (b) his legal advisor,
    (c) a medical adviser to the subject,
    (d) a combination of (b) and (c) above.

The court may hear the evidence in camera if convinced that the evidence would be damaging to the patient.

(4) Duty to society
It is regarded as ethical (but not in all countries) for the doctor's duty to society to override his duty to maintain his patient's confidence. This occurs when a patient reveals that he has committed or is about to commit a grave crime:

> Dr H Edgell became aware, during an interview with a patient at a special hospital, of information indicating dangerousness. This information was not available to the Mental Health Review Tribunal. Against the wishes of the patient and the patient's solicitor Dr Edgell gave the information to the Tribunal. The Court of Appeal ruled that Dr Edgell was right to do so. (W v Edgell, Court of Appeal 8.11.89)

It may also occur when the police ask for access to personal medical information which will help them with their enquiries. In general, the doctor should seek, if possible, to persuade the patient to disclose or give permission for the information to be released. Failing this, the doctor must decide on his own conscience what action to take. In difficult cases, the doctor should consult the BMA or his defence organization. Should he reveal the information he should know that he may have to justify his decision to the General Medical Council or to a court of law. Sometimes, a patient will ask whether the doctor will treat confidentially information about a crime. No absolute assurance can be given.

In America, an important rule was established by the Tarasoff decision[13]. A patient, Poddar, told his therapist of a plan to kill Tatiana Tarasoff. The therapist, realizing the dangerousness of the situation, consulted colleagues and recommended involuntary detention. The agents of detention, in that State, were the police. They detained Poddar, then released him as he appeared rational and promised to stay away from Tarasoff. Poddar then broke off treatment. Two months later he murdered Tarasoff. The relatives sued the therapist and the police claiming that Tarasoff should have been warned of the danger. The suit was initially dismissed but was upheld on appeal to the Californian Supreme Court. The ruling, initially that the therapist had a duty to protect Tarasoff (i.e. a duty to warn) was later modified to place a duty on the therapist to use reasonable care to protect the victim, e.g. by simply hospitalizing the patient. Versions of the ruling were adopted in several States. As yet there is no such ruling in Britain. All sorts of problems arise from such a ruling. How is the therapist to judge which threats are real threats and must be acted upon and what effect will all this have on the patient's readiness to confide in his therapist?

(5) For the purposes of medical research

Information about a patient may be used in research approved by a research ethics committee. Whether it is appropriate to seek consent from the patient depends on the nature of the research, e.g. a simple count of the outcome of treatment might not require the consent of the patient. On the other hand, special enquiries taken directly from the patient for research purposes would require consent as would an experimental trial of treatment. The Royal College of Psychiatrists[14] urge that great care be taken with detained patients and 'incompetent' patients. Detention may affect a patient's ability to give free consent. There should be no suggestion, for example, that compliance will lead to release. The patient should be allowed a period of time to consider quietly the carefully explained and discussed proposal. Similar arrangements should stand for prisoners. Where the subject has no capacity to give consent, research is still possible if the patient does not resist inclusion and relatives have been informed and given consent. If there are no relatives a suitable independent person who knows the patient should be consulted. A judgement has to be made as to whether the patient would be likely to consent if he had the capacity. When information in the form of a case history is published in a scientific paper it is normal not to obtain consent but to disguise details to hide the identity of the patient.

(6) Information for the Mental Health Review Tribunal

Tribunals must be held by law at certain stated intervals on each detained patient (see Chapter 4). The responsible medical officer must give, even without the patient's consent, a report which will disclose details obtained in the therapeutic relationship. Furthermore, the case notes will be made available to the tribunal members (normally only the medical member). The doctor is not only expected to act as a professional witness and to give an account of his patient but is also expected to act as an expert witness in the sense of giving an opinion. The report of the doctor will normally be made available to the patient through his solicitor unless the doctor has some quite outstanding reason which convinces the tribunal that it would be harmful for the patient to see the report. It is good practice, therefore, for the doctor to discuss his report with the patient beforehand, indicating what his views to the tribunal will be and the reasons for them.

(7) Information to the hospital managers

At present, on renewal of a section, the managers, after seeing the responsible medical officer and receiving his reason for continuing detention, do not consult the patient except at the patient's request. The patient should be informed of the right to see the managers. The information given to the managers (who are usually three lay persons) will have been obtained within the doctor–patient relationship but will be confined to essentials. The patient's consent is not required.

(8) Information to the Home Office on restricted patients

The Home Office expects regular reports on restricted patients and full reports when the requests are made to alter conditions relating to the restriction order. In this situation it is normal not to obtain a patient's consent before sending these reports but it must remain good practice to explain to the patient what has been said and the reasons for any opinion. There is no doubt that this situation can be a difficult one because a patient may have no insight into his condition and therefore not appreciate the doctor's reasons for failing to support the patient's wish to be released.

(9) Information to the Advisory Board to the Home Office

The members of the Advisory Board (see Chapter 4) expect, on visiting a patient, to have full access to the medical records although they may be laymen. They need to do this in order to prepare a report for the Home Office on restricted patients who have been nominated as patients of particular dangerousness who need the consideration of the Board. It is not normal for the patient's consent to be obtained for this information to be revealed. Furthermore, the report of the committee is not made available either to the responsible medical officer or to the patient.

(10) Information to the Mental Health Act Commission

The Mental Health Act Commissioners are entitled to review case records and may do so without the patient's consent, from time to time, when a visit is made to a hospital to check on the care of detained patients, even though the commissioners may not be medically qualified. When a problem of consent to treatment arises with a detained patient, the Mental Health Act Commission sends an appointed practitioner to give a second opinion. That doctor will expect to have access to the medical notes. The consent of the patient would not be required.

The ethics of the control of detained patients

In looking after detained patients there are various situations in which staff may be obliged to physically hold or contain a patient, e.g. during a violent outburst or during a determined attempt to abscond. Clearly, the rights of staff in this situation must be understood as well as there being a code of behaviour for the staff to follow.

Rights of staff

Staff receive legal protection from a charge of assault when in the course of their duty they have to do such things as use physical force, give injections without consent, seclude or prevent a patient absconding. They are protected by both common law and the Mental Health Act 1983. The common law allows the imposition of treatment without consent when given to prevent a criminal act occurring or to save life or prevent a serious harm, (e.g. treating an unconscious patient). Before the present Mental Health Act, if a patient felt aggrieved about his treatment by staff he could not bring the matter to court unless he first convinced a judge in chambers that the staff member had not acted in good faith. This arrangement was criticized as giving too much protection to staff. The present Mental Health Act modified the arrangement so that, now, no civil proceedings may be brought without leave of the High Court, and no criminal proceedings except by or with the consent of the Director of Public Prosecutions in respect of an act purporting to be done as part of the duty arising out of the Mental Health Act (section 139, Mental Health Act 1983). For such proceedings to succeed, the court must be satisfied that the person accused acted in bad faith or without reasonable care. Jones[15] in his annotation of section 139 states that the House of Lords held that treatment may necessarily involve the exercise of discipline and control.

The ethics of physical control

Guidelines are needed to indicate when physical control should be used including seclusion lest it be used arbitrarily. The Code of Practice[1] outlines the different sorts of behaviour by patients which cause management problems, including uncooperative behaviour and behaviour which is threatening or dangerous. It outlines ways to minimize such behaviour: keeping patients informed and attending to their complaints; having defined personal space for patients; ensuring open space and access to facilities such as a telephone, structured and energetic activities, having trained staff.

Restraint is defined as anything from mild instruction to seclusion. Health authorities should have clear policies on the use of restraint. Physical restraint should be used as a last resort, in an emergency to prevent significant harm being done. The advice given on how to actually physically restrain whilst proper enough, has been overtaken by the use of 'control and restraint' methods developed in the prisons and transplanted into hospitals. Staff are taught various key holds (potentially painful) which effectively immobilize the subject with the minimum chance of staff or patient being injured. There must be careful monitoring of the use of physical restraining to ensure that it is not abused and is always reasonable in the circumstances. The Code states that a senior manager should be informed if restraint lasts for more than two hours. The manager should then contact the patient and check if the patient has any complaints.

Seclusion is defined as the supervised confinement of a patient alone in a room which may be locked. Seclusion should be used as little as possible. It is only indicated as a last resort to contain severely disturbed behaviour which is likely to cause harm to others. It should never be used to control the suicidal or merely because equipment is being damaged. In fact there is a clear move to abandon it altogether. Clinical experience is beginning to suggest that it might be avoided, even in secure units, if suitable levels of staffing, training and facilities are provided, i.e. a small ward or area given over to the very intensive care of the very disturbed[16].

If seclusion is used then a doctor should attend immediately. A nurse should be within sight and sound of the seclusion room at all times. A documented report (with reasons for the seclusion and its continuance) should be made every 15 minutes by the nurse and countersigned by the doctor and nurse manager. If the seclusion continues then there must be a review every two hours by two nurses, every four hours by a doctor, and at eight hours (or after a total of 12 hours intermittently in 48 hours) by a team of RMO, nurses and others not directly involved in the patient's care. If they cannot agree then the unit manager should become involved.

The secure room should be properly heated, lit, ventilated and safe. Continuous observation should be possible whilst offering privacy from other patients. There must be a regular review, by the managers, of the use of seclusion.

Treatment by programmes of behaviour modification

Following a scandal in the use of behavioural methods, a Department of Health joint working party[17] was set up to formulate ethical guidelines for the conduct of programmes of behaviour modification. The term 'behaviour modification' was used to refer to programmes in which attempts were made to apply to practical issues, management and treatment, the principles and techniques which have been developed from systematic and experimental studies on human and animal behaviour.

The problems of using such techniques on detained patients include the risk of abuse, either by excessive zeal or ignorance of untrained staff. There may be a loss of flexibility, loss of compassion and loss of respect for the rights of patients. This problem (and the problem of 'time out' and other psychological treatments) has been addressed in the Code of Practice[1]. No treatment should deprive a patient of food, shelter, water, warmth, a comfortable environment, confidentiality or reasonable privacy.

Managers have a responsibility to see that behaviour modification programmes are clearly set out and understandable. The programme and the patient should be monitored by a person with sufficient skills. A programme must be part of an agreed treatment plan and not a sudden reaction to unwanted behaviour. Patients and relatives must be fully informed. A patient's consent should be sought, if possible. However, if consent cannot or is not obtained, the treatment can be used if the responsible medical officer (RMO) consults with a suitably trained person who is not part of the team responsible for the patient. If the treatment then goes ahead, the RMO should notify the management. The RMO is responsible for seeing that the staff involved in the therapy have the necessary skills.

Duty of care

When a doctor has accepted responsibility for treating a patient he takes on a duty of care which is shared by his team. The BMA point out that the doctor has a responsibility for continuing care until the patient is handed on to another doctor.

The ethics of medical care in prison

Ethical problems can arise in the case of all prisoners but particularly with the mentally abnormal offender. The following points have caused concern:

(1) Prisoners cannot choose their own doctor. It is particularly important, therefore, that the prison medical officers accept the responsibility of providing a professional relationship with their patient which shall be as good as that of a doctor working outside prison. Access to a second opinion should be easy.

(2) The conditions and standard of care (reflecting different skills and staffing levels) in prison healthcare centres for the care of the mentally ill may fall far below that in psychiatric hospitals.

(3) The prison doctor has a duty to the patient but he also has a duty to the institution. This could cause a conflict of interest[18] but as Gunn[19] points out, the doctor's first responsibility must always be the welfare of the patient within the framework of the institution. The prison doctor may be required to comment on the prisoner's fitness to face disciplinary charges in prison and to state whether a mental disturbance accounts for offending behaviour. If the prisoner is mentally unfit it is normal to be excused punishment and for the doctor to take over his care. Gunn[19] points out that this activity is no different from psychiatrists assessing offenders for the court.

(4) The prison doctor may be required to comment on a prisoner's fitness for punishment. Prison doctors in England restrict themselves to commenting on the inmates' fitness for adjudication. The United Nations' standard minimal rules for the punishment of prisoners allow close confinement and reduction of diet providing it is not calculated to damage health. The BMA advise that doctors should not be associated with any dietary restriction (or other punishment) which would damage health. The doctor, therefore, has a role in deciding if a procedure is excessive or dangerous to the prisoner's health. If it is, then the doctor should make a written report and refuse to be further associated with the procedure. The doctor should not be associated with corporal punishment or incarceration in a dark cell. Some have argued that a doctor should have nothing to do with *any* punishment. However, medical integrity may be better preserved by trying to excuse sick people from adjudication for such punishment than by refusing to examine them at all[19].

(5) The prison doctor may prescribe drugs but this has to be with the prisoner's consent as prison hospitals are not covered by the Mental Health Act. However, in cases of emergency, under common law, medication may be given without consent if it is to save life, to restrain a violent prisoner who is violent because of his clinical condition, or to prevent irretrievable deterioration. Otherwise, if a patient is very disturbed and refuses treatment, seclusion may be the only option available.

(6) The secrecy of the prison service is such that there is no independent professional monitoring of standards within the prison medical service (though prisons and their medical services are independently

inspected by Her Majesty's Chief Inspector of Prisons). This leaves the service vulnerable when charges of unethical behaviour are made.

(7) The doctor, bound by the Official Secrets Act, may find himself unable to oppose and having to condone what would be, in other settings, unacceptable standards of care.

Because of all these difficulties it has been argued and is now recommended that the personal medical care of patients should be in the hands of doctors contracted in from outside the prison, though there is little evidence that this would alter the ethical problems[18].

Doctors and torture

Torture is the deliberate infliction of severe and excruciating pain in hatred, revenge or for extortion or control, etc. A doctor should have nothing to do with it.

It is agreed that, despite the extreme dangers, the doctor has a duty to expose it, especially when his own patients are victims. The doctor may also come across torture directly or from seeing injured patients. The perpetrators may be acting for the State or on their own.

Britain is a signatory to the European Convention of Human Rights of which Article 3 says that no one shall be subjected to 'inhuman and degrading treatment or punishment'[20]. Inspectors from the Convention will make *ad hoc* visits to places where people are detained, e.g. prisons, police cells, psychiatric hospitals and nursing homes. The purpose is to expose deficiencies and bad practice and bring them to the notice of governments in the expectation that they will be corrected. The findings will clarify and modify ethics in this area. If the corrections do not occur the findings will be published.

References

(1) Department of Health and Welsh Office (1993) *Code of Practice: Mental Health Act 1983*. HMSO, London.

(2) Special Committee on Unethical Psychiatric Practises (1992) Ethical issues concerning psychiatric care in prison. *Psychiatric Bulletin* **16**, 241–2.

(3) British Medical Association (1993) *Medical Ethics Today: Its Practice and Philosophy*. British Medical Journal Publishing Group, London.

(4) Ewing, C.P. (1983) Dr Death and the case for an ethical ban on psychiatric and psychological predictions of dangerousness in capital sentencing proceedings. *American Journal of Law and Medicine* **8**, 407–28.

(5) Bottoms, A.E. (1982) Selected issues in the dangerousness debate. In Hamilton, J.R. and Freeman, H. (eds) *Dangerousness: Psychiatric Assessment and Management*. Gaskell for the Royal College of Psychiatrists, London.

(6) Bowden, P. (1983) Madness or badness? *British Journal of Hospital Medicine* 388–94.

(7) Gostin, L. (1977) *A Human Condition*, Vol 1. MIND, London.

(8) Clare, A. (1979) Ethics in Psychiatry. In Gaind, R.N. and Hudson, B.L. (eds) *Current Themes in Psychiatry* Vol. 2. The Macmillan Press Ltd, London and Basingstoke.

(9) Campbell, R.J. (1985) Lessons for the future drawn from United States legislation and experience. In Roth, M. and Bluglass, R. (eds) *Psychiatry, Human Rights and the Law*. Cambridge University Press, Cambridge.

(10) Legal correspondent (1984) Consent to treatment: the medical standard reaffirmed. *British Medical Journal* **288**, 802–3.

(11) Brahams, D. (1989) Sterilisation of a mentally incapable woman. *Lancet* **i.** 1275–6.

(12) Royal College of Psychiatrists (1985) *Confidentiality and Forensic Psychiatry*. (Unpublished paper.)

(13) Roth, L.H. & Meisel, A. (1977) Dangerousness, confidentiality, and the duty to warn. *American Journal of Psychiatry* **134**, 508–11.

(14) Royal College of Psychiatrists (1990) Guidelines for research ethics committees on psychiatric research involving human subjects. *Psychiatric Bulletin* **14**, 48–61.

(15) Jones, R.M. (1991) *Mental Health Act Manual*. Sweet and Maxwell, London.

(16) Cope, R. (1993) Management of patients at the Raeside Regional Secure Unit without seclusion. Personal communication.

(17) Royal College of Psychiatrists (1977) *Report of the Joint Working Party to Formulate Ethical Guidelines for the Conduct of Programmes of Behaviour Modification*. Unpublished paper.

(18) Bowden, P. (1976) Medical practice: defendants and prisoners. *Journal of Medical Ethics* **2**, 163–72.

(19) Gunn, J. (1985) Psychiatry and the prison medical service. In Gostin, L. (ed.) *Secure Provision*. Tavistock Publications, London and New York.

(20) Harding, T.W. (1989) The application of the European Convention of Human Rights to the field of psychiatry. *International Journal of Law and Psychiatry* **12**, 245–62.

Chapter 17

Management of Patients within Secure Psychiatric Institutions

Introduction

This chapter will give a description of the following institutions which contribute to the care of the forensic psychiatric patient:

(1) Special hospital
(2) Regional secure units
(3) Locked wards in local hospitals (intensive care wards)
(4) The penal system – there is little scientific work in this area but there are clinical descriptions of present practice.

Ethnic Minorities and the Institution

Offenders from the ethnic minorities are found at frequencies greater than expected by population ratios in forensic institutions. In 1989 16% of prisoners were from the ethnic minorities compared to a general population ratio of 5.6%. The percentage imprisoned is greatest for the Afro-Caribbean group (nearly 10 times the expected number) and only slightly increased for the other groups (see Chapter 5). Studies of sentencing reveal that less use was made of cautioning and non-custodial penalties for the ethnic minorities. This may reflect:

(1) Racial prejudice
(2) A different quality in the crimes committed by the ethnic minorities.
(3) A refusal of the ethnic minorities to plead guilty, reflecting their mistrust of the system (thus preventing the use of cautioning).
(4) The effects of having greater social deprivation and consequently less social support.

The situation is not clear. The custodial excess of Afro-Caribbean also occurs in secure psychiatric institutions. This may reflect:

(1) A raised incidence of psychosis in the Afro-Caribbean group.
(2) An expectation that the Afro-Caribbean group will be more violent or uncooperative when psychotic[1,2].

Again, the research is conflicting.

The special hospitals (Broadmoor, Rampton, Ashworth)

History and Purpose

The background has been reviewed by Parker[3]. In the Middle Ages it became lawful in England to incarcerate a dangerous lunatic in his own home or in the local brideswell for everyone's protection. In the eighteenth century two Vagrancy Acts (1714 and 1744) empowered two Justices of the Peace or more to direct that 'furiously mad and dangerous' wandering lunatics be kept safely locked up – though recognizing that a friend or relative could take the lunatic into their own protection. It was further recognized that the lunatic might be cured during the period of restraint so that he could then be released. In 1800 James Hadfield, under the influence of delusions (though not appearing 'furiously mad') fired at King George III. He was charged with treason but was found not guilty by reason of insanity. Ordinarily this would have led to his release but because of his potential dangerousness he was returned to Newgate Prison. The 1800 Criminal Lunatic Act was then promptly passed to allow for the detention in safe custody of insane persons charged with offences of treason, murder or felony and acquitted on the grounds of insanity or found insane on arraignment. They were to be detained under His Majesty's Pleasure and became known as HMP cases. However, no specific accommodation was provided.

A select committee in 1807, studying the problems of lunatics in general, recommended that there should be one institute for HMP cases as well as county asylums for ordinary pauper lunatics. Only the latter suggestion was initially taken up and resulted in the 1808 County Asylums Act which permitted (but did not enforce) the building of public asylums for:

(1) Those detailed under the 1744 Vagrancy Act.
(2) HMP cases.
(3) Pauper lunatics.

By chance, the Bethlem Hospital was negotiating a move to Southwark at this time and agreed that part of the new hospital would be a criminal asylum. The male and female wing were completed in 1816. By this time (1815) an amending act to the Criminal Lunatic Act of 1800 dealt with the question of admission and discharge of patients to the asylum and introduced the need for a medical certificate. In 1818 an act was passed (strengthened in 1838 and 1840) to allow the transfer of prisoners who had become insane during their sentence. Thus, by the first quarter of the nineteenth century the basis of modern legislation was laid.

However, some HMP cases and insane prisoners were still being kept in prison. The Bethlem Hospital could only take a proportion of them and counties did not all have asylums. As a result, the Bethlem agreed to enlarge its criminal asylum in 1838. In 1840, in order to reduce the number of mentally ill in prison, an act was passed to allow insane prisoners, lunatics or dangerous idiots, before or after sentence, to be transferred to a county asylum.

The development of the county asylum ('counties') system and its regulation through the lunacy commission (following the 1845 Lunacy Acts) although generally an enormous reform failed to provide for the criminal lunatic. The Bethlem wing overflowed to Fisherton House near Salisbury. The counties complained that their facilities were inadequate to look after the criminal lunatic, particularly the ones from prison who were disruptive and difficult. The commissioners pressed for a separate asylum. The 1860 Criminal Lunatics Acts made possible the building of the first one, Broadmoor Hospital, to be run by the Home Office. It was eventually agreed that it would accept HMP cases (a group of patients who in general were easy to look after) and convicted prisoners who had become insane subsequent to conviction (a group of patients who were in general regarded as very disruptive and dangerous). The emphasis at that time in regard to the care of patients in asylums in general was the humane, decent containment within the institution. John Connolly from the Hanwell Asylum and experience from the Lincoln Asylum before that, had shown that individual mechanical restraints were not necessary though the establishment itself was secure. Staff could be fined heavily for letting a patient escape.

Inevitably, Broadmoor – which took both male and female patients – became full despite enlargements. Special temporary arrangements had to be made for insane prisoners within the prison and a part of Parkhurst Prison was set aside as the Parkhurst Criminal Lunatic Asylum in 1900. In 1912 Rampton Hospital was opened as a second criminal lunatic asylum also run by the Home Office.

The 1913 Mental Deficiency Act allowed for the care of mental defectives. By this time, a Board of Control had replaced the Lunacy Commission and taken over the supervision of county asylums as well as institutes for the mental defectives. Moss Side Hospital opened in 1919 for dangerous male and female defectives admitted under the Deficiency Act. During the First World War the number of detained criminally insane requiring security fell and they could all be detained in Broadmoor Hospital. Rampton Hospital became free and as it was larger than Moss Side it changed its function to become the state institute for mental defectives taking the Moss Side patients. However, Rampton and Broadmoor again became full and Moss Side was reopened as an institute for the defective in 1933.

In 1948, after the National Health Service was set up (1946), the three institutions passed to the ownership of the Ministry of Health. The control of admissions and discharges of Broadmoor patients (HMP and insane prisoners) remained in the hands of the Home Office. The 1959 Mental

Health Act brought the mentally ill and mentally defective under the same act and obliged the Minister of Health to provide institutions of special security for those patients requiring it on the grounds of dangerous, violent or criminal propensities. It became possible then to admit non-offender patients under the Act to all three special hospitals – the name given to Moss Side, Rampton and Broadmoor. The Ministry of Health (now the Department of Health) became the managers of the hospitals and controlled admission. The Home Office has retained control of discharge in the case of restricted patients. There the matter rested for some years until gross overcrowding of Broadmoor – the special hospital which dealt principally with mental illness – led to the setting up of Park Lane Hospital in 1984, placed in grounds next to Moss Side Hospital. In 1989 Moss Side and Park Lane were amalgamated into one, Ashworth Hospital, under the newly formed Special Hospitals Service Authority. The functions of the two hospitals were retained in Ashworth (south) and Ashworth (north) respectively.

The current purpose of the special hospitals is stated in section 4 of the National Health Service Act 1977 which requires the Secretary of State for Health to provide special hospitals for patients subject to detention who require treatment under conditions of special security on account of their dangerous, violent or criminal propensities. This is interpreted by the Department of Health as being of a nature such that the patient is an immediate grave danger to others – either to the public outside the hospital because of persistent, determined absconding associated with dangerous behaviour or to patients or staff within the hospital. In both cases, the severity of the behaviour disorder must be such that it requires the security of a special hospital.

Buildings and security in special hospitals

Hamilton[4] has given a description of the special hospitals. The buildings of the special hospital vary from the old, worn buildings of Victorian Broadmoor (soon to be replaced), to the ultra-modern in Park Lane. There are, however, some common features. In all there is a secure perimeter wall or fence, sufficiently high to prevent absconding. Electronic detectors are incorporated in the perimeter security in the most recent developments. The entrance to the hospitals is an 'airlock' system with an outer and inner door which in the most modern arrangement will be electronically operated. All movements in and out of the building are monitored and recorded by staff at the entrance. Having secured the perimeter, the hospitals themselves consist of locked wards or villas within which there is a variable degree of freedom depending on the estimate, by the staff, of the patient's dangerousness and clinical state. Movement between the locked wards will be carefully monitored with the patients normally moving only with an escort. Each ward will, as far as possible, provide single room accommodation which will be furnished according to the estimated dangerousness of the patient. The more modern rooms will be provided with full sanitation and all will be normally locked at night and only unlocked when sufficient staff are present. On each ward there will be day rooms with the normal facilities for leisure (television, radios, snooker tables, etc.) though access may be restricted for the very dangerous patient who may have to be confined to his room. Within each ward there will also be a special secure room to contain the patient during any brief periods of disturbed behaviour.

Within the perimeter wall will be workshops, education centres, social rooms, gymnasiums, swimming pool, gardens, sports fields, hospital shops, etc. Movement to and from these facilities will be carefully regulated and monitored and most patients escorted. The tendency in modern design is to incorporate security equipment like television scanning cameras and unbreakable glass.

Maintaining security involves a regular count of patients, checks on equipment (knives, forks, workshop tools, etc.) random spot checks on patients' rooms, parcel checks, and checks on goods brought in by visitors. Nevertheless, security depends also on staff knowing patients well and remaining vigilant. There is no substitute for creating an atmosphere of understanding, sympathy and acceptance. The more acceptable the hospital, the less will patients strive to abscond.

Staffing levels

The staff at the special hospitals are drawn from the normal hospital disciplines. There are no special security staff or discipline staff. However, the tradition of the Home Office days lingers on and male staff in some hospitals still wear a uniform similar to that of a prison officer and some of the nursing staff of the hospital are still represented, at the union level, by the Prison Officers' Association who negotiate their pay and conditions. The staffing levels are improving but are still considered too low. The consultant to patient ratio is about 1:60. Overall nurse to patient ratio is about 1:1, psychologist to patient ratio is again about 1:60–1:50. The staff will also include psychiatrists in training, visiting psychotherapists, social workers, occupational officers, administrative and clerical staff, teaching staff, librarians, chaplains, physiotherapists, catering and domestic staff, etc.

The patients

The special hospitals admit some 170–200 patients annually and have a total population of 1700 patients.

Broadmoor and Ashworth (north) patients suffer principally (75%) from mental illness, mainly schizophrenia, and the rest from psychopathic disorder. All the patients are detained, none are informal. The majority (80%) will be on court orders (section 37), of which most will also have a restriction order. Less than 10% will be on treatment orders (section 3) and slightly more than 10% will have been transferred from prison (section 46–48). Of those sent by the court, 30% will have committed homicide. Other violent offences and arson account for nearly 55%. Sex offences only account for 3%. The rest are criminal damage, theft, burglary, etc. Half the patients have been there five years or more and the average length of stay is around six years. Very short stays, as seen in acute psychiatric wards, are very unusual.

Rampton and Ashworth (south) patients also suffer principally from mental illness as a first diagnosis (30–40%) but they also have a substantial number of patients with mental impairment as a first diagnosis (20%) and severe impairment (15%). Some 25% of the patients have psychopathic disorder. The patients with mental illness in these two hospitals often also have mental impairment and in that way the patients differ from those in Broadmoor or Park Lane hospitals. Just over 50% of the patients are on court orders and up to 30% are on treatment orders (section 3). Amongst the offences, sexual offences are more frequent (around 10%) than at Broadmoor, and homicide less (around 10%). Violence and arson account for 60%, arson being a commoner offence amongst the Rampton/Ashworth (south) patients than at Broadmoor/Ashworth (north). Lengths of stay at Rampton and Ashworth (south) follow the same medium- to long-stay pattern.

Treatment and management of patients

The treatment offered to patients in special hospital is on the same lines as in other psychiatric hospitals given the limitations which the need for security imposes. Patients stay longer in special hospitals partly because their condition is one which will not be easily controlled and because of anxiety about their prognosis; it's particularly true of psychopathy[5]. There is always the anxiety that apparent improvement may not be sustained. Special hospitals appear to have an ability to cope with and bring under control behaviour that is not tolerable or manageable elsewhere. It seems as though this ability is linked to the setting and routine. At best this provides a regular, stable environment in which staff react with firmness and fairness to unwanted behaviour. The traditions by which staff manage violent patients are in themselves a source of security to the staff who must remain in control of what could otherwise be an extremely dangerous situation. Most dangerous patients are placed on wards where staffing ratios are sufficiently high to engender confidence in the staff. Nevertheless assaults on staff (particularly nurses) and patients are regular occurrences, though they tend to be committed by a small minority of patients. Injuries were moderate or severe in two-thirds of cases. High density of patients and lack of privacy are provoking factors[6]. A study of prison officers suggests that the more experienced officers learn to avoid incidents[7]. As the patient improves so he can be moved to wards which are less controlling and less heavily staffed.

Educational facilities are provided from the most basic subjects to Open University and occupational facilities offer training in a wide range of skills. The hospitals have been criticized for a lack of rehabilitation schemes but they are endeavouring to improve this. They are inhibited (though not completely) from offering experience beyond the perimeter walls because of the political pressure arising from the fear of a patient absconding. Other criticisms (see below) have risen from the tendencies of such institutions to become rigid, interned and isolated but again there has been a very active attempt to put this right. The hospitals are monitored by the Mental Health Act Commission.

Interaction with other psychiatric facilities

Admission to the secure hospitals is obtained by applying to the admission panel at each special hospital (see Chapter 15 and Chapter 1). When a patient becomes well enough to leave the hospital, the responsible medical officer contacts the doctor in the catchment area hospital or regional secure unit to whom he wishes to refer the case. Some patients will be fit enough to return directly to the community – perhaps with outpatient care – whilst others will need to go to a hospital setting. It is argued from various surveys that up to 50% of the patients in special hospital do not actually require to be there. They could be managed in lesser security if long-stay beds with medium security were provided in the regions. At present such facilities do not exist though the Reed Committee recommended their development[8].

The transfer of patients, apart from these long-term ones, has not always worked very well[9], and transfers have been delayed for months or even years. It has been found that the chances of a patient leaving special hospital are much increased if the appropriate consultant and his team take up the invitation to see the patient in the special hospital.

Outcome studies of special hospital patients

Bowden[10] has reviewed the principal follow-up studies. The studies cover a very heterogeneous group of people varying in age, previous criminality and diagnosis. The studies also differ in their length of follow-up. Overall, 50% of those released from special hospital re-offended within five years although the new offences will be mostly trivial. Some 10% will be involved in a serious violent offence and 1% will commit homicide. On the other hand, nearly 60% will be in the community, 20% recalled to special hospital and the rest divided between prison and ordinary psychiatric hospital. Conditionally discharged patients, particularly the mentally ill, do better than those absolutely discharged[11]. Those who did worst had a diagnosis of psychopathic disorder or mental handicap. They also had more previous hospital admissions and more previous offences, and tended to be younger (see also Chapter 14).

In comparison, Home Office figures for all psychiatric hospitals show, for restricted patients with mental illness, an overall five-year reconviction rate for grave offences of 2% compared with 11% for psychopathic disorder. Amongst these patients, those originally admitted to special hospital were nearly twice as likely to re-offend as those restricted patients admitted directly to other hospitals. Psychopaths were also younger and had committed more previous offences.

The future of the special hospitals

The hospitals have experienced two damaging enquiries (1980 and 1992) arising out of allegations of improper care of patients[12, 13]. The problems can be seen as being linked to institutionalization and pockets of anachronistic attitudes, as well as to problems arising from staffing levels and physical difficulties. It is also now recognized that about half of the patients, although needing long-term hospital care, do not require the care to be in the high-security of the special hospitals. The committee of enquiry into Ashworth Hospital concluded that the only solution was the closure of the hospitals. A recent working group[8] recommended that the hospitals be retained for the time being but those 50% of patients who no longer need the high security should be moved to new accommodation to be provided in the regions. This reduction in population should make the hospitals more manageable as will their attainment of self managing trust status under new NHS arrangements. If the reduction in patients was sufficiently large then closure of one of the hospitals would become a possibility.

Regional secure units

History and purpose

As local psychiatric hospitals abandoned physical security and became increasingly open from the 1950s onwards, so it was felt that there would be a need for a special regional arrangement to look after those patients who were too difficult or dangerous to be coped with in an open setting but not so disturbed as to require a special hospital.

The first official suggestion came from the Royal Commission in 1957[14] and this was made more explicit in 1961 by the Working Party on Special Hospitals[15]. That working party recommended regional secure units which would become centres for the care of difficult and dangerous patients – psychopathic and otherwise – a centre for forensic psychiatry, education and research. The recommendation was taken up by the then Department of Health and Social Security (DHSS) and the regional health authorities were asked to provide them. Only two attempted to do so but neither survived as such. The Northgate Clinic in North-West Thames region became an adolescent unit, and the secure unit at South Ockenden Hospital (Cyprus Villa) was abandoned after a hospital enquiry revealed the bad practices which had evolved (excessive repression, lack of therapeutic programmes, individual attention or therapeutic input). No further attempts to construct a regional secure unit occurred despite continuing DHSS circulars.

In 1974 the interim report of the Committee on Mentally Abnormal Offenders (the Butler Committee) was published[16] and the report from the Working Party on Security in the National Health Service (NHS) (the Glancy Report) was circulated[17]. Both had studied the increasing problems arising from patients being refused treatment by psychiatric hospitals because of the lack of proper facilities to cope with difficult or dangerous patients. Such patients were therefore being sent to prison, held too long in special hospital or simply not cared for. Both reports concluded that regional secure units would be the answer though they differed radically about the number of beds required. Butler recommended 2000 while Glancy recommended 1000. The DHSS accepted the lower recommendation and urged the regional health authorities to provide them. When it became clear that the regional health authorities were not going to hurry, the DHSS made funds available to promote the scheme asking that interim arrangements be made quickly whilst designs for definitive units were drawn up. Now, most regions have either an interim unit or have moved into a definitive regional secure unit. There has, however, been considerable variation in the interpretation of the various guidelines as well as considerable variation in the sums which regions have allocated to the schemes to top up the initial DHSS grant. Some regions have provided more beds than the recommended norm from the DHSS of 20 beds per million whilst others have provided just rather more than half. Bluglass[18] and Treasaden[19] describe the development of and practice in the units.

Buildings and security

The interim arrangement that most regions made was to convert a ward or villa in a psychiatric hospital into a secure ward with individual bedrooms, day-rooms and occupational therapy facilities. The units varied considerably in the level of security provided. The amount was often dictated by political rather than clinical pressures. In one urban area there was enormous opposition to the unit being opened and it was only tolerated provided that it appeared quite secure. Airlock door systems, high perimeter fence and tight security practices were adopted. At the other end of the scale, in a rural setting, a unit was only accepted by the staff representatives on condition that it would be essentially community orientated, open as much as possible, (though with the possibility of locking it) and no perimeter fencing[20]. Staff would have to know their patients well and be able to anticipate disturbed behaviour or absconding and intervene in time. High physical security, it was argued, would (1) lead to a false sense of security and tempt the unit to accept patients who should really have been in a special hospital, and (2) lead at times of low staffing to an unacceptable authoritarian, repressive regime. Fortunately, this unit was in a community which was willing to accept the scheme.

The first interim units were opened in 1976–77 and the first definitive regional secure units from the early 1980s. The definitive units have varied as much as the interim units, in terms of physical security and size. In many regions there is one central regional secure unit. In others there are two or three small ones. In the South-East Thames there is one larger (30-bedded unit) with four smaller (15-bedded) units within the region. The South-West Thames region has encouraged the development of 'intensive care' wards within catchment area hospitals, and plans a small central regional secure unit. The West Midlands, on the other hand, will have a 100-bedded central regional secure unit and no peripheral units. Not only has the size and pattern varied but, as with the interim units, the level of physical security has varied considerably.

The apparent difference in physical security between the units, however, seems to be of far less importance than first appeared. The physical features which all the units have in common are:

(1) The capacity to contain safely a very disturbed patient in a secure area or room.
(2) The capacity (using a combination of locked doors and escorted parole) to contain all their patients safely within the building and its immediate grounds.

All the units, however, have an Achilles heel in their security arising from the need to rehabilitate the patients to make them well enough to return to the community or catchment area hospital. All the units, therefore, have developed a parole system as part of their rehabilitation. At some stage the patients have freedom to move unaccompanied outside the perimeter of the unit. Once this stage is reached the security is breached and all units have some patients abscond at this point.

The experience of the interim unit and regional secure units taught that wards should not be larger than 15 single bedrooms. Above that level it becomes difficult for the staff to be aware of what is going on. The total size of the unit may turn out to be important. Smaller units are much easier to manage as communications are easier which has an effect on patient management and staff morale. It has been suggested that 50 beds is a good maximum size but the advantages of larger units (up to around

100 beds) include better staffed departments e.g. occupational therapy. Because the regions have not provided all the beds originally requested by the DHSS the total number of beds provided by the system will be only 800 places. The Reed Committee[8] has pressed for a substantial increase.

Staffing

When the interim secure units were set up and the regional secure units were being planned it was possible, because of the desire of the DHSS to set up the units, to press successfully for much higher staffing levels than hitherto had been the case in psychiatric units. It became possible, perhaps for the first time, to approach really adequate levels of staffing for treating difficult patients. This allowed a much more therapeutic approach to be taken.

Consultant to inpatient ratios range between 1:7 to 1:16. Nurse to patient ratios overall to provide 24 hour cover and community care average about 2.5:1. Psychologist to inpatient ratios lie between 1:7 and 1:30, social worker ratios between 1:7 and 1:30, occupational therapists average 1:12. When it became apparent that some patients would become day patients of the units, community nursing services were developed. In addition, the units have clerical, domestic and administrative staff. Pharmacy services and other services tend to be provided by the parent hospital in which the unit is placed. A problem will arise when parent hospitals close (as part of the national scheme) leaving the regional secure units isolated as may happen at a number of sites.

Patients

Patients in most secure units suffer principally from mental illness (mostly schizophrenia) whilst the remainder will suffer from psycho-pathic disorder. Very few will be mentally impaired and none severely mentally impaired except in the regional unit for mental impaired in the Oxford region. Patients are referred from NHS hospitals (25%), special hospitals (20%), courts and remand prisons (40–50%) and the community services (up to 10%) and ordinary prisons (1–2%).

Most patients will either be on a hospital order with or without restrictions or treatment orders reflecting their source of referral. A few may be informal (e.g. ex-inpatients re-admitted voluntarily because of a brief breakdown). Personal violence (or threats of it) will be the main precipitant leading to referral (80%) and fire raising or other destructive behaviour will occur in 10–15%. The patients will usually have had previous offences and previous admissions to other hospitals.

The length of stay has varied between units quite markedly depending on the policy of the unit. In 1976–80, the average stay in the Wessex Interim Unit was six months whereas the equivalent stay in the North-

West region was 12 months. There have been changes in policy and types of patient as experience has been gathered and whether this difference in length of stay still holds is unclear. There are factors outside the unit which will affect the length of stay. The current cautious approach of the Home Office to the release of restricted patients will increase their length of stay as will the decreasing lack of facilities in catchment area hospitals to cope with difficult, chronically ill patients.

Treatment and management of patients

There is, at present, no study comparing styles of care in the different units. Some may be more authoritarian than others, lengths of stay may differ, aftercare facilities may differ. Nevertheless, the units that have opened have continued on an optimistic, therapeutic note. Multi-disciplinary approaches are the norm. The high staffing levels have made it possible to devise individual programmes for each patient as appropriate and also to give much more personal attention than is normal. This attention should provide any necessary controls as well as warm and rapid attention to anxieties. As patients recover from their most disturbed phase, so genuine attempts at individual rehabilitation can be begun. The success of any unit requires high staff morale and the proper interaction of all disciplines without destructive rivalries. Achieving this requires considerable attention to personnel and administrative problems. The attention paid to solving staffing problems substantially affects the care of patients.

The types of treatment offered by the units do not differ from the treatments given on ordinary wards. However, the nurses become skilled at tactfully managing the disturbed patient and the staffing levels and security make it possible to easily detain disturbed patients who would otherwise abscond. Medical staff become accustomed to dealing with psychoses which have failed to respond to conventional doses of drugs; psychologists and nurses become skilled at devising nursing programmes for the manipulative, emotionally draining patient or the very disturbed. Occupational therapists, art therapists and social workers adapt their skills to assist in the rehabilitation of patients whose lives have become totally chaotic. Thus, the skills acquired are developments of normal practice.

Interaction with other units

Admission to the regional secure unit is controlled by the responsible medical officer and staff of the unit. Usually an assessment of the patient is made at the request of the patient's doctor before admission in order to plan the patient's care. Similarly, when the patient is sufficiently improved in the regional secure unit, the catchment area hospital consultant will be invited to assess the patient with a view to his returning to his own hospital. Originally, it was expected that regional secure units would be able to return all their inpatients to the care of the catchment area team. However, some patients were refused re-admission by the area team either because of their reputation or because of differences of opinion between the team and the regional secure unit about the patient's dangerousness. Some patients formed a strong bond to the secure unit and their condition remained so fragile that it seemed sensible for the personnel of the regional secure unit to provide the aftercare. A number of regional secure units now provide accommodation such as a group home in the community as well as a day and outpatient service.

The units have been criticized, particularly the small ones which are often full, for being unable to offer prompt admission. The units have tended to exclude, to a large extent, those with psychopathic disorder and mental impairment. Because of their small size the units have not been able to provide the educational and occupational facilities seen in the larger special hospitals.

Secure wards in catchment area hospitals

History and purpose

Wards have been opened at local levels (known as 'intensive' or 'special care' wards) with high staffing levels to provide for patients presenting disruptive or dangerous behaviour which cannot be coped with in ordinary wards. These wards have been developed sporadically on local initiative. Descriptions of such wards have been given by Woodside *et al.* in Edinburgh[21], Carney and Nolan in Shenley Hospital[22] and Goldney *et al.* in Adelaide[23]. Such wards often meet a degree of opposition at first, as occurred in Edinburgh, because other staff fear that the ward represents a return to old, repressive, locked wards. Their value is quickly appreciated, however, and they become an established part of the psychiatric hospital service. The usual pattern is for the wards to accept patients briefly to get them over an acute disturbance before returning them to the original ward. In both Edinburgh and Shenley it has become clear, however, that a number will be chronic patients. In Edinburgh, a ward for chronically disturbed patients had to be set up to support the intensive care ward. There has been no assessment of the extent to which such wards have been developed throughout the country. The work of such wards obviously overlaps with that of the regional secure unit and some have felt[24-28] that they will be an essential part of the total forensic service if the regional secure units are not to become hopelessly jammed. Indeed, it was thinking of this sort which promoted the south-west regional scheme mentioned above. This need is also recognised by the Reed Committee[8]

Buildings and security

Intensive care wards are commonly wards converted for the purpose, though standards of conversion tend to be lower than that for an interim secure unit. Individual bedrooms may be provided and there may be access to a fenced garden. The extent of physical security varies but commonly the ward will be permanently locked and use may be made of unbreakable glass.

Staffing levels

These are lower than in a regional secure unit but higher than in a normal hospital. In Edinburgh, it was arranged that five nurses would be present on a day shift to look after 15 inpatients; in Shenley nine nurses look after 48 beds in two locked wards; in Adelaide there are 3 nurses on a day shift for eight patients. The wards usually represent only part of the work of the consultant psychiatrist. Occupational therapists and psychologists also devote much less time to the ward than would be available in a regional secure unit.

Patients and their management

The patients are admitted from the main hospital because the normal ward is unable, temporarily, to manage the patient. It is usually expected that the referring psychiatrist will keep in contact with the treatment of the patient – which will have passed to the care of the psychiatrist in charge of the intensive care ward – and accept the patient back when he is well enough. The interaction of staff and patients in the units appears to be similar to that in a regional secure unit. Supportive, attentive staff giving individual attention and involving the patient in his own care are common themes. The main difference between patients in the intensive care ward and the regional secure unit lies in the forensic history which is much commoner in a regional secure unit. The stay in intensive care wards is much shorter, lasting from a few days to a few weeks. This may reflect the fact that these patients have disorders less resistant to treatment or that the staff are less anxious about their dangerousness because of the lack of forensic history.

Psychiatric Care in the Private Sector

In recent years there has been a steady expansion in the private sector hospitals (e.g. Kneesworth House, St Andrews, Stockton Hall) specializing in the secure psychiatric care of patients, including mentally abnormal offenders for whom there are no suitable facilities in the patient's district.

This growth began before regional secure units were developed and provided regional secure unit type facilities for those regions which were late in developing the service. At the same time, these hospitals developed units for brain-damaged patients, personality disordered patients, and disturbed adolescents. The patients are paid for by their district health authority. The admissions are arranged by the patient's doctor and the private hospital in conjunction with the district health authority.

The units adapt a token economy regime around a structured and varied day which certainly benefits some patients[25]. Apart from meeting a need for a group of very difficult patients they also provide an interesting alternative regime to the standard approach in the National Health Service. It remains to been seen whether this approach has therapeutic advantages. It certainly uses staff more economically and can produce an atmosphere of high morale and enthusiasm.

Psychiatric Care in the Penal System

Introduction

The development of the prison medical service is described by Gunn[26]. The medical service for the prisons began in the eighteenth century to preserve the health of prisoners. Legislation in 1808, 1816 and 1840 allowed the transfer of insane prisoners to a county asylum[1]. Other arrangements within the prisons had to be made for mental defectives (housing them in particular prisons) until legislation in 1867 permitted their transfer to the county asylums. Later legislation (Mental Deficiency Acts 1913 and 1927) set up special institutions for the defective. An attempt was made to deal with inebriates by the Inebriates Act (1898) which enabled courts to send them to reformatories. This system was abandoned by the 1920s.

In the 1920s there was increasing interest in the possibility of using psychotherapy within the prisons to treat some offenders whose offending could be understood to have a neurotic basis. Dr Norwood East (prison medical officer) and Dr W. de Hubert (visiting psychiatrist) recommended in 1939 the setting up of a penal institution for: (1) medical investigation and criminological research into treatment for selected prisoners, and (2) a colony for offenders who could not adapt to ordinary life. This recommendation eventually resulted in the setting up of Grendon Prison (opened 1962), a prison with a psychiatrist as governor and using psychotherapeutic methods with psychopathic offenders (see Chapter 10).

The doctors of the prison medical service are employed directly by the Home Office. There are 130 working full-time and 130 part-time; the full-time doctors are part of the prison staff (see Chapter 1).

Psychiatric disorder amongst prisoners

Various psychiatric surveys of convicted prisoners have been summarized by Coid[25, 27]. There are considerable difficulties with definitions of disorders, particularly of neurosis, and personality disorders, and considerable variation in percentages. Serious mental illness (psychoses and affective disorder) did not, Coid concluded, occur in a significantly higher incidence than in the general population (rates about 3–4%), neither did neurosis. There was evidence of a raised incidence of subnormality (some reported over 14%) and epilepsy (up to 1.5 times normal). The common diagnoses were psychopathic disorder (up to 80%), alcoholism (up to 50%) and drug abuse (up to 25%). The most recent survey (1991) in England and Wales of sentenced prisoners[28] gave results within these limits (37% having a psychiatric disorder) – closely resembling a similar study in 1972. An attempt was made to assess the treatment needs of the population using normal clinical judgement. Only some 3% needed hospital treatment (mainly psychoses); 10% needed treatment in prison (mainly neurotic disorder, personality disorder, substance abuse); 5% needed treatment in a therapeutic community (mainly personality disorder and substance abuse). There was uncertainty in 1%, and 77% did not require psychiatric treatment.

Whether the incidence of serious mental illness is as low as appears has also been brought into question by Taylor's study of 183 life-sentenced people[29] in which the incidence of schizophrenia was 9%, and affective disorder 13%. Coid draws attention to the difference between illnesses and disorders which were present before the offence, and psychiatric morbidity and behavioral disorder which occur, apparently, as a response to imprisonment. The latter is a contentious matter; there is evidence that prison does not have a deleterious effect – indeed that people appear to mature while imprisoned[30]. Nevertheless, clinically one does see individuals who appear to react badly.

Special problems in prison

The combination of committing a dreadful offence or being arrested and charge, separated from normal surroundings, imprisoned and facing the uncertainties of a trial and sentencing, naturally increases tension and feelings of dysphoria and depression. A good prison regime (based on human decency, consideration for the individual, sensible surroundings and interesting occupation) will do a lot to counteract these baleful effects[31]. In all prisons, but especially where the regimes are poor (inconsiderate staff with corresponding inmate hostility, lack of occupation, poor surroundings) it is more likely that the prisoner will show some adverse psychological reaction e.g. depression/anxiety/tension. There are also behaviours which seem particularly associated with imprisonment which the doctor may be asked to deal with. These include:

(1) Suicide attempts.
(2) Food refusal.
(3) Self-mutilation.
(4) Sleep disturbance.
(5) Malingering.

Suicide attempts
Suicide rates have been increasing in prison (121% over 15 years) and are estimated to be higher than in the community as a whole[32] though there are methodological difficulties in assessing this (getting a proper control group). Higher rates in prison are especially associated with the first few stressful weeks on remand, long-term imprisonment and committing violent or destructive offences. The suicides seem associated with isolation, guilt, remorse, depression and despair, though a proportion are associated with psychosis. One-third will have had previous psychiatric contact. Unfortunately, there are no control studies to confirm whether these developments are solely a reaction to the stress of prison and loss of family, etc. or a feature of unstable prisoners. A ten-year-follow-up study of conscripts to the Swedish Army, for example, found a suicide rate more than three times normal amongst those with some features of antisocial personality[33].

The increased death rate from suicide in prisoners is mirrored by the increased death rate in ex-prisoners (five times normal) and violent offenders where the principal causes of death are poisoning from drug abuse and violence[34].

The prison service has responded by trying to make staff more aware of the problem and able to identify 'at risk' inmates. Support schemes for distressed inmates are evolving including support by other inmates. Medical care is also moving to hospital standards for the mentally ill and suicidal.

Food refusal
Inmates may refuse food, and sometimes drink. Two forms may be recognized[35].

(1) A minority who are seriously mentally ill: Their food refusal may well be coupled with fluid refusal. They are characterized by generally (though not always) being unable or unwilling to give a reason. They require urgent transfer to a psychiatric hospital.
(2) A majority who use the food refusal in an argument with authority: 'I will refuse to eat until ...'. The majority will not have serious psychiatric disorder. Some will have psychopathic disorder and one or two may also be psychotic or depressed.

Prisons have a routine of having all food-refusers psychiatrically assessed so that those who are psychiatrically ill can be identified and treated. Those who are normal usually respond to counselling and support. Rarely, a determined psychiatrically normal inmate will starve to death to make a political point.

Self-mutilation

Here inmates cut or burn themselves (e.g. superficial repeated cuts to the arms; burns with cigarette ends) in reaction to feelings of tension and despair. Where the levels of tension are high in a prison, self-mutilation can acquire an almost infectious quality as the behaviour spreads in the institution. Emotional instability and immaturity are frequent features of those inmates. Some believe, on clinical grounds, that a high proportion of female self-mutilators have also been victims of serious sexual abuse.

Sleep disturbance

Increased levels of tension and alleged sleep disturbance lead to requests for sedation. Prison doctors are likely to find themselves being pressed by inmates, especially by the personality disordered or those with a history of drug abuse, for sedatives and hypnotics. It requires considerable judgement to get the right balance between over- and under-prescribing. It may be useful for the doctors to agree a guidance policy for this situation, perhaps in consultation with an outside psychiatrist experienced in these matters.

Malingering

Clinically, serious malingering appears to be quite rare, both for physical and psychiatric illness. It is usually done in order to escape from an intolerable situation within the prison (threat by other prisoners) or to escape from prison:

> An inmate mysteriously lost weight rapidly and presented as 'ill'. A move to a local general hospital for investigation became necessary. He escaped from there but was later re arrested. His mysterious weight loss began again and continued to an extreme degree. Every effort was made to check that he was truly eating his food as he claimed but such was his cunning that it was many months before it could be shown that he was disposing of his food through the bars to the prison dogs. He then gave up and ate normally.

Psychiatric treatment in prisons

The legal and ethical difficulties and the administrative constraints on practising psychiatry in prison have been discussed in Chapter 16. Treatment has been discussed in Chapter 1. Despite all the difficulties arising from both the ethical and administrative problems, the medical staff see it as their task to provide a medical care to the same personal standard as within the service outside prison.

The core team within a prison consists of the prison medical officer assisted by healthcare officers (discipline officers who have had special training in basic nursing but with very little psychiatric training) and, increasingly, trained nurses employed either as nurses or as healthcare workers. There are also visiting psychiatrists who will have the task of assessing and treating inmates both by psychotherapy and medication if the patient will accept these voluntarily. Some personality disordered and neurotic prisoners appear clinically to benefit (though scientific evidence is lacking of long-term effectiveness) from psychological treatments, such as social skills training and drama therapy conducted by probation or education officers attached to the prison. Psychologists may be involved directly or as supervisors. Some workers have developed particular interests in particular groups, e.g. sex offenders. The extent of these services depends on the size of prison, with some prisons or youth custody centres taking a particular interest in psychiatrically disturbed prisoners and some in sex offenders. What has also become clear is that a humane regime, of which these therapies may be part, leads to a much better prison atmosphere – which must be beneficial to all involved[31].

References

(1) Noble, P. & Rodgers, S. (1989) Violence by psychiatric inpatients. *British Journal of Psychiatry* **155**, 384–94.

(2) Cope, R. & Ndegwa, D. (1990) Ethnic differences in admission to a regional secure unit. *Journal of Forensic Psychiatry* **1**, 365–78.

(3) Parker, E. (1985) The development of secure provision. In Gostin, L. (ed.) *Secure Provision*. Tavistock Publications, London and New York.

(4) Hamilton, J.R. (1985) The special hospitals. In Gostin, L. (ed) *Secure Provision*. Tavistock Publications, London and New York.

(5) Dell, S. & Robertson, G. (1988) *Sentenced to Hospital: Offenders in Broadmoor*. Oxford University Press, Oxford.

(6) Caldwell, J.B. & Naismith, L.J. (1989) Violent incidents on special care wards in a special hospital. *Medicine, Science and the Law* **29**, 116–23.

(7) Davies, W. & Burgess, P.W. (1988) Prison officers' experience as a predictor of risk and attack: an analysis within the British prison system. *Medicine, Science and the Law* **28**. 135–38.

(8) Department of Health and Home Office (1992) *Review of Health and Social Services for Mentally Disordered Offenders and Others Requiring Similar Services*. (Chairman: Dr. John Reed). Cm. 2088. HMSO, London.

(9) Dell, S. (1980) The transfer of special hospital patients to the National Health Service hospitals. *Special Hospitals Research Unit Report No. 16*. Department of Health and Social Security, London.

(10) Bowden, P. (1985) Psychiatry and Dangerousness: a counter renaissance. In

Gostin, L. (ed.) *Secure Provision*. Tavistock Publications, London and New York.

(11) Baily, J. & MacCulloch, M. (1992) Patterns of reconviction in patients discharged directly to the community from a special hospital: implications for aftercare. *Journal of Forensic Psychiatry* **3**, 445–61.

(12) *Report of the Review of Rampton Hospital*. (1980) Cmnd. 8073. HMSO, London.

(13) *Report of the Committee of Inquiry into Complaints about Ashworth Hospital*. (1992) Cmnd. 2028 HMSO, London.

(14) *Report of the Royal Commission on the Law Relating to Mental Illness and Mental Deficiency 1954–57*. Cmnd. 169. HMSO, London.

(15) Ministry of Health (1961). *Special Hospitals. Report of Working Party*. HMSO, London.

(16) Home Office and Department of Health and Social Security (1974). *Interim Report of the Committee on Mentally Abnormal Offenders*. Cmnd. 5698. HMSO, London.

(17) Department of Health and Social Security. (1977) *Revised Report of the Working Party on Security in National Health Service Hospitals*. Unpublished.

(18) Bluglass, R. (1985) The development of regional secure units. In Gostin, L. (ed.) *Secure Provision*. Tavistock Publications, London and New York.

(19) Treasaden, I.H. (1985) Current practise in regional interim secure units. In Gostin, L. (ed.) *Secure Provision*. Tavistock Publications, London and New York.

(20) Faulk, M. (1979) The Lyndhurst Unit at Knowle Hospital. *Bulletin of the Royal College of Psychiatrists* **3**, 44–46.

(21) Woodside, M., Harrow, A., Basson, J.V. & Affleck, J.W. (1976) An experiment in the management of sociopathic disorders. *British Medical Journal* **2**, 1056–59.

(22) Carney, M.W.P. & Nolan, P.A. (1978). Area security unit in a psychiatric hospital. *British Medical Journal* **1**, 27–8.

(23) Goldney, R., Bowes, J., Spence, N., Czechowicz, A. & Hurley, R. (1985). The psychiatric intensive unit. *British Journal of Psychiatry* **146**, 50–4.

(24) Faulk, M. (1985) Secure facilities in local psychiatric hospitals. In Gostin, L. (ed.) *Secure Provision*. Tavistock Publications, London and New York.

(25) Coid, J.W. (1991) A survey of patients from five health districts receiving special care in the private sector. *Psychiatric Bulletin of the Royal College of Psychiatrists* **15**, 257–62.

(26) Gunn, J. (1985) Psychiatry and the prison medical service. In Gostin, L. (ed.) *Secure Provision*. Tavistock Publications, London and New York.

(27) Coid, J. (1984) How many psychiatric patients in prison? *British Journal of Psychiatry* **145**, 78–86.

(28) Gunn, J. Maden, A. & Swinton, M. (1991) Treatment needs of prisoners with psychiatric disorder. *British Medical Journal* **303**, 338–41.

(29) Taylor, P.J. (1986) Psychiatric disorder in London's life-sentenced offenders. *British Journal of Criminology* **26**, 63–78.

(30) Coker, J.B. & Martin, J. (1985) *Licensed to Live*. Blackwell, Oxford.

(31) Grapendaal, M. (1990) The inmate culture in Dutch prisons. *British Journal of Criminology* **30**, 341–57.

(32) Dooley, E. (1990) Prison suicide in England and Wales 1972–87. *British Journal of Psychiatry* **156**, 40–5.

(33) Allebeck, P., Allgulander, C. & Fisher, L.D. (1988) Predictors of completed

suicide in a cohort of 50 465 young men: role of personality and deviant behaviour. *British Medical Journal* **297**, 176–8.

(34) Harding-Pink, D. (1990) Mortality following release from prison. *Medicine, Science and the Law* **30**, 12–16.

(35) Larkin, E.P. (1991) Food refusal in prison. *Medicine, Science and the Law* **31**, 41-4.

Chapter 18

The Civil Courts and Forensic Psychiatry

Introduction

This chapter describes civil law and civil courts. The psychiatrist's involvement is subsequently described. In practice a lot of civil work is carried out by a few general and forensic psychiatrists who have taken an interest in this field. Nevertheless requests for reports may occasionally fall to any psychiatrist.

The civil law and the courts

The civil law deals with citizens rights. It involves seeking redress for injury, wrong doing, fraud, etc., as well as settling claims and disputes between people (e.g. deciding on the legality and disposition of a will) and protecting those at risk (e.g. children, battered wives, the mentally disordered).

Civil cases are disposed of mainly by county courts, sometimes by magistrates' courts (in minor domestic cases such as maintenance payments), and more serious cases set up in the high courts set up around the country and including the High Courts of Justice in London. Cases in the high courts and county courts are generally heard before a single judge. A jury is only used in special cases. The judge is therefore deciding issues of fact and law. The high court, as part of its concern with the law to protect the individual, is the first court of appeal for the Mental Health Review Tribunals and the Mental Health Act Commission.

The high court is divided into three divisions. These are the:

(1) Queen's Bench Division: The majority of common law cases concerning contracts and damages between people are dealt with here.
(2) Chancery Division: Deals with trusts, wills, companies and tax and other financial matters.
(3) Family Division: Deals with adoption, wardship and divorces.

Appeals from these courts are heard at the Court of Appeal. The House of Lords acts as the final UK court of appeal on points of law. The European

Court of Justice can act as an appeal court on points of European law including points concerning citizens' rights.

The role of the psychiatrist in civil law

As in the criminal courts, the adversarial system is used. The injured party is known as the plaintiff or complainant and the other the defendant. Nevertheless, there is contact between the two sides and where compensation is an issue there will be attempts to reach settlement to avoid going to court. At this stage evidence held by one side need not be shown to the other. However, all the expert reports to be presented at the trial have to be disclosed beforehand so that both sides can be sure of the issues. Frequently an agreement or settlement is reached before court, even in the moments right up to the appearance in court. The case may not need then to proceed to a judgement in the court. If settlement is reached once the court is sitting, the court may simply check and ratify the agreement.

The psychiatrist's job will be to prepare a report to answer the questions asked by the lawyer instigating the report. It is necessary to clarify the questions the lawyer wants answered. It is wise to check before handing in the report that the questions have been addressed. This report will be used, if suitable, to assist the case of the lawyer. The psychiatrist should not, however, take sides with the lawyer, but present a balanced and carefully researched report.

Frequently, especially in cases of compensation, non-psychotic conditions may be the basis of the claim. These can be (and are) simulated or exaggerated. It is important to get as much objective evidence as possible, and be prepared to be surprised. Sometimes a private detective is more revealing than a psychiatrist:

> A psychiatrist wrote a report supporting the claim of the complainant who appeared to have developed a paraplegia due to 'hysterical dissociation' following a road traffic accident. Happily the psychiatrist was saved embarrassment in court. Before the psychiatrist's evidence was called, the defendant showed a detective's video film of the complainant, believing himself to be unobserved, walking normally.

It may be helpful to try and classify the situations in which a psychiatric opinion may be required in civil law cases.

(1) *Where the mental fitness of a subject, suspected of having mental disorder, is being questioned:* the psychiatrist may be asked to comment on the state of mind of a patient or individual in relation to a contract or statement, e.g. to show whether the patient could reasonably enter into a contract, have the ability to make a will or be held responsible for a libel. On the other

hand, the subject may be claiming his freedom or recovery from mental disorder and fitness to be released, e.g. at a Mental Health Review Tribunal (see Chapter 4).

(2) *Where the psychiatric damage caused to a subject is being considered:* the psychiatrist may be asked to consider whether a particular act (e.g. a traumatic event or medical treatment) or omission committed by a defendant has caused a psychiatric disorder in the complainant sufficient to justify the payment of compensation. The complainant is said to be seeking a 'remedy' in law to an alleged injury, physical or psychological. The psychiatrist may be instructed by the defendant or the complainant. Victims of criminal acts may seek compensation from the Criminal Compensation Board (a government body). Reports may be required by the complainant or the Board:

> A long-term prisoner developed a psychosis and features of brain damage as a result of being battered by a brick in an assault by another prisoner. A report was required by the Compensation Board to confirm the extent of the injuries and psychosis and to give an indication of the prognosis (in this case, poor). The sum awarded reflected the loss of earning power in the future as well as the pain and injury he received and adjusted (reduced) to allow for the amount being 'given' to the prisoner in the way of free board and lodgings in prison!

(3) *Where a psychiatrist's practice is being questioned.*

(4) *The psychiatrist may be involved in the placement of children in Care Proceedings, custody of children decisions, adoption decisions, and possibly marital decisions.* (Descriptions of these activities are beyond the scope of this book.)

General principles of report preparation

As in the preparation for reports for criminal cases, it is essential to collect all the appropriate evidence. In civil cases, more than in criminal, especially where large sums of money are involved, there seems to be a much greater tendency for lawyers to fail to disclose material damaging to their case until full disclosure is demanded when the case finally appears in court. It is also said that there is much greater chance of the complainant exaggerating, elaborating, or downright lying than in criminal cases.

It is often said that where compensation is involved, the lawyers appear to be playing a complicated game, each group trying to get the best for their client. The defendants' lawyers will try to get the complainant to settle for a smaller sum out of court (before the case reaches court). The complainants' lawyers, unless offered a suitable sum, will recommend going to court to get a better result. However, there is a risk. If the court makes an award which is the same or smaller than the sum already offered by the defendant, then the complainant must pay the costs of the case.

When the case comes to court the lawyers will do their best to discredit the evidence of the psychiatrist. They will look for evidence of sloppiness in accruing the evidence. They will challenge the findings. They may use detectives to check the complainant's behaviour. Finally, the diagnosis of the psychiatrist may be challenged and its interpretation. Many recommend that diagnosis should be derived from the ICD or DSM where there are clear criteria to be met:

> 'Mr. Brown's symptoms (give a list) meet the criteria for a diagnosis of post traumatic stress disorder as defined in the Diagnostic and Statistical Manual, 1990'.

Be aware of variations and do not be afraid to speak from clinical experience.

> 'Although not typical of the symptoms of depression, in my experience such symptoms are occasionally seen in this condition'.

The form of the report will be similar to that seen in criminal cases (see Chapter 15). There should be the same introduction covering the evidence and an account of the time spent with the client. Then should follow an account of the history. It will be clear from the above that as much as possible should be supported by evidence other than the client's own account. It should be made clear where the client's account cannot be substantiated, either because of the lack of evidence or the presence of conflicting evidence. The timings of the various episodes in the history are particularly important to points at issue, particularly the timing of the development of symptoms in relation to any trauma. The court wants to know, first, if the complainant's symptoms are genuine and second, what the prognosis is likely to be. The report should be structured to deal with these points as well as any others the lawyers wish to be addressed.

Where the question of mental fitness of the subject is the issue

Contracts

A contract requires free full consent. If the subject is of unsound mind at the time of the contract, the contract is regarded as void. Compulsorily detained patients in hospital (as a result of mental disorder) are permitted to execute deeds and similar documents provided the responsible medical officer in that hospital certifies that the nature of the contract is understood by the patient. Mentally disordered patients can similarly contract for necessities (e.g. food or clothing) if the contract is appropriate to their needs.

Testamentary capacity

This refers to the ability to make a will which requires a 'sound disposing mind'. Illness itself is no bar. Based on the judgement of *Banks* v *Goodfellow* (1870) the following points of guidance were given. To be of sound disposing mind a person should have:

(1) The ability to understand the nature of a will and its consequences.
(2) The ability to recall the nature and extent of the subject's property, though not necessarily the details.
(3) The ability to recall the names of all near-relatives and their claim on his bounty.
(4) The absence of a morbid state of mind which might pervert the natural feelings of the testator and influence his decisions.

The question will be brought up either at the time of making the will (when the solicitor may seek professional reassurance about the subject's ability) or when the will is challenged by the relatives after death. In the latter case, the psychiatrist would have to build up a picture from medical and psychiatric notes and interviews with the relatives[1].

In the former case the subject must be carefully examined with regard to the four points and proper regard paid to other medical evidence – especially if there is a mental illness present. It is necessary to get objective evidence to check if what the subject says about the family and property is true and not influenced, for example, by delusions, affective disorder, dementia or mental retardation.

Inability to consent and surgical operation

It has been ruled by the House of Lords (see Chapter 16) that an application to the High Court (Family Division) should be made in the case of someone unable, through mental disorder, to give proper consent and where the operation is serious and irreversible, as in the operation of sterilization. The application would need to be supported by psychiatric reports which would need to describe the mental disorder and the problems of consent as well as describe the reasons for the application and the benefit to the patient:

> A female patient, F, suffering from severe mental subnormality was living with a male patient with similar problems. It was argued successfully in court (using psychiatric evidence) that the patient could not have cared for a child but should not be denied the comfort of her relationship. At the same time her understanding was such that she could not give proper consent to the operation. The court ruled that the operation should be carried out.

Any similar cases in the future would similarly have to seek the court's permission[2].

Marriage

This comes under the terms of contracts, i.e. a person who has such a mental disorder so as not to appreciate the nature of the contract may not become involved in the contract of marriage.

A marriage may be annulled if any of the following can be shown that:

(1) A partner had a mental disorder at the time so as not to appreciate the nature of the contract:
(2) One partner suffered from at least one of the following undisclosed diseases:
    (a) epilepsy;
    (b) communicable venereal disease.
(3) Either of the parties was under the age of 16 at the time of the marriage.
(4) There was non-disclosure of pregnancy by another man at the time of the marriage.
(5) There was non-consummation, i.e. no intromission of the penis.
(6) One of the partners was forced under duress to agree to the marriage.

Tort

A tort is a civil wrong to the person, reputation or the estate of an individual, e.g. libel, slander, fraud, or trespass. A mentally disordered patient is considered incapable of committing a tort unless it can be shown that, at the time, the disorder did not preclude the person from understanding the nature and probable consequences of the act.

The insane as witness

A mentally disordered person may give evidence if the judge has determined that he is fit to give evidence and can understand the nature of obligations of the oath. Medical evidence may be called about the witness before he is sworn. The jury has to decide how much weight or importance has to be put on the witness's evidence. A mentally disordered person can make a written statement, and similarly a medical report may be required about the witness's capacity to do so.

Certificate of sanity

This certificate or report may be required:

(1) If the patient wants to support his claim to sanity to the Mental Health Review Tribunal.
(2) After compulsory detention in order to prove the patient's capacity to make a will or sign a legal document.

(3) In some cases to rescind a receivership.

Where the question of psychiatric damage to the complainant is the issue

1. Physical trauma and psychiatric damage

The courts recognize that psychiatric disturbance can occur from physical trauma. However, normal emotional reactions to stress are not eligible for compensation, e.g. normal sadness or grief following loss, but 'psychiatric damage' (or 'nervous shock') – the legal terms for psychiatric sequelae – does provide a basis for compensation. The courts also recognize that people vary in their vulnerability to traumatic events. Some people may have a very thin skull. In such a case, the defendant must take the plaintiff as he finds him. The fact that the victim has a thin skull is no defence against the accusation of fracturing it.

The sum awarded for compensation (known as the quantum for damages) will involve an assessment of loss of earning, pain and suffering, physical inconvenience, social discredit, mental distress and loss of society of spouse or child. The psychiatrist may be expected to comment on the extent to which the trauma caused these things.

An attempt must be made to try and estimate the effects of the different traumas present in the situation. Clearly, injury to the brain sustained in a catastrophe, could lead the victim to have neurological and neurologically based psychiatric symptoms. At the same time, the experience of being in a potentially lethal situation may also cause psychological symptoms quite separate from those which are due to brain damage.

(i) Psychiatric symptoms after head injury

This subject has been reviewed by Lishman[3] and McClelland[4]. Long-term psychiatric sequelae are common after severe head injury and can lead to a great deal of social and psychological impairment. Severe injuries will be associated with neurological symptoms which will tend to improve with time. Mild injuries may be associated with dizziness, transient disturbance or concussion with no later evidence of gross neurological damage.

Following a period of concussion, there will be a period of confusion from a few seconds to weeks depending on the severity of the injury and the physical condition of the subject (worse for the elderly, the arteriosclerotic, and alcoholics). In the confusional period there may be lethargy or irritability and perplexity, disturbed orientation, misinterpretations, depression or boisterous behaviour, and there may be hysterical, aggressive or paranoid traits with delusions and hallucinations. Memory may be patchy or absent (post-traumatic amnesia). Violent behaviour can occur. Crimes can be committed in this state and can appear, superficially at least, to be highly motivated just as sportsmen, following a blow to the head, can complete the game with no memory for it after the blow.

Post-traumatic (anterograde) amnesia may be complete or patchy. The length of the post-traumatic amnesia is a guide to the severity of the injury and the prognosis. Post-traumatic amnesia longer than one week indicates a poor prognosis with invalidism up to one year.

Retrograde amnesia is the amnesia which occurs before the blow and is generally very brief (seconds or minutes). In very severe brain injury there may be a retrograde amnesia of days or weeks. The length of the retrograde amnesia may shrink with time. Long retrograde amnesias with minor head injuries suggest elaboration and deception.

Psychiatric symptoms following head injuries vary considerably and owe something to organic factors, mental constitution and something also to psychogenic ones, including those arising from environmental and legal problems. Symptoms include:

(1) Headaches, dizziness, fatigue, impaired concentration and irritability.
(2) Neuroticism (phobias, anxiety states, depression) sometimes following quite trivial injuries (as well as with serious ones). These are perhaps associated with other life difficulties and seem to be more psychogenic rather than organic. Careful history taking may reveal their presence before the injury.
(3) Major affective psychosis.
(4) Schizophrenic psychosis.
(5) Intellectual impairment and memory impairment (reflecting the severity of the injury).
(6) Wide ranging changes (deteriorations) in personality, commonly after severe head injuries and including frontal lobe syndrome, temporal lobe syndrome and basal syndrome.
(7) Sexual dysfunction.
(8) Epileptic phenomenon.

Prognosis will be worse the older the patient (perhaps due to the deteriorating ageing brain and any co-existent disease). Features of inadequacy and neurosis will worsen the prognosis, as will emotional features arising from the incident (fear etc.). The domestic and occupational problems which face the patient after the injury also influence recovery. Medicolegal issues, the opportunity for compensation and extended litigation, are also said to worsen matters producing anxiety in their own right and prolonging the symptoms acquired after the injury.

(ii) Post-concussional syndrome

ICD 10 describes the syndrome as one following a head injury usually after concussion. It is characterized by headaches, dizziness, fatigue, irritability, difficulty with concentrating and performing menial tasks, impairment of memory, insomnia, and reduced tolerance to stress, emotional excitement or alcohol. Anxiety and depression are often present. Headaches and dizziness may persist in over half for some months but only 1% will have the symptoms at one year and in the majority of those, neurological examination will reveal no abnormality.

The evidence about the relative role of organic and psychogenic factors in the persistence of symptoms is contradictory[5]. It has been asserted that the symptoms merely reflect the desire for compensation. Some surveys found the strongest association with previous constitution, social class, nature of the accident and litigation. Other surveys and follow-ups suggest an association with early neurological symptoms (diplopia, anosmia, length of post-traumatic amnesia). Lishman suggests that the symptoms begin organically and generally resolve but can be maintained by psychological factors. In a prospective study, a mixture of causes (organic and social) was found for the persistence of symptoms but a desire for compensation was not a factor[6].

Medicolegal considerations
The court will want to know:

(1) Are the symptoms genuine?
(2) Was the head injury a contributing cause of the symptoms?
(3) If so, to what extent did the head injury contribute (would the symptoms have occurred anyway)?
(4) What is the prognosis?

The court will recognize the fact that a more vulnerable person will suffer more from an injury than will a robust person.

(iii) Accident neurosis (compensation neurosis) and malingering

Malt[7] followed-up 107 adults who had been accidently injured. Nearly a quarter had some psychiatric disorder in the two year follow-up period. At one year some 17% had non-organic symptoms (anxieties, affective disorder, adjustment disorder) and at two years only 9% had such symptoms. Litigants after injury may complain of such symptoms as well as having complaints of pain and weakness, headache, dizziness and fatigue, perhaps in conjunction with conversion hysteria. Such symptoms may seem organically unrelated to the precipitating trauma. The question of whether they have an unconscious psychological cause (eligible for compensation) or are due to deliberate malingering (not eligible) will arise. It has been said that such cases represent a spectrum with the majority of the complainants towards the malingering end. It was believed[8] that the desire for compensation sustained the symptoms which were said to disappear promptly when the case was settled. The situation seems more complex than this. In some studies the litigation group did not clear up after settlement[9]. The persistence of severe hysterical symptoms in those cases may owe something to the legal situation (desire for compensation) but also something to the role of the family in believing, supporting and adapting to the disabled complainant who would lose face if he 'recovered'. On the other hand, another group of litigants with psychiatric symptoms[10] involved in industrial and motor vehicle accidents showed a steady improvement both before and after the time that the compensation claims were settled and most eventually had substantial remission of psychological symptoms. Nevertheless, there was a clear association between delay in getting the case settled and prolongation and exacerbation of the symptoms.

True malingering certainly occurs. Insurance companies have increasingly used detectives to demonstrate how allegedly handicapped people behave normally when they believe that they are not being observed. Complex frauds involving families across the country were described in Australia with family members coaching each other to simulate illness (e.g. whiplash injury) after organized trivial car accidents. It can be almost impossible for an average physician or psychiatrist to detect such frauds especially when the differential diagnosis includes a conversion syndrome or neurotic condition. The best protection is a very careful history with probing of details and gathering of information from other sources, especially the notes of the general practitioner:

> A child was killed in a road traffic accident whilst crossing the road. Her mother was told of the death by the police. The mother subsequently claimed damages on the basis that she was suffering from a severe depression as a result of the accident. When seen, at the request of the solicitors, some two years after the accident, the mother painted a picture of social withdrawal and depression. Checking some of the medical facts with the general practitioner revealed evidence of an active and flourishing social life quite incompatible with her story.

(iv) Victims of torture and psychiatric symptoms

Torture may be followed by a whole range of symptoms. These include impaired memory and concentration, headache, anxiety, depression, sleeplessness with nightmares and other intrusive phenomena, emotional numbing, sexual disturbances (especially after sexual torture), rage, social withdrawal, lack of energy, apathy and helplessness, somatic pain and chronic hyperventilation[11]. In formal diagnostic terms this would include post-traumatic stress disorder, anxiety states, hyperarousal, and depression (associated with loss of sense of self and survivor guilt) and somatoform disorders[12]. Cognitive impairments occur, partly due to brain injury (blows, anoxia, malnutrition) but also due to psychological factors. The psychological effects will permeate the whole family including the children of the victim.

A problem for the psychiatrist lies in gaining the trust of these victims who will tend to be very guarded following their previous experience with authority. A clear description of their sufferings and symptoms is required, however, in helping persuade authorities of their need for asylum and refugee status.

2. *Psychological trauma and psychiatric damage*

Following any psychological shock (sudden loss, threat to life etc.), there may be a 'normal emotional reaction' likely to be covered by such diagnosis as 'acute reaction to stress' or 'adjustment reaction'. A normal emotional reaction, however, is not accepted as the basis for compensation. A successful plea requires that:

(1) There is 'psychological damage' (also known in the courts as 'nervous shock') to the plaintiff usually taken to mean a psychiatric disorder such as depression or prolonged anxiety state. Post-traumatic stress disorder and pathological grief are now accepted by the courts as examples of psychiatric damage.
(2) The defendant has shown a breach of duty.
(3) Causation is established from the event to the injury.

A catastrophe such as an air crash, major explosion etc. may, through its physical effects, have any of the traumatic physical effects mentioned above. It is also likely that it will have psychological effects due to the threat to life, the shattering of the subject's sense of inviability or the horror of seeing people injured or killed.

There are, however, a wide variety of psychological responses to a catastrophe. There may actually be an improvement in self-esteem and maturity following the experience or the subject may be unaffected either way. Most, however, will suffer a variety of pathological states. The main pathological reactions include:

(1) An anxiety state or other neurotic state (such as panic states, phobias, conversion syndromes).
(2) An affective state (mania or depression).
(3) A post-traumatic stress disorder.
(4) A personality change possibly associated with antisocial behaviour.
(5) A psychosis (rare).

Of these post-traumatic stress disorder (recognized in the present form only since 1980) has received a good deal of attention in recent years but the other conditions should not be forgotten.

(i) Post traumatic stress disorder (PTSD)

It has long been recognized that very distressing situations can lead subsequently to psychological and physical symptoms. Victims of railway accidents in the nineteenth century developed nervous symptoms which were accredited to the effects of the 'spinal shock' sustained in the incident. Soldiers who developed symptoms in war were said to have 'battle fatigue' (American Civil War), 'psychasthenia' (1909), or 'shellshock' (World War I). Initially, the symptoms were accredited to physical causes (trauma of the spine in railway accidents or the effects of blast in war). As evidence was collected it became clear that the cause was psychological, the symptoms occurring in the absence of actual blast or relevant physical injury. There has been a reluctance on the part of the authorities – partly because of the financial implications – to recognize the extent to which victims can be affected. The question of malingering is always raised.

Compensation has been sought for psychological symptoms arising from trauma since the late nineteenth century. In modern times, the Korean war, and more importantly the Vietnam war, raised awareness of the condition. Follow-up studies on a series of disasters has also shown that symptoms occur in a large number of survivors and their rescuers and these symptoms can be disabling in a number of cases. PTSD has now been described in all ages, in a wide variety of circumstances including being a victim or a rescuer. War veterans, victims of violence, firefighters, survivors of major accidents, rescuers attending major incidents, relatives of homicide victims, prisoners exposed to trauma, child witnesses to homicide and rape victims[13, 14] have all been described as being susceptible to developing PTSD.

Definition of PTSD
The DSM IIIR requires for a diagnosis of PTSD that there should be:

(1) A stressor severe enough to cause significant symptoms of distress in almost any one.
(2) At least one symptom involving the mental reliving of the trauma (intrusive thoughts or recurrent dreams or sudden feeling that it was recurring).
(3) At least three symptoms of persistent avoidance of stimuli associated with the trauma or numbing of responsiveness, such as avoidance of thoughts or feelings associated with the trauma, significantly diminished interest in activities, feelings of detachment and constricted affect.
(4) Persistent symptoms of increased arousal as indicated by two of the following – sleep disturbance, irritability, angry outbursts, hypervigilance, exaggerated startle responses, or physiological reactivity upon exposure to events which symbolize or resemble the traumatic event.
(5) Duration of the disturbance of at least one month.

The condition is recognized as being acute or chronic or delayed in form. The ICD 10 has a similar definition. The disorder should generally only be diagnosed if the symptoms appear within six months of the event though there may be exceptions.

Incidence of PTSD after a catastrophe

The lifetime prevalence rate for PTSD in a normal community was found to be 1.3%[15]. The incidence varies widely (20%–90%) in different studies following major catastrophes. Apart from any methodological problems of research (definitions, methods of assessment, timing of the assessment), this may reflect the differing exposure trauma, the morale and support offered to the subjects, and their social situation. Cambodian refugees emigrating to the USA after experiencing war, loss and torture still had a PTSD rate of over 80% some years after experiencing the trauma[16]. British soldiers returning from the successful Falklands War had a rate of 20% for the fully developed syndrome[17]. Police officers carefully briefed beforehand and supported by senior officers during the event were able to handle the dead bodies after an oil rig disaster without significant morbidity, though of course, the officers were not themselves exposed to a life threat[18].

Symptoms generally occur quickly after the event. The onset of symptoms can, however, be delayed for some months. The onset of the symptoms may then be precipitated by further stress or a reminder of the original trauma. They may have been postponed due to preoccupation with a concurrent physical illness or due to excellent early support[13].

PTSD may occur not only in the victims but also in onlookers, and rescuers especially if exposed to fatigue, danger and disturbing sights.

Factors affecting the development of symptoms

There has been considerable discussion over the years about pathogenic factors. How much is due to the victim's personality or previous experience and how much due to the catastrophe? All three factors are influential. The severity of the symptoms depends not only on what happens but how it is perceived. The event will be more stressful and produce more symptoms and features of guilt if the victim blames himself or feels that he could have done more to have controlled it, as shown in a study of the *Herald of Free Enterprise* ferry disaster[19].

A study which would clarify this would, ideally, include all the people exposed to the trauma, it would be prospective and data about the subjects' previous personality and life experiences would be already known. There would also have to be a control group to show the underlying rate of psychiatric symptoms as measured by the instruments used. No study reaches this quality and judgements have had to be made on less rigorous studies. These have been biased in a number of ways including not having the whole population and having to use retrospective data and lacking proper controls. Studies of the Vietnam war survivors support the hypothesis that PTSD reflects the severity of the combat experience. The soldiers' symptoms reflected the extent to which they faced combat stress[20]. Other psychiatric symptoms were also commoner in soldiers exposed to greater combat stress[21].

Studies of Australian bush fire fighters support the opposite hypothesis. It was found that previous personality problems (introversion and neuroticism) and family history of psychiatric disorder coupled with a severe subjective perception of the trauma distinguishes those with a more severe reaction to stress[22]. People who had a similar trauma (fractured limbs) from different causes were compared. It was found that the subjects' subjective view of the trauma (rather than the actual severity of the trauma) distinguished those who got psychiatric symptoms[23]. A study of a normal community found a strong association between PTSD and other psychiatric disorders as well as with increased incidence of adverse childhood experiences[15].

The nature of the biological basis for the symptoms has been considered. The role of depleted endorphins and blunted adrenocorticotrophic responses to corticotrophin-releasing hormone has been questioned without clear results. Part of the difficulty lies in getting a 'pure' PTSD population[13].

Assessing the complainant
Begin by reading the statements and background to clarify in detail the trauma experienced by the victim. Obtain a careful, thorough history from the client and from a relative. Check with the general practitioner (obtain his notes if necessary). Obtain an account of the victim's behaviour and work from his work place for the period before and after the trauma. Be able to offer support from all this data for any opinion you may give.

Prognosis of PTSD
The majority of people with PTSD symptoms improve over the subsequent months. Some however, are much more handicapped by the symptoms. Up to 46% will have chronic symptoms though many will learn to live with them and not complain[15, 24, 25].

Litigation has been suspected of prolonging symptoms. However, those victims of a disaster who went to litigation did not do better after settlement than those who did not go to law, though both groups improved after the settlement which may have more to do with the whole community coming to terms with the event[23].

Treatment of PTSD
After the stress immediate post-stress counselling is the approach of first choice for which there should be an organization of trained person-

nel[26, 27]. The victims should be brought together and encouraged to give an account of their experiences. Some recommend that this should be very detailed and others that it can be quite brief. In part this must depend on the state of the subject at the time. The subjects should be advised of the reactions they may experience and the offer made to them of continued follow-up, either as a routine for support or only if symptoms develop. Where there are symptoms a number of treatments have been used varying from individual counselling and simple debriefing and attribution therapy[19] to group work, behavioural therapy (desensitization) and even intensive complex residential treatment as has been carried out with Service personnel with post-traumatic symptoms[28]. Some have been helped by antidepressants (tricyclics, serotonin re-uptake inhibitors and monoamine oxidase inhibitors), anxiolytics (beta-blockers, benzodiazepines) and lithium[29]. However, it is not yet clear which treatment is the most effective[26].

PTSD and the courts

The diagnosis of PTSD has been accepted since 1989 (following the case arising from the *Herald of Free Enterprise* disaster) as an example of 'nervous shock' or 'psychiatric damage' being eligible for the compensation. However, there may be difficulties in convincing lawyers and the courts of the seriousness of the symptoms. Confusion may also be created by having several psychiatric reports arriving at different conclusions[30].

It is obvious that symptoms developing in a person who was actually subject to the trauma would be eligible for compensation. Less obvious is the case of a person who developed symptoms after seeing the trauma happen to a close relative or to a stranger. Less obvious still is the case of a person developing symptoms after seeing the trauma (to a relative or stranger) broadcast on the television or radio or hearing about it from a third person (e.g. the police).

At the time of writing, the ruling (following the Hillsborough disaster) appears to be that symptoms are eligible for compensation if they result from:

(1) Being directly subjected to the trauma.
(2) Seeing, in real life, a close relative (spouse, parent, child, sibling) being killed.
(3) Seeing the killing of a close relative on a television broadcast.
(4) Hearing about it from a third person, e.g. a policeman.

Compensation was refused when the symptoms arose when the victim was a distant relative (nephew, fiancée), or the news has been learned from the radio or the recording of a television programme.

(ii) Other psychiatric disorders following psychological trauma

Clinical features
Neurotic states, affective disorders, substance abuse, personality change and (rare) psychosis may be seen after traumatic events. Some 22% of people admitted to a surgical department after an accident were found to have developed psychiatric symptoms related to the accident – mainly anxiety and depression – at some time in the subsequent two years. Only 4% had PTSD[7]. Following the trauma of war, those soldiers who faced greater war stress developed higher rates of neurotic symptoms than those who had faced lower stress[21]. Others developed a personality change characterized by irritability and antisocial acts[31] related in some to unresolved guilt for acts committed or the guilt of surviving when others had died. What is seen is a change in behaviour. People, who previously had been easy-going and law-abiding, become irritable and difficult. They may also become involved in criminal behaviour of a major or minor nature. All this may be complicated by the abuse of alcohol or drugs.

Prognosis
The majority of people will have lost their symptoms by one year. In Northern Ireland, 71% of a group of victims of violence on tranquillizing medication, no longer needed the medication by one year and the majority were back at work[32].

Treatment
Treatment will consist of a mixture of psychological approaches as in PTSD (immediate de-briefing, support and more intensive treatment if required) plus medication as appropriate.

Prophylaxis
It may be possible to psychologically prepare people who are going to be exposed to trauma (police, rescuers) by alerting them to the sort of things they are likely to see and experience, as well as the sort of emotional responses they may have[33]. Combining this with informal support and limiting the hours worked seemed to reduce the stress for police who had to retrieve bodies from the Piper Alpha oil rig disaster.

(iii) Psychological reactions and grief

The feelings of bereavement which follow the death of a close person are regarded as 'normal' (grief, sadness or distress) and therefore do not attract compensation in their own right even though the death may be the fault of the defendant. It might be possible to make a claim if it can be shown that the death had led to some impoverishment of the complainant or to some other situation eligible for compensation (see above). From a psychological point of view compensation would only become relevant when a pathological state occurred, such as depression or pathological grief reaction. The complainant would then be seeking a 'remedy' in law for an alleged injury, in this case psychological illness:

> A mother developed a deep depression as a psychological reaction to her son being killed by a run-away fork lift truck. She neither saw the accident nor was she present at her son's death. Nevertheless, it was agreed that she had developed a depressive illness as a result of the death. 'She had failed to contain the ordinary emotions of grief and a reactive depression had set in.'

Damages were awarded against the defendant (responsible for the truck) as her illness had been caused by his breach of duty. (*Ravenscroft* v. *Rederiaktiebologet Transatlantic. Times Law Report* 17 April 1991).

When the question of psychiatric negligence is the issue

Definition

When considering negligence it has to be shown that the psychiatrist had a duty of care to the plaintiff, that there was a breach of duty, and that some damage resulted. The standards by which the psychiatrist will be judged are those of his peers. The amount of damages (the quantum) awarded will reflect the extent to which the negligence has led to any physical, medical or psychiatric condition. The cost of any care the litigant has had to have will be taken into consideration as will any loss of work. The subjective distress of the plaintiff will also be taken into account particularly where it amounts to special suffering, to 'nervous shock'.

Typical problems

The commonest cause for litigation is the suicide of the psychiatrist's patient. The grounds for complaint may rest on:

(1) Failure of assessment.
(2) Failure of management.

The notes will show whether the diagnosis was made and recorded. Good practice requires that this information be transmitted to the nursing staff, that there should be a good operational policy in the unit for dealing with this situation and sufficient staff to carry it out. The question to be asked is: 'Was there proper care in this case, would proper care have prevented it?'

The second commonest cause for litigation is drug toxicity. The doctor may be regarded as negligent if:

(1) The wrong drug was prescribed.
(2) The drug was not properly monitored.
(3) The patient was not given proper warning.
(4) Proper consent procedures had not been followed.

The third commonest cause for complaint about professional practice is failure to diagnose an organic condition. In this case, the notes would have to be scrutinized to see if 'reasonable' care had been taken. A judgement has to be made to compare the doctor's care with those of his peers in that situation.

References

(1) Spar, J.E. & Garb, A. (1992) Assessing competency to make a will. *American Journal of Psychiatry* **149**, 169–74.
(2) Brahams, D. (1989) Incompetent adults and consent to treatment. *Lancet* **i**, 340.
(3) Lishman, W.A. (1987) *Organic Psychiatry* (2nd ed.). Blackwell Scientific Publications, Oxford.
(4) McClelland, R.J. (1988) Psychosocial sequelae of head injury – anatomy of a relationship. *British Journal of Psychiatry* **153**, 141–6.
(5) Lishman, W.A. (1988) Physiogenesis and psychogenesis in the post concussional syndrome. *British Journal of Psychiatry* **153** 460–80.
(6) Fenton, G., McClelland, R., Montgomery, A., MacFlynn, G. & Rutherford, W. (1993) The postconcussional syndrome: social antecedents and psychological sequelae. *British Journal of Psychiatry* **162**, 493–7.
(7) Malt, U. (1988) The long-term psychiatric consequences of accidental injury. *British Journal of Psychiatry* **153**, 810–18.
(8) Miller, H. (1961) Accident neurosis. *British Medical Journal* **i**, 919–25; 992–8.
(9) Tarsh, M.J. & Royston, C. (1985) A follow-up of accident neurosis. *British Journal of Psychiatry* **146**, 18–25.
(10) Binder, R.L., Trimble, M.R. & McNiel, D.E. (1991) The course of psychological symptoms after resolution of lawsuits. *American Journal of Psychiatry* **148**, 1073–75.
(11) Turner, S. & Gorst-Unsworth, C. (1990) Psychological sequelae of torture. *British Journal of Psychiatry* **157**, 475–80.
(12) Ramsay, R., Gorst-Unsworth, C. & Turner, S. (1993) Psychiatric morbidity in survivors of organised state violence including torture. *British Journal of Psychiatry* **162**, 55–9.
(13) Loughrey, G. (1990) Post traumatic stress disorder. *Current Opinion in Psychiatry* **3**, 262–6.
(14) Mezey, G.C. (1990) Victims and survivors. *Current Opinion in Psychiatry* **3**, 739–44.
(15) Davidson, J.R.T., Hughes, D., Blazer, D.G. & George, I.K. (1991) Post-

traumatic stress disorder in the community: an epidemiological study. *Psychological Medicine* **21**, 713–21.

(16) Carlson, E.B. & Rosser-Hogan, R. (1991) Trauma experiences, post-traumatic stress, dissociation and depression in Cambodian refugees. *American Journal of Psychiatry* **148**, 1548–51.

(17) O'Brien, L.S. & Hughes, S.J. (1991) Symptoms of post-traumatic stress disorder in Falkland veterans five years after conflict. *British Journal of Psychiatry* **159**, 135–41.

(18) Alexander, D.A. & Wells, A. (1991) Reactions of police officers to body-handling after a major disaster. *British Journal of Psychiatry* **159**, 547–55.

(19) Joseph, S.A., Brewin, C.R., Yule, W. & Williams, R. (1991) Causal attributions and psychiatric symptoms in survivors of the *Herald of Free Enterprise* disaster. *British Journal of Psychiatry* **159**, 542–6.

(20) Green, B.L., Grace, M.C., Lindy, J.D., Gleser, G.C., & Leonard, A. (1990) Risk-factors for PTSD and other diagnoses in a general sample of Vietnam veterans. *American Journal of Psychiatry* **147**, 729–33.

(21) Jordan, B.K., Schlender, W.E., Hough, R., Kulka, R.A., Weiss, D., Fairbank, J.A. & Marmor, C.R. (1991) Lifetime and current prevalence of specific psychiatric disorders among Vietnam veterans and controls. *Archives of General Psychiatry* **48**, 207–15.

(22) McFarlane, A.C. (1988) The aetiology of post-traumatic stress disorders following a natural disaster. *British Journal of Psychiatry* **152**, 116–21.

(23) Feinstein, A. & Dolan, R. (1991) Predictors of post-traumatic stress disorder following physical trauma: an examination of the stressor criterion. *Psychological medicine* **21**, 85–91.

(24) Green, B.I., Lindy, J.D., Grace, M.C., Glesser, G.C., Leonard, A.C., Korol, M. & Winget, C. (1990) Buffalo Creek survivors in the second decade: stability of stress symptoms. *American Journal of Orthopsychiatry* **60**, 43–54.

(25) Home Office (1989). *British Crime Survey*. Home Office Research Study No. 111. HMSO, London.

(26) Editorial (1989) Psychiatric intervention after a disaster. *Lancet* **ii**, 138.

(27) The Psychiatric Division of the Royal Airforce Medical Service (1993) The management of hostages after release. *Psychiatric Bulletin* **17**, 35–7.

(28) Brandon, S. (1991) The psychological aftermath of war. *British Medical Journal*, **302**, 305–6.

(29) Davidson, J. (1992) Drug therapy of post-traumatic stress disorder. *British Journal of Psychiatry* **160**, 309–14

(30) Fowlie, D. & Alexander, D. (1992) Collective actions following major disasters. *Journal of Forensic Psychiatry* **3**, 321–9.

(31) Sparr, L., Reaves, M. & Atkinson, R. (1987) Military combat, post-traumatic stress disorder and criminal behaviour in Vietnam veterans. *Bulletin of the American Academy of Psychiatry and Law* **15**, 141–62.

(32) Kee, M., Bell, P., Loughry, G.C., Roddy, R.J. & Curran, P.S. (1987) Victims of violence: a demographic and clinical study. *Medicine, Science and the Law* **27**, 241–7.

(33) Raphael, B. Meldrum, L. & O'Toole, B. (1991) Rescuers' psychological responses to disasters. *British Medical Journal* **303**, 1346–7.

Index

Aarvold Committee, 66
Abnormality of mind, 49
Abortion, 103
Absconding, 161
Absent minded offending, 90
Absolute discharge, 17
Accident neurosis, 361
Accusatorial system, 13
Actual bodily harm, 103
Actus reus, 12
Acquisitive offences (*see* property
    offences), 84–93
Adolescent Units, 267
    behaviour modification, 267
Advisory Board to the Home Office, 66, 325
Affective Psychosis (*see also* depression and
    mania)
    acquisitive offence, 89
    crime, 153–4
    definition, 153
    medicolegal, 154
Aftercare, 8, 164
Aggression (*see* violence)
Alcohol (*see also* substance-induced
    organic disorder)
    acquisitive offence, 90
    defence, 52, 187–90
    mental effects, 187–90
    violence, 110
Amnestic syndrome, 190
Amnesia
    as a defence, 51, 190
    organic, 190
    psychological, 51
Antisocial personality, 195–6
Anxiety, 87
Any other disorder or disability of mind,
    30
Appeal system, 54–6
Arson (*see* property offences), 84, 93–9
    assessment of offender, 98
    classification, 94–98
    court, 99
    dangerousness, 98

definition, 84
outcome in court, 99
psychiatric disorder, 93
psychiatric report, 99
schizophrenia, 150
sexual excitement, 97
tension and depression, 97
Ashworth Hospital, 4, 224, 335
Assaults
    indecent, 138
    types, 103
Assessment of offenders
    disposal, 161
    missed cases, 160
    over-referral, 159
    problems, 159
    rates of remand, 159
    screening process, 159
Attendance Centre Order, 21, 23
Attention deficit disorder with
    hyperactivity, 73, 186
Attorney General, 55
Automatism, 12, 50, 115, 120
    epilepsy, 181
    insane, 50
    sane, 50
    sleep disorders, 190–91

Bail, 14, 165
Bail hostel, 27
Battered wives, 126–8
Behaviour modification, ethics of, 328
Behaviour therapy, 199, 219, 244–5
Benperidol, 248–9
Bethlem Hospital, 333
Binding over, 17
Blackmail (*see* property offences), 83
Borderline personality, 196
Brain damage, 89, 184
British Crime Survey, 68, 105
Briquet's syndrome, 256
British Medical Association, 315
Broadmoor, 4, 333–9
Buggery, 133

Burglary, 83
Butler Committee
  interim report, 5
  mental retardation, 224
  psychopathic disorder, 193–4
  regional secure units, 339
  report, 193

Camberwell delinquency study, 75–7
Cambridge-Somerville Study, 208, 265
Care order, 25
Care Programme, 8
Carstairs Hospital, 5
Castration, 247
Certificate of Sanity, 358
Child abuse, 128, 139–44
Child destruction, 103
Child Guidance Clinic, 267
Child killing, 261–3
Child stealing, 259–60
Children
  criminal responsibility, 16
  protection from sex offenders, 143
  sex offenders, 141–3
  witnesses, as, 269
Children and Young Persons Acts (1933),
  24
Children Act (1989), 25
Chromosomal defects, 74–75
Civil Courts, 298, 353
Civil Law:
  role of psychiatrist, 354
  report preparation, 355
Clerk of the court, 14, 298
Code for Crown Prosecutors, 93, 71
Code of Practise for psychiatry, 64, 315
Cognitive therapy, 209
Combination order, 18, 24
Committee on Mentally Abnormal
  Offenders (*see* Butler Committee)
Community home, 266
Community nurse, 164, 167, 342
Community service order, 18, 21
Compensation, 17, 359
Compensation neurosis, 361
Compulsive states, 87
Concealment of birth, 103
Conditional discharge, 17
Confessions, 52–3
Confidentiality, 322–6
Connolly, John, 334
Consent to treatment rules, 64–5, 320
Consent to surgery, 357
Contingent negative variation, 73
Contracts, 356
Coroners courts, 16, 298
Corporal punishment, 329
Cortical excitability, 73

Court of Appeal, 15, 54, 298
Court procedures, 298
Crime
  definition, 67
  effect on victim, 81
  patterns, 69
  prognosis, 70
  rates, 68–9
Criminal bankruptcy order, 17
Criminal damage, 84
Criminal Justice Act (1991), 16, 24
Criminal Lunatics Act, 48, 333
Criminal Procedure (Insanity and
  Unfitness to Plead) Act (1991), 46, 48,
  50
Criminal responsibility, age of, 16, 67
Criminality (*see* delinquency)
Crown Courts, 15, 288, 298
Crown Prosecution Service, 11, 288
Curfew Order, 19, 24
Custody for life, 22
Cyproterone acetate, 249

Dangerousness, 271–85
  arson, 98
  behaviour in prison or hospital, 281–2
  childhood factors, 278
  clinical assessment, 277–85
  definition, 271
  estimation, 161, 274–6
  ethics, 318
  mental abnormality and violence, 111
  mental illness, 161
  mental state, 283–4
  mentally disordered offenders, 276–7
  occupational history, 279
  offence, 282–3
  personality, 279
  psychiatric history, 280–81
  reconviction prediction score, 272
  sexual history, 278
  sexual offending, 144
Death of infants, 102
Delinquency
  attention deficit disorder, 73
  Camberwell Study, 75
  chromosome abnormalities, 74–5
  conditioning, 73
  electroencephalogram, 72
  family effects, 75–7
  films and TV, 79
  inheritance, 71
  intelligence, 74, 76
  labelling, 78
  neurophysiological factors, 72–4
  parenting effects, 76
  physical characteristics, 77
  protecting factors, 79–81

racial background, 77
school, 78
serotonin, 74
theories of causation, 70–71
town, 77
Delirium, 176
Delusional jealousy, 151–153
Dementia, 174–176
  clinical features, 174
  law, 175–6
  older offenders, 176
  property offences, 89
Depression
  acquisitive offence, 86
  adolescent, 154
  alcoholism, 154
  arson, 154
  homicide, 153
  infanticide, 153
  personality disorder, 154
  puerperal, 121
  sexual offence, 131, 154
  shoplifting, case history, 170
  theft, 153
Destructive offences (*see* property offences
    and arson), 84, 93–9
Detention in a Young Offenders
    Institution, 24
Detention during Her Majesty's Pleasure,
    24, 25
Detention, ethics of, 320
Determinate prison sentence, 19
Diminished responsibility, 13, 49–50, 115,
    119, 120, 175, 201, 217, 319
Director of Public Prosecutions, 11
Disability in relation to trial (*see* fitness to
    plead)
Dissocial personality disorder, 195–6
Disqualified from driving, 17
Diversion schemes, 7, 43
Driving offences, 104–5
Drugs (*see also* substance-induced organic
    disorder)
  acquisitive offence, 90
  defence, 52
  mental effects, 187–90
  violence, 110
Due legal process, 322
Dundrum Hospital, 4
Duty of care, 328
Duty to society, 323
Duty to warn, 324

East, Norwood Dr, 346
Electroencephalogram and crime, 70,
    182–3
Emergency treatment, 65

Endocrine disorder, 91
Epilepsy
  acquisitive offence, 89
  assessment, 183
  automatism, 178, 181
  behaviour, 177–81
  behaviour between fits, 179–81
  behaviour disorder in children, 179
  crime, 181–82
  Criminal Procedures (Insanity and
      Unfitness to Plead) Act (1991), 181
  disturbances of consciousness, 177–8
  fetishism and transvestism, 181
  forms, 177
  insane automatism, 50
  law and Mental Health Act, 181, 183
  mental illness like state, 180, 183
  mental retardation, 180
  personality disorder, 179, 184
  prison rate, 182
  sexual dysfunction, 181
  Sullivan case, 181
  violence, 182–3
Episodic dyscontrol syndrome, 185
Ethics, 315–30
  assessing responsibility, 319
  behaviour modification, 328
  confidentiality, 322–6
  consent, 320–22
  definition, 315
  detaining patients, 320, 326–7
  duty of care, 328
  medical care in prison, 328–30, 349
  physical control, 326
  prediction of dangerousness, 318–19
  psychiatric report, 316–18
  torture, 330
Ethical committee, 322
Ethnic minorities, 332
European Convention of Human Rights,
    330
Exclusion Order, 18
Execution, 21, 319
Exhibitionism, 236–7
Expert witness, 316

Facultative sexual disorder, 228
False confessions, 52
Family Proceedings Court, 25
Feltham Youth Custody Centre, 225, 268
Female offenders (*see* women offenders)
Fetishism, 234–5
  temporal lobe focus, 181
Fillicide, 261
Fine, 17
Firesetting (*see* Arson)
Fisherton House, 325
Fitness to stand trial, 45

Fitness to plead
  consideration of, 117, 169, 190, 217
  definition, 45–7
  homicide, 117
Food refusal, 348–9
Forensic psychiatric services, 1–9, 332–50
  attitudes to patients, 162
  definition, 1
  diversion schemes, 7–8
  interconnection of services, 8–9
  local hospital in-patient units, 6–7, 344–5
  out-patient services, 7
  penal system, 1–3, 346–50
  private hospitals, 6, 345–6
  regional secure units, 5–6, 339–44
  special hospital, 4–5, 333–9
Forgery (*see* property offences), 84
Fraud (*see* property offences), 84
Frustrated-drive hypothesis, 107
Functional psychosis and crime, 148–55
  classification, 148

Ganser syndrome, 158
Glancy Committee, 5, 224, 331, 340
Glen Parva Youth Custody Centre, 225, 268
Glenthorne Youth Treatment Centre, 267
Goserelin acetate, 250
Grendon Underwood Prison, 205, 346
Grief, 368–9
Grievous bodily harm, 103
Guardianship Order, 26, 34–5
  effects, 35
  medical treatment, 35
  requirements, 35

Hadfield, James, 333
Handling stolen goods (*see* property offences), 84
Hanwell Asylum, 334
Head injury, 186, 359–60
Health care service for prisoners, 2
Henderson Hospital, 207
Her Majesty's Chief Inspector of Prisons, 330
Herstedvester Treatment Centre, 205
High Court, 354
Holloway Prison, 257
Home Office
  confidentiality, 325
  restriction orders, 37–9, 166, 167, 169, 325
Home Secretary (*see* Home Office)
Homicide (*see also* murder, manslaughter)
  aftermath, 122–3
  classification, 101–4
  mental abnormality, 115–21
  multiple, 212–2
  psychiatric assessment, 116–21

  rate, 106
  women, 260
Homicide Act (1957), 28, 49, 119
  definitions, 49
Homosexuality, 241–2
Hospital Order, 33–4
  effects, 33
  rate, 7
  requirements, 33
Hospital, psychiatric
  children's wards, 267
  forensic psychiatry, 6
  mentally ill offenders, 162–4
  mental retardation, 223
  secure wards, 344–5
  treatment of psychopaths, 206
House of Lords, 15, 298
de Hubert, W. Dr, 346

Incest
  definition, 139
  genetics, 141
  incidence, 139
  types, 139–41
Incorrigible rogue, 203
Indecent assault, 138
Indecent exposure, 138–9
Indictable offences, 12
Infanticide, 51, 102, 115, 120, 261
Infanticide Act (1938), 51, 120
Inpatient Care, 162–4
Insane as a witness, 358
Insane automatism, 50
Insanity defence (*see* McNaughten Rules), 118
Instinct hypothesis, 107
Intelligence
  arsonists, 216
  delinquency, 74, 76, 216
  sex offenders, 216
Intent
  absence, 84, 90–91
  basic, 188
  incapacity to form, 188
  meaning, 12
  specific, 84, 188
Intensive care ward, 7, 162, 344–5
Interim Hospital Order, 36
  effects, 36
  requirements, 36
Interim regional secure unit, 340
Intoxication, 187
  involuntary, 188
  pathological, 188

Jealousy, delusional and pathological, 151–3
Judge (*see* Crown Court, Court of Appeal)

Juvenile delinquency (*see* delinquency),
  70–81
  custodial facilities, 266–9
  non-custodial facilities, 23–4
  sentences of the court, 23–6
Juvenile justice bureau, 27

Korsakoffs psychosis, 190
Kleptomania, 87

Learned response hypothesis, 108
Life sentence, 20
  mandatory, 20
  discretionary, 21, 310
Lincoln Asylum, 334
Lipman case, 188
Lombroso, Professor, 70
Lord Chancellor, 56

McNaughten, Daniel, 48
McNaughten Rules, 47–8
  affective disorder, 154
  dementia, 175
  epilepsy, 181
  homicide, 118
  mental retardation, 214
  schizophrenia, 168
Magistrate (*see* Magistrates' Court)
Magistrates' Court, 13, 288, 289
Malingering, 158, 160, 203, 349, 361
Managers of the hospital, 63
Mania, 154
Mania a Poitu, 188
Manie sans delire, 193
Manslaughter, 102
Marriage contract, 358
Masochism, 239–40
Matricide, 150
Medea syndrome, 261
Medical research, ethics of, 324
Medroxyprogesterone acetate, 250
Mens rea, 12, 50
Menstruation, 255, 258
Mental abnormality
  defences in court, 44–51
  definition, 28, 49
  diminished responsibility, 49, 119
  relation to violence, 111–14
Mental capacity and consent, 65
Mental Deficiency Acts (1913, 1927), 71,
  193, 334, 346
Mental disorder (*see* mentally disturbed)
  court, 30
  definition, 28
  home, in the, 42
  homicide, 115–16
  prisoners, 347–9
  probation, 43

  property offences, 86–93
  public place, 42
  sexual offending, 131–2
  violence offences, 111–13
Mental Health Act Commission, 63–66,
  167, 321, 325
Mental Health Act (1983)
  definition of disorders, 28–30, 194
  sections:
  Section 2 (observation), 165
  Section 3 (treatment), 165
  Section 35 (remand for report), 31, 124,
    125, 165, 168
  Section 36 (remand for treatment), 32,
    166, 168, 169
  Section 37 (hospital order), 33, 120, 121,
    125, 167, 170, 175, 202, 220, 296
  Section 37 (guardianship), 34
  Section 38 (interim hospital order), 36,
    125
  Section 39, 36
  Section 41 (restriction order), 37, 120,
    125, 167, 170, 175, 204, 297
  Section 42, 39
  Section 43, 39
  Section 44, 39
  Section 46, 39
  Section 47 (transfer of convicted), 40, 219
  Section 48 (transfer criminal/civilian),
    48, 166, 169
  Section 49, 41, 166, 219
  Sections 50–53, 41–2
  Section 135, 42
  Section 136, 42, 165, 176
  Special Hospital, 334
Mental Health Review Tribunal, 56–62
  criticism, 62
  definition, 56
  ethical aspects, 320, 324
  no access to tribunal, 62
  patients under Criminal Procedure Act
    (1964), 62
  procedures, 57, 298
  rights to a tribunal, 58–62, 167, 169, 202
  structure, 56
Mental illness (*see also* mental abnormality
    and disorder)
  crime, 148
  definition, 29
  disposal of offenders, 161
  prosecution decisions, 148
  substance abuse as a cause, 187
  treatment and management in offenders,
    162–4
Mental impairment (*see* mental
    retardation, 29–30
  acquisitive offence, 90
  regional secure unit, 224

retardation, 213–14
  severe, 29
Mental retardation (*see also* mental
  disorder and mental impairment,
  213–26
  borderline subnormal, 215
  case histories, 217–23
  classification, 213
  clinical features, 213
  definition, 213
  diminished responsibility, 217
  fitness to plead, 217
  insanity, 217
  medicolegal assessment, 216–17
  Mental Health Act, 214
  mental impairment, 216–17
  offending, 215–16
  treatment and management facilities,
  223–5
  unreliable historian, 217
Mentally disturbed (*see* mental disorder)
  civil law, 356–9
  contracts, 356
  court, 27
  marriage, 358
  prison, 40–41
  public place, 42
  testamentary capacity, 357
  tort, 358
  witness, 358
Mood disorder (*see* affective psychoses,
  depression, mania), 153–4
Moral deficiency, 193
Moral insanity, 193
Moss Side Hospital, 3
Multiple personality disorder, 155
Munchausen syndrome by proxy, 263
Murder
  aftermath, 122–3
  assessment, 116–21
  defences, 115
  definition, 102
  mental abnormality, 115–22
  multiple, 121
  objective test, 102
  serial, 122
  subjective test, 102
  women, 260
Mute defendants, 52

National Health Service Act, 334, 335
Negligence, 369–70
Neonaticide, 261–2, 263
Nervous shock, 359
Neuroses
  acquisitive offence, 86–8
  alcohol, 157
  arson, 157

crime, 155–8
crime incidence, 156
definition, 155
homicide, 156
imprisonment, 157
medicolegal aspect, 158
sexual offences, 157
theft, 157
types, 155–7
Non-accidental injury, 128–9
Not fit to plead (*see* fitness to plead)
Not fit to stand trial (*see* fitness to stand
  trial)
Not guilty by reason of insanity (*see*
  McNaughten Rules), 13, 47–9
Nursing, 163, 164, 199, 336, 342, 345, 350

Observation and assessment centre, 266
Oestrogen therapy, 247–8
Offences, 12
Offences against the person, 101–45
  criminological details, 105–7
Organic brain disorder, 174
Oral evidence in court, 297
Organic personality syndrome, 184–6
  behaviour, 184
  clinical features, 184
  law, 184–5
Organic psychoses, 186–90
Orgasmic re-conditioning, 244
Othello syndrome, 151

Paedophilia, 197, 237–9
Paranoid disorders, 151
Park Lane Hospital, 3
Parkhurst Prison 'C' Wing, 206
Parole, 20
Parole score, 272
Passive avoidance learning, 73
Parricide, 260
Pathological jealousy, 151
Penal system
  chief inspector, 330
  ethics of medical care, 328–30
  mentally retarded, 224
  prison, 1
  problems – clinical, 347–9
  psychiatric care, 349–50
  psychiatric disorder in prisoners, 347
  psychopathic disorder, 205–6
  young offenders institutions, 1
Penrose's Law, 276
Personality
  severely inhibited, 132
  undercontrolled and overcontrolled, 105
  violence, 105
Personality disorder
  aggressive, 134, 139, 195

borderline, 196
  inadequate, 96
  inhibited, 132, 134
  sadistic, 135, 197
  sociopathic or dissocial, 195
  unstable, 196
Physical control, 326
Poisoning, 103–4
Police and Criminal Evidence Act, 217
Pornography, 132
Post-concussional syndrome, 360–61
Post-traumatic stress disorder, 170, 363–7
Powers of the Criminal Courts Act (1973), 26
Premenstrual syndrome, 255, 258
President of Tribunal, 56, 298
Prison (*see* penal system)
Prison Medical Service, 2, 329, 346, 350
Prison Officers' Association, 336
Private medium secure units, 6, 345–6
Probation, 26–7
  bail hostel, 27
  condition of treatment, 18, 23
  hostels, 27, 208
  probation order, 18, 23, 43
Property offences
  acquisitive, 84–93
  clinical assessment, 91
  definition, 83
  destructive, 93–9
  management of mentally disordered offenders, 92
  non-psychiatric motives, 85
  prosecution, 93
  psychiatric disorders, 86–92
Prosecution of offenders, 11, 14
Prostitution, 258
Provocation, 115
Pseudo-dementia, 158
Psychiatric damage, 359
Psychiatric illness (*see* mental illness and mental disorder)
Psychiatric reports, 14, 287–314
  admission to Special Hospital, 308–10
  automatism, 300
  ethics, 316–18
  form of report, 292–7
  homicide, 299
  Home Office re: restricted patients, 304–7
  hospital managers, 302–4
  infanticide, 299
  Mental Health Act Commission, 313–14
  Mental Health Review Tribunal, 300–2
  oral evidence, 297–8
  prison doctor, 2, 310–11
  psychiatrists' requests, 311–12
  transfer of prisoners to hospital, 307–8
Psychological trauma, 363, 368–9

Psychopathic disorder, 195–210
  alternative terms, 195
  acquisitive offence, 90
  case histories, 201–4
  classification, 195–7
  clinical features, 195–7
  definitions, 30, 193
  incest, 139–40
  incidence, 194
  medication, 209–10
  medicolegal, 200–1
  Mental Health Act, 194
  Mental illness, 197–8
  primary, 73, 195
  psychotic episodes, 198, 203
  sadism, 132, 204
  secondary, 195
  self-mutilation, 198–200
  sexual offences, 132
  treatment, 205–10
  violence, 111–13
Psychophysiological testing, 137, 244
  psychopathic disorder, 209
  psychoses and crime, 148–55
  sexual deviations, 243
  supportive, 92

Quantum for damages, 359

Rampton Hospital, 5, 224, 333–9
Rape, 133–8
  assessment of rapist, 136
  classification, 134
  definition, 133
  homicide, 135
  management, 136–8
  mental disturbance, 134
  prognosis, 136
  psychopathology, 133–4
  victims, 137
Reactive psychoses, 155
Reality therapy, 208
Reconviction Prediction Score, 272–4
Reconviction rate, 70
Reed Committee, 5, 8
Regional Secure Unit, 5, 207, 224, 339–44
  buildings and security, 340–42
  history, 339
  interaction, with services, 343
  patients, 342
  staffing, 342
  treatment and management, 343
Remand Centre, 2, 268
Remand in custody, 14, 166
  on bail, 14, 27
  for young people, 25
Remands to hospital (*see* Mental Health Act)

for report, 31
for treatment, 32
Reports (*see* psychiatric reports)
Responsibility, 12, 319
  juveniles, 16, 67
Restraint, 327
Restriction Order (*see* Mental Health Act)
  effects, 37
  problems, 38
  requirements, 37
Rights, of patients, 320, 326–8
Rights, of staff, 326
Robbery (*see* property offences), 83
Royal College of Psychiatrists, 315, 316, 322
Royal Commission (1957), 339

St Charles Youth Treatment Centre, 267
Sadism, 240–41
Schizoid personality disorder, 197
Schizophrenia, 149–51
  acquisitive offence, 88
  arson, 150
  crime, 149–51
  dangerous behaviour, case example,
    165–8
  definition, 149
  matricide, 150
  medicolegal aspects, 151
  not guilty by reason of insanity, case
    example, 168–9
  relationship to offending, 111, 149
  unfit to plead, case example, 169–70
  violence, 112–14
Seclusion, 163, 327
Seclusion room, 327, 336, 341
Secretary of State for Home Affairs (*see*
  Home Office), 37
Secure Hospital Working Party, 5
Secure room (*see* Seclusion room)
Secure training order, 25
Secure wards, in local hospitals, 344–5
  buildings and security, 345
  history, 344
  patients and their management, 345
  staffing levels, 345
Security, 335, 340, 345
  relation to admission, 162
Self-mutilation, 198–200, 349
Sentences
  adults, 17–21
  courts and sentencing, 16–26
  medical disposal, 26
  mentally abnormal offender, 26
  mitigation, 13
  offenders under 18 years, 22–5
  young adults, 21–2
Serotonin, 74, 97, 110–11
Sexual abuse of children, 139–44

Sexual disorders, 227–50
  aetiology, 229–33
  classification, 228–9
  descriptions, 233–42
  psychopathy, 197
  sexual offending, 125
  treatment, 235–43
Sexual offences, 129–45
  against children, 141–3
  classification, 130–32
  definition, 129
  incidence, 130
  mental disorder, 131–2
  pornography, 132
  prognosis, 144
  protection of children, 143
  retardation, mental, 216, 218
  specific offences, 132–43
Shoplifting (*see* property offences), 85–93
Sleep disorder, 50, 120, 190
Sleep disturbance, 349
Social group
  effect on delinquency, 77–8
  effect on violence, 109
Social Services, 223
Social skills training, 219, 246
Social workers
  after-care, 164
  restriction orders, 37, 167
  secure institutions, 336, 342
Sociopathy (*see* psychopathy)
Special Hospitals, 4, 333–9
  admission, 4, 338
  buildings and security, 335–6
  future of hospitals, 339
  history, 333
  interaction with services, 338
  mental retardation, 224
  outcome studies, 338
  patients, 336–7
  psychopath treatment, 207
  staffing levels, 336
  treatment and management, 337–8
Special Hospital Services Authority, 4
Substance abuse (*see* alcohol, drugs)
Substance-induced organic disorders,
  187–90
  crimes of basic intent, 188
  crimes of specific intent, 188
  definition, 187
  intoxication, 18
  law, 187–9
  Lipman case, 188
  medication, 188
  mental illness, 189
  types, 187
  withdrawal disorders, 189
Suicide in prison, 348

Suicide pact, 115
Sullivan case, 181
Summary offences, 12
Supervision order, 23, 25
Suspended sentence, 20

Tarasoff case, 323–4
Testamentary capacity, 357
Theft (*see* property offences), 83
Time out, 318
Tort, 358
Torture, 330, 362
Transfer direction
    convicted and civil, 40
    unconvicted prisoners, 40
Transsexualism, 233
Transvestism, 234–5
Trauma
    physical, 359
    psychological, 363, 368
Triable either way, 12

Under disability (*see* fitness to plead)
United Nations Standard Minimal Rules,
    prison, 329

Vagrancy Acts, 333
Van der Hoeven Clinic, 207
Victimology, 110
Victims
    battered wives, 110
    effect of crime, 81, 123
    murder, 110, 123
    paedophilia, 239
    rape, 137–8
    torture, 362–3
    violence, 110
Violence
    assessment and disposal of lesser
        offenders, 124–9

crime rates, 105–7
    environment factors, 110
    management, 162–4, 206–10, 242–50
    medication, 162–3, 209–10, 246–50
    medicolegal aspects of mental
        abnormality and violence, 114
    mental abnormality, 111–14
    modifying factors, 108–11
    physiological and biochemical factors,
        110–11
    theories of causation, 107–11
    victims, 110, 137–8
Voyeurism, 237

Wernicke's encephalopathy, 190
Witness, child, 269
Wolfenden Committee, 129
Women offenders, 253–64
    aetiological factors, 254
    associated offences, 258–64
    family history, 254
    homicide, 260
    incidence of crime, 253
    medicolegal aspects, 257–8
    premenstrual syndrome, 257
    in prison, 256
    psychiatric disorder, 256–7
Working Party on Security in the NHS (*see*
    Glancy Committee)
Wounding, 103

Young Adults, sentences, 21–2
Young, Graham, 66
Young offenders, 264–9
Young offender institution, 22, 25, 268
Young persons and children, sentences,
    22–6
Youth courts, 16
Youth treatment centre, 267